Atlas of
Gynecologic and Obstetric
Diagnostic Histopathology

Atlas of
Gynecologic and Obstetric
Diagnostic Histopathology

N. A. Janovski, M.D., F.C.A.P.
Commander, Medical Corps, United States Navy Reserve,
Chief, Anatomic Pathology Division,
Laboratory Department, U.S. Naval Medical School,
National Naval Medical Center, Bethesda, Maryland

Viktor Dubrauszky, M.D.
Professor of Obstetrics and Gynecology,
Head of the Gynecological Histopathology Laboratory,
University Women's Clinic,
Julius-Maxmilian University,
Würzburg, Germany

The Blakiston Division McGRAW-HILL BOOK COMPANY
New York   Toronto   Sydney   London

To Our Mothers

Preface

Modern pathology began with Morgagni as a descriptive science dealing with the seat and origin of disease. The horizons of Morgagni's dissections and gross descriptions were enlarged by Virchow and his successors to include cellular pathology. Refinements in the light microscope further assisted in the development of histopathology or morbid anatomy as we know it today. In recent decades the development of the electron microscope has enabled us to take the first steps beyond the conventional limits of histopathology into the pathology of the cell.

Pathology, having been borne in the Age of Reason, remains *au fond* an empirical discipline. It is founded on anatomic description, its limits and variations, and to it can be added as interpretations only those inferences which may be legitimately drawn from anatomic specimens and the context in which they are collected.

It is customary to teach medical students pathology in terms of a set of slides supplemented by such gross specimens and photomicrographs as the lecturer may have available or select to emphasize specific features. No one or two, or even half a dozen instances can present a fully rounded picture of a given lesion in all its manifold variations. We tend to teach pathology much in terms of an isolated view of a single frame in what is really a continuous reel of motion picture film. In this method, much of the visual emphasis is on the surface details. It is left to the student's imagination to fuse these details into a meaningful and coherent form of the disease process.

Needless to say, pathology does not consist of a series of visual impressions; this is an artefact of certain aspects of our didactic methodology. There is little profit in having a correct visual picture, even making an accurate histopathologic diagnosis, if it is not accompanied by an understanding of the nature of the process, its biologic behavior and implications, its natural history.

In theory, the art of pathologic description should be practiced by morbid anatomists with such a high degree of skill that another reader could reconstruct the original specimen from reading the description. Pleasant as this ideal is to contemplate, the exigencies of life and the lack of articulacy among many pathologists render it unrealizable. In actuality, the photomicrograph has replaced the carefully written, well-worded microscopic description.

In recent years visual aids have been emphasized. It is purely in this contemporary spirit that this Atlas has been put together. The authors have had the privilege of studying and collecting many choice specimens relating to the pathology of the female reproductive organs. Apart from whatever didactic value they may have to any reader, they have a certain beauty as objects in themselves. This Atlas has been planned chiefly as an *aide-memoire*, and as a survey rather than an implementation. Circumstances arise in which identification is an important first step. The authors do not pretend to deal with any individual lesion in depth or "in the round." Proper identification of pathologic specimens is a starting point from which further study begins. However, without it, further study will probably be along false leads. Diagnostic ability and sound clinical judgments are based on understanding of microscopic pictures of the disease entity.

This Atlas is designed for the medical students, residents in pathology, obstetrics, and gynecology, gynecologists, pathologists, and anyone interested in or practicing the healing art of the diseases of female reproductive organs. Each chapter begins with several photomicrographs of the normal histologic appearance of the organ under discussion. This is necessary in order to refresh the readers' memory with the normal histologic appearance of tissue prior to exposing him to various pathologic entities. We have chosen 1,692 photomicrographs selected from a large number of specimens to represent problems of interest. The interpretation of this material is colored by our experiences in the clinic, at the bedside, and in the laboratory.

We sincerely hope that this Atlas will be a source of stimulation to its readers to search for better explanations, new pathways and solutions to problems presented. In doing so, our efforts in writing this Atlas will be rewarded.

We are grateful to Dr. H. Naujoks for contributing, as a supplement, a chapter on chromosomal aberrations in gynecology. It is planned for beginners in this interesting and new field so important to the practicing gynecologist.

The authors acknowledge with gratitude the following persons from whom histologic slides and/or photomicrographs and helpful suggestions were received:

vii

R. G. Bunge, M.D.
University Hospital, Iowa's Medical Center, Iowa City, Iowa (Figs. 911 and 912)

C. P. Douglas, M.D.
University of West Indies, Mona, Kingston, Jamaica (Fig. 28)

Franz Enzinger, M.D.
Armed Forces Institute of Pathology, Washington, D.C. 20305

František Horálek, M.D.
Professor of Pathology, Institute of Pathological Anatomy, Masarikova Universita, Brno, Czechoslovakia (Figs. 829, 830, 831)

F. O. Huhn, M.D.
University Women's Clinic, Köln, Lidenthal, Germany (Fig. 1287)

Raymond H. Kaufman, M.D.
Assistant Professor, Baylor University, College of Medicine, Texas Medical Center, Houston, Texas (Fig. 1138)

T. R. Kazancigil, M.D.
Professor of Obstetrics and Gynecology, 1st Clinic of Obstetrics and Gynecology, University of Istanbul, Istanbul, Turkey (Figs. 149 and 240)

Mr. Harold J. Kerr
American Registry of Pathology, Armed Forces Institute of Pathology, Washington, D.C. 20305

H. Knolle, M.D.
Institute of Pathological Anatomy, Martin Luther University, Halle-Württenberg, Germany (Figs. 1419 and 1420)

Mr. Victor R. Landi
Medical and scientific photographer, Arlington, Virginia

Walter F. Lever, M.D.
Professor of Dermatology, Tufts University School of Medicine, Boston, Massachusetts (Fig. 195)

K. G. Ober, M.D.
Professor of Obstetrics and Gynecology, Friedrich Alexanders University, Erlangen, Germany (Figs. 392, 399, 401, 402, 403, 406, 851, 852, 1218, 1219)

William B. Ober, M.D.
Director of Laboratories, Knickerbocker Hospital, New York, N.Y.

Lars Santesson, M.D.
Professor of Pathology, Institute of Radiopathology, Radiumhemmet, Stockholm, Sweden (Figs. 942, 967, 968, 989, 990)

Edmund F. Schuller, M.D.
Buffalo General Hospital, Buffalo, New York (Fig. 579)

Roger B. Scott, M.D.
Professor of Obstetrics and Gynecology, Western Reserve School of Medicine, University Hospitals of Cleveland, Cleveland, Ohio (Fig. 415)

Robert E. Scully, M.D.
Pathologist, Massachusetts General Hospital, Boston, Massachusetts (Figs. 681, 682, 927)

Bruce H. Smith
Captain, MC, USN, Deputy Director, Armed Forces Institute of Pathology, Washington, D.C. 20305

G. Strauss, M.D.
University Women's Clinic, Johanes Gutenberg University, Mainz, Germany (Fig. 38, Color plate VII)

Gunter Stuttgen
Professor of Dermatology, Goethe University, Frankfurt am Main, Germany

Gunnar Teilum, M.D.
Professor of Pathology, The University Institute of Pathological Anatomy, Copenhagen, Denmark (Figs. 1043, 1062, 1150, 1151, 1152, 1153)

Jerzy Teter, M.D.
The Endocrine Department, The First Clinic of Obstetrics and Gynecology, Medical Academy, Warsaw, Poland (Figs. 1097, 1098, 1099, 1100, 1101)

D. H. Wright, M.D.
Department of Pathology, Makerere University College, Kampala, Uganda (Fig. 1157)

The authors also thankfully acknowledge the following publishers for permission to reproduce illustrations previously published by the authors:

Janovski, N. A.:

Am. J. Clin. Pathol., 39(3): 273–283, 1963. (Figs. 4, 5, 7, 8, 11)

Am. J. Clin. Pathol., 39(4): 383–388, 1963. (Figs. 4, 5, 6)

Am. J. Obstet. Gynecol., 82(4): 909–912, 1961. (Fig. 5)

Am. J. Obstet. Gynecol., 82(5): 1186–1191, 1961. (Figs. 1, 2, 3, 4)

Am. J. Obstet. Gynecol., 83(1): 105–108, 1962. (Figs. 2, 3)

Am. J. Obstet. Gynecol., 84(2): 179–181, 1962. (Fig. 1)

Am. J. Obstet. Gynecol., 84(3): 382–389, 1962. (Figs. 1, 2, 3)

Am. J. Obstet. Gynecol., 84(4): 523–536, 1962. (Figs. 1, 3, 4)

Am. J. Obstet. Gynecol., 84(5): 682–686, 1962. (Figs. 1, 2)

Am. J. Obstet. Gynecol., 85(7): 919–925, 1963. (Fig. 3)

Am. J. Obstet. Gynecol., 85(7): 926–939, 1963. (Figs. 3A, 6A)

Bull. Sloane Hosp. Women, 8(2): 65–76, 1962. (Figs. 2, 5)

Bull. Sloane Hosp. Women, IX(2): 44–47, 1963. (Figs. 1, 2)

Gynaecologia, 153:354–368, 1962. (Figs. 6, 7, 8. 9, 10, 11, 14)

J. Pediatrics, 63(2): 211–216, 1963. (Figs. 2, 3, 4)

Med. Ann. District Columbia, 32(4): 134–137, 1963. (Figs. 4, 5)

Neurology, 13(9): 788–792, 1963. (Figs. 1, 3, 4, 5, 6, 7, 8, 9)

N.Y. State J. Med., 63(10): 1463–1487, 1963. (Figs. 3, 5, 6, 8, 9)

Obstet. Gynecol., 18(2): 206–212, 1961. (Figs. 4, 5, 6, 8, 9)

Obstet. Gynecol., 18(4): 385–402, 1961. (Figs. 1, 3, 4, 7, 9, 12)

Obstet. Gynecol., 19(1): 77–80, 1962. (Fig. 2)

Obstet. Gynecol., 20(2): 227–231, 1962. (Figs. 1, 2)

Obstet. Gynecol., 20(3): 384–393, 1962. (Figs. 3, 4)

Obstet. Gynecol., 21(3): 363–367, 1963. (Figs. 1, 4, 5)

Obstet. Gynecol., 21(4): 471–476, 1963. (Figs. 1, 5, 6)

Obstet. Gynecol., 21(4): 481–485, 1963. (Figs. 4, 5)

Obstet. Gynecol., 22(2): 246–252, 1963. (Figs. 7, 9, 10)

Obstet. Gynecol., 22(4): 461–467, 1963. (Figs. 3, 4)

Obstet. Gynecol., 22(6): 697–708, 1963. (Figs. 3, 7, 8, 13)

Dubrauszky, Viktor:
"Grundriss der pathologischen Anatomie und Histologie der weiblichen Geschlechtsorgane: 1–347: mit 285 teils farbigen Abbildungen," Johann Ambrosius Barth, Munich, 1954.

Arch. Gynaekol., 176:726–745, 1949. (Figs. 7, 8, 9)

Arch. Gynaekol., 179:594–602, 1951. (Figs. 1, 2, 3, 5, 6, 8, 9)

Arch. Gynaekol., 179:603–614, 1951. (Figs. 2, 5)

Arch. Gynaekol., 187:650–660, 1956. (Figs. 2, 3, 4, 5)

Arch. Gynaekol., 191:212–223, 1958. (Fig. 7)

Geburtsh. Frauenheilk., 12:596–601, 1952. (Figs. 3, 4)

Geburtsh. Frauenheilk., 13:914–921, 1953. (Fig. 4)

Geburtsh. Frauenheilk., 15:940–945, 1955. (Figs. 2, 4)

Gynakologia (Basel), 133:145–155, 1952. (Figs. 2, 5, 11, 15)

Gynakologia (Basel), in press. (Figs. 1, 2)

Zentr. Gynaekol., 82:558–562, 1960. (Fig. 2)

Z. Geburtshilfe Gynaekol., 134:213–226, 1951. (Fig. 6)

Z. Geburtshilfe Gynaekol., 847:82–88, 1957. (Figs. 2, 6)

The following histological material for black and white illustrations has been obtained from the files of AFIP, Washington, D.C.

Fig.	AFIP Acc.	Fig.	AFIP Acc.	Fig.	AFIP Acc.	Fig.	AFIP Acc.	Fig.	AFIP Acc.
46	#829927	178	#938924	436	#490342	1017	#972742	1426	#736951
59	#810027	179	#949477	437	#490342	1018	#972742	1427	#736951
60	#810027	180	#949477	442	#749466	1019	#972742	1428	#109034
63	#939980	187	#949477	589	#811161	1020	#972742	1429	#109034
64	#939980	188	#949477	590	#811161	1141	#1126564	1430	#109034
66	#916752	191	#286245	591	#811161	1142	#1126564	1460	#789329
67	#916752	212	#522444	637	#749185	1148	#1002987	1461	#789329
68	#916752	263	#1116402	638	#749185	1149	#1002987	1462	#984142
94	#932843	264	#515008	639	#749185	1154	#1065083	1463	#984142
95	#932843	268	#192565	640	#749185	1155	#1065083	1465	#1127170
99	#269300	283	#512989	665	#1181310	1176	#903273	1466	#1127170
100	#269300	284	#512989	666	#1181310	1255	#1121317	1467	#1127170
108	#522444	285	#512989	702	#984142	1256	#1121317	1468	#1127170
118	#910121	286	#512989	777	#916306	1257	#1121317	1474	#1109813
129	#678906	287	#551982	778	#916306	1357	#1004908	1475	#1109813
130	#678906	299	#542757	897	#664882	1358	#1004908	1480	#960035
135	#482355	356	#1170870	898	#664882	1359	#1004908	1481	#960035
155	#824382	357	#878116	903	#1063279	1360	#1004908	1537	#695268
156	#824382	358	#878116	904	#1063279	1424	#736951	1538	#695268
177	#938924	359	#878116	905	#1044255	1425	#736951		

The following color material has been obtained from the files of AFIP, Washington, D.C.

Fig.	AFIP Acc.	Fig.	AFIP Acc.	Fig.	AFIP Acc.	Fig.	AFIP Acc.	Fig.	AFIP Acc.
20	#582727	33	#218754	47	#494965	79	#577456	100	#218754
21	#865667	34	#515904	48	#956850	86	#306188	101	#528667
24	#218754	35	#493294	54	#1060050	89	#330204	102	#294207
27	#302915	43	#499239	60	#370652	90	#330204	104	#218754
28	#218754	44	#499239	65	#490325	92	#319414	106	#298098
31	#533500	45	#194508	66	#502878	99	#218754–	110	#573309
32	#322313	46	#496421	69	#514253		351		

All photomicrographs are the property of the authors, unless otherwise acknowledged.

N. A. Janovski

Viktor Dubrauszky

Special Acknowledgment

The authors wish to extend sincere and warm thanks to the following, without whose help the completion of this Atlas would have been impossible:

Joe M. Blumberg
Major General, MC, USA
The Director
Armed Forces Institute of Pathology
Washington, D.C. 20305
For his understanding and interest in the field of gynecologic and obstetric pathology from which came his constructive criticisms and suggestions. We further thank him for granting us permission to use material from the files of the Armed Forces Institute of Pathology.

Herbert B. Taylor, M.D.
Chief
Obstetric, Gynecologic, and Breast Pathology Branch
Armed Forces Institute of Pathology
Washington, D.C. 20305
For his cooperation, assistance, and advice in selection of materials.

Miss Aiko Noda, H.T. (A.S.C.P.)
Armed Forces Institute of Pathology
Washington, D.C. 20305
For her free time, efforts, and skill given to the preparation, filing, arranging, and indexing of material used.

N. A. Janovski
Viktor Dubrauszky

Foreword

The authors have set out to publish an atlas of gynecologic and obstetric diagnostic histopathology based on their vast personal experiences, believing that there is a need for such an atlas to serve both clinicians and pathologists. When one considers that in the average active general hospital today malignant tumors of the female reproductive tract account for about 35 per cent of all cancers in women and that specimens from obstetric and gynecologic services may account for over 50 per cent of all surgical specimens received in a hospital laboratory, then it can be seen that there is a need for an atlas of this type. No one text or atlas will give all the answers, but since pathology began as a gross descriptive science and has progressed to the microscopic level, this atlas should have a place in the study of diseases of this area. The pathologist has a responsibility today more than ever in the improvement of patient care and the lowering of its cost. A part of this can be brought about through correct diagnosis early, so that proper treatment can be initiated, the length of time lost from illness reduced, and the incidence of mortality from these gynecologic diseases lowered.

In the main, this represents collections of cases actually seen by the writers. One of the authors (N. A. Janovski) served in the Army in my unit overseas in Japan and later was a member of the staff of the Armed Forces Institute of Pathology. I have been aware of his long-term interest in collecting the material that has gone into this publication, and I know that he has presented material in which he has had a personal interest and that he has seen the patient as well as the pathologic specimen.

Although not every subject may be fully covered, the physician should be led to further study and reading. The histologic characteristics of an entity may vary from case to case; by presenting these differences, this atlas can assist the physician to realize the wide variability of the same disease from one individual to another. The authors are aware of their limitations, but I know that they feel that this collection is worthy of passing on to others. It is felt that if the book is used in the spirit intended it will assist many in learning more of surgical pathology.

Joe M. Blumberg
Major General, MC, USA
The Director
Armed Forces Institute of Pathology
Washington, D.C. 20305

Contents

Part 1   Gynecologic Histopathology

1   *Diseases of the Vulva*   1

2   *Diseases of the Vagina*   83

3   *Diseases of the Cervix Uteri (Exocervix and Endocervix)*   105

4   *Diseases of the Endometrium*   157

5   *Diseases of the Myometrium*   213

6   *Diseases of the Oviduct*   245

7   *Diseases of the Ovary*   275

8   *Diseases of the Uterine Ligaments and Parametrium*   407

9   *Diseases of the Pelvic Peritoneum, Omentum, Retroperitoneum, and Pelvic Lymph Nodes*   425

10   *Diseases of the Adrenals of Gynecologic Interest*   453

Part 2   Obstetric Histopathology

11   *Placentation and Morphologic Alterations Encountered in Pregnancy*   457

12   *Abortion, Puerperal Infection, and Ectopic Pregnancy*   477

13   *Diseases of the Placenta and Membranes*   493

14   *Diseases of the Umbilical Cord*   519

15   *Hydatidiform Mole, Chorioadenoma Destruens, and Choriocarcinoma*   523

16   *Complications of Pregnancy*   541

Part 3   Chromosomal Aberrations in Gynecology

17   *Chromosomes and Their Aberrations*   559

1

Diseases of the Vulva

1 Normal skin of the mons veneris in a woman of reproductive age
Normal skin from the mons veneris shows a large amount of fat tissue. The patient is a woman of 35 years. (H&E. ×7)

2 Normal skin of the external surface of the labium majus in a woman of reproductive age
The epidermis shows prominent stratum corneum. There are several hair shafts and sebaceous, sweat, and apocrine glands. (H&E. ×15)

3 Normal sebaceous gland of the labium majus in a woman of reproductive age
High magnification of Fig. 2. Alveoli are formed by polyhedral cells with fine granular fat droplets. The nuclei are centrally placed. There is a holocrine type of secretion resulting from destruction of epithelial cells. (H&E. ×62)

4 Normal sweat eccrine glands of the labium majus in a woman of reproductive age
High magnification of Fig. 2. Note the coiled tubular glands with ducts. Secretion is of the eccrine type. (H&E. ×100)

5 Normal apocrine sweat glands of the labium majus in a woman of reproductive age
High magnification of Fig. 2. Apocrine glandular structures. Cells arranged on the basement membrane in a single layer. Myoepithelial cells are scattered on the basement membrane. The epithelial cells contain granular cytoplasm, and there is protrusion of protoplasm from the free surface of the cells. Functional changes of the epithelial cells consisting of enlargement are observed in the premenstrual period. Marked regressive changes occur after the menopause. (H&E. ×150)

6 Normal labium minus in a woman of reproductive age
A cross section of the labium minus of a woman of 22 years is shown. Absence of fat tissue and marked vascularity are noted. The sebaceous glands are numerous without relation to hair follicles (so-called free sebaceous gland). (H&E. ×5)

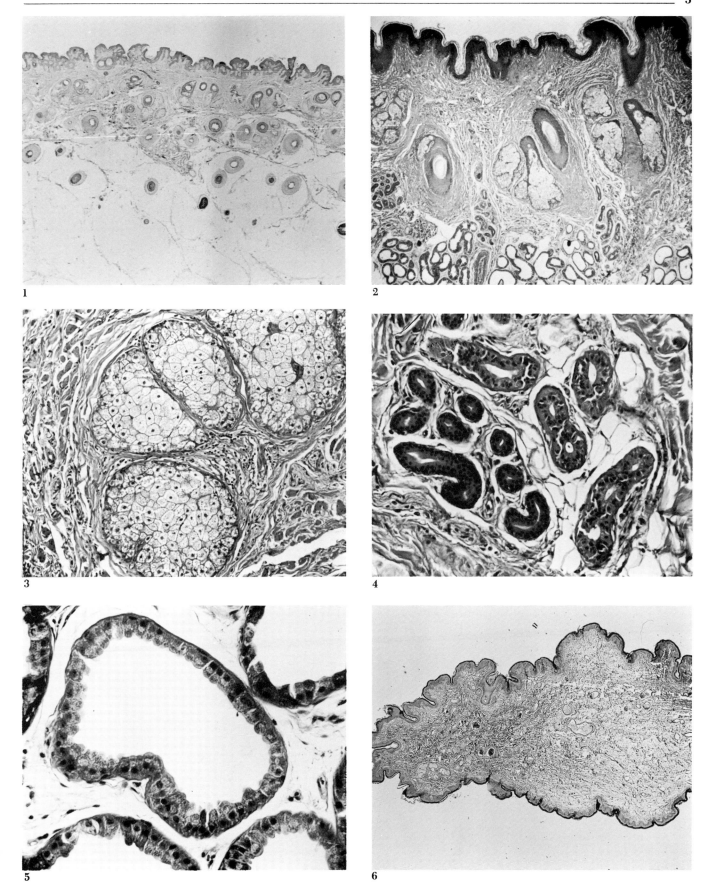

1

2

3

4

5

6

7   Normal Bartholin's gland in the left lateral wall of the vestibule in a woman of reproductive age

The tuboalveolar terminal portions are lined by mucus-producing cells. The duct on the left shows flattened epithelial cells. Involutory changes are observed after the thirty-fifth year. (H&E. ×80)

8   Normal corpus cavernosum of the clitoris in a woman of reproductive age

A cross section of erectile cavernous bodies is shown. The vascular spaces are lined by endothelial cells. (H&E. ×24)

9   Pacinian corpuscle of the clitoris in a woman of reproductive age

The corpuscle is located in the subcutis of the clitoris with various other nerve endings. (H&E. ×62)

10   Normal urethral meatus

The fold of mucous membrane is lined by stratified squamous epithelium. (H&E. ×50)

11   Normal paraurethral glands (Skene's glands) of the urethral meatus

Glandular acini are made of cuboidal mucin-producing cells. The lumens may be dilated and contain colloidlike material. (H&E. ×120)

12   Normal imperforated hymen in a woman of reproductive age

Stratified squamous epithelium is seen on both surfaces, with a thin, vascularized connective tissue core. (H&E. ×15)

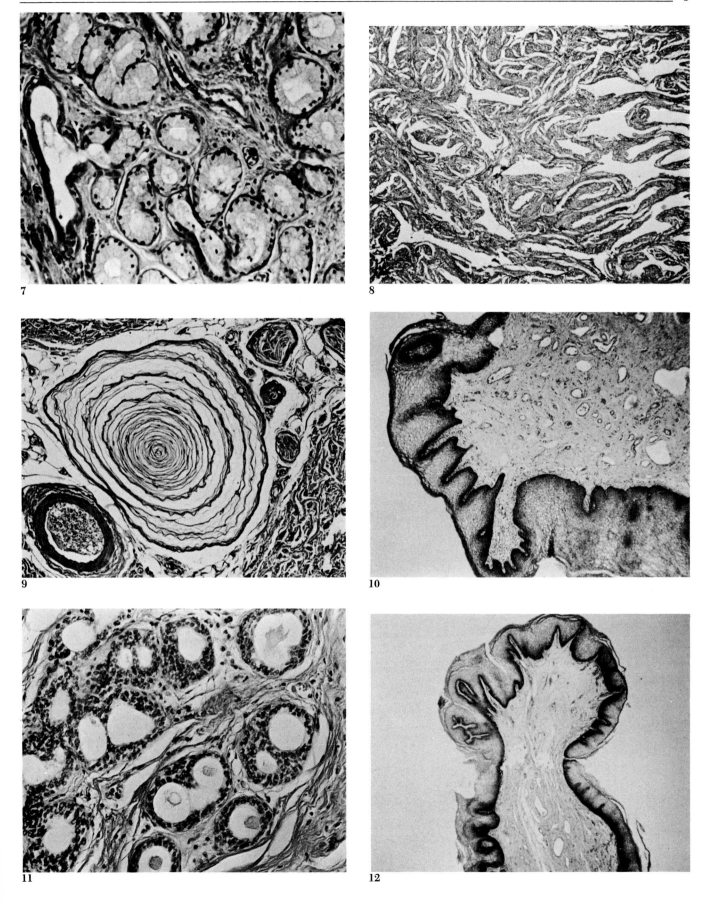

13 Varicose vein of the labium majus
Irregular fibrosis of the vascular wall and thinning of the muscle coat of the vessel are seen. The lumen of the vessel shows ramification. The likelihood of thrombosis is great. (H&E. ×24)

14 Lymphangiectasis of the vulva
There is dilatation and tortuosity of the lymph vessel. Long-standing chronic inflammation, cicatrization, tumors, and other obstructive conditions may bring about lymph stasis and produce lymphangiectasis. (H&E. ×80)

15 Elephantiasis of the vulva
Hypertrophy and hyperplasia of connective tissue are associated with marked edema. All dermal appendages (hair follicles, eccrine and apocrine sweat glands, and sebaceous glands) have been obliterated. There is dilatation of lymphatic channels with perivascular round cell infiltration. In the late stages, there is marked sclerosis of the connective tissue. (H&E. ×70)

16 Acute nonspecific vulvitis of the labium majus
The upper dermis is infiltrated predominantly with acute inflammatory cells. There is marked dilatation of vessels and moderate edema of the connective tissue. There is migration of the inflammatory cells through the epidermis. (H&E. ×50)

17 Chronic nonspecific vulvitis of the labium majus
Note the slight hyperkeratosis of the epidermis. The stratum germinativum shows vacuolar degeneration. The upper dermis is focally infiltrated with chronic inflammatory cells. (H&E. ×125)

18 Chronic nonspecific hyperkeratotic vulvitis of the labium majus
Long-standing nonspecific inflammatory process of the labium majus is shown. There is marked hyperkeratosis and acanthosis. The upper dermis is diffusely infiltrated with chronic inflammatory cells. Note the disappearance of dermal appendages. (H&E. ×50)

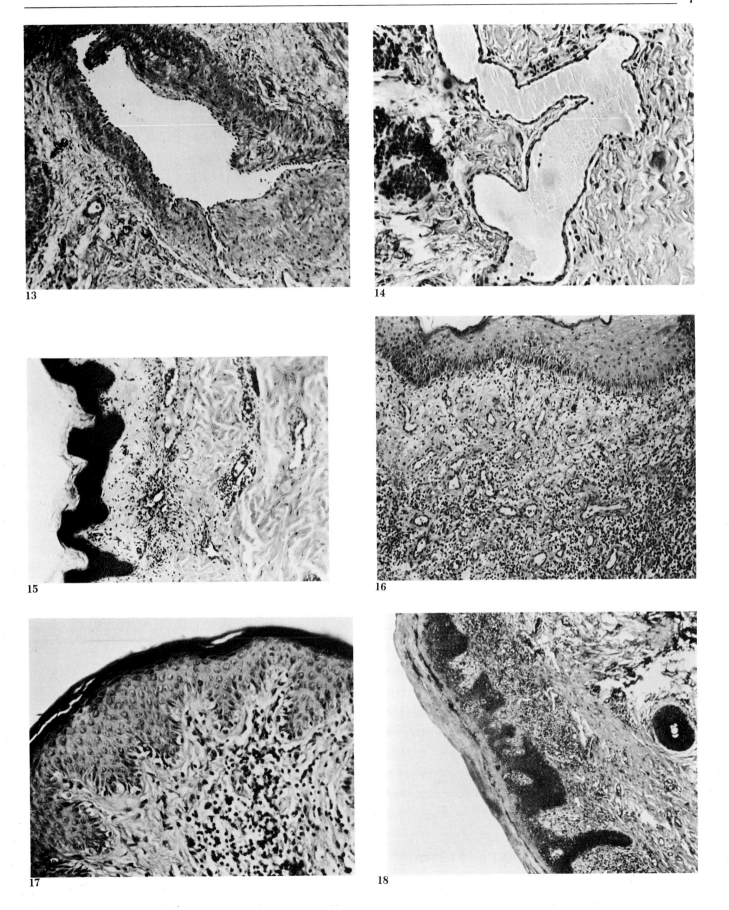

13

14

15

16

17

18

19   Diabetic vulvitis of the labium majus
There is hyperkeratosis and atrophy of the epidermis. Infiltration of histiocytes and lymphocytes of the upper dermis is seen. There is focal hyalinization of collagen. (H&E. ×125)

20   Folliculitis and perifolliculitis of the skin of the vulva
The perifollicular infiltrate consists of acute and chronic inflammatory cells. This perifollicular cellulitis may terminate in suppuration and abscess formation. This condition is caused by staphylococci. (H&E. ×24)

21   Impetigo herpetiformis of the skin of the vulva
Intraepidermal accumulation of numerous neutrophilic leukocytes is seen. There is migration of the inflammatory cells through the epidermis and a moderate inflammatory reaction of the upper dermis. The onset often occurs during the last trimester of pregnancy. The cause is unknown. (H&E. ×80)

22   Granuloma pyogenicum of the skin of the vulva
The lesion represents vegetation of exuberant granulation tissue formed by capillaries and young edematous connective tissue cells interspersed by leukocytes, plasma cells, and mast cells. (H&E. ×50)

23   Ecthyma of the skin of the vulva
There is destructive dermatitis with formation of an ulcer which is partly covered by a crust. The pronounced polymorphonuclear infiltration led to the formation of abscesses. The causative agent is *beta-hemolytic streptococcus*. (H&E. ×24)

24   Lupus vulgaris (tuberculosis cutis luposa) of the skin of the vulva
Through the entire dermis and partly in the subcutis, typical granulomatous inflammation with central caseation and conglomeration is seen. It is a result of infection of the vulvar skin by *Mycobacterium tuberculosis*. (H&E. ×25)

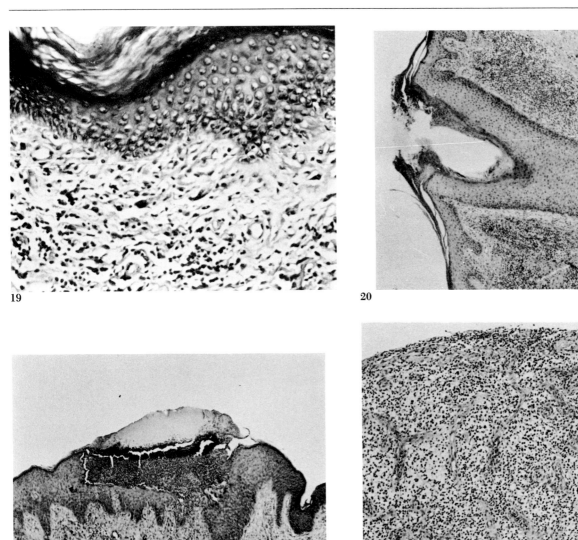

19

20

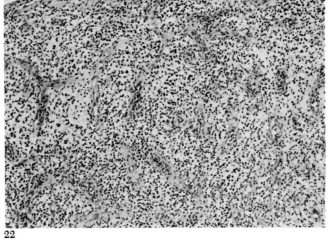

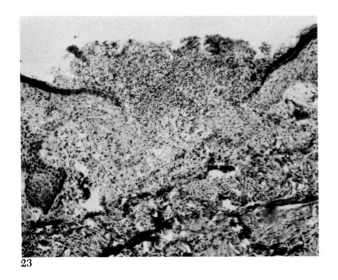

21

22

23

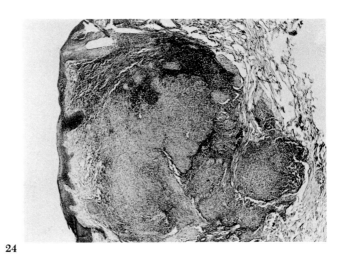

24

25   Lupus vulgaris (tuberculosis cutis luposa) of the skin of the vulva

There is granulomatous inflammation in the upper dermis with formation of a tubercle. The tubercle is formed by nests of epithelioid cells, Langhans' giant cells, lymphocytes, and plasma cells. (H&E. ×120)

26   Granuloma inguinale (donovanosis) of the skin of the labium majus

Note the marked pseudoepitheliomatous hyperplasia and severe infiltration of the dermis with plasma cells, histiocytes, and polymorphonuclear leukocytes. Numerous microabscesses are formed. The number of lymphocytes as a rule is small. (H&E. ×25)

27   Granuloma inguinale (donovanosis) of the skin of the labium majus

High magnification of Fig. 26. Formation of a microabscess and destruction of the epidermis are seen. (H&E. ×120)

28   Granuloma inguinale (donovanosis) of the skin of the labium majus

The diagnosis of granuloma inguinale rests upon demonstration of intracytoplasmic inclusions called Donovan bodies. Numerous bodies may be observed in a macrophage. They are caused by *Donovania granulomatis,* a gram-negative bacterium. (Wright's stain. ×800)

29   Chancroid (ulcus molle) of the fourchette of the vulva

The ulcer shows undermined, irregular edges. The base of the ulcer shows necrotic tissue surrounded by inflammatory exudate and edematous tissue. (H&E. ×25)

30   Chancroid (ulcus molle) of the fourchette

High magnification of Fig. 29. The granulomatous reaction consists of plasma cells, lymphocytes, and polymorphonuclear leukocytes. There is proliferation of the endothelial cells within the capillaries. Giemsa's stain is useful in demonstrating gram-negative *Hemophilus ducreyi.* (H&E. ×200)

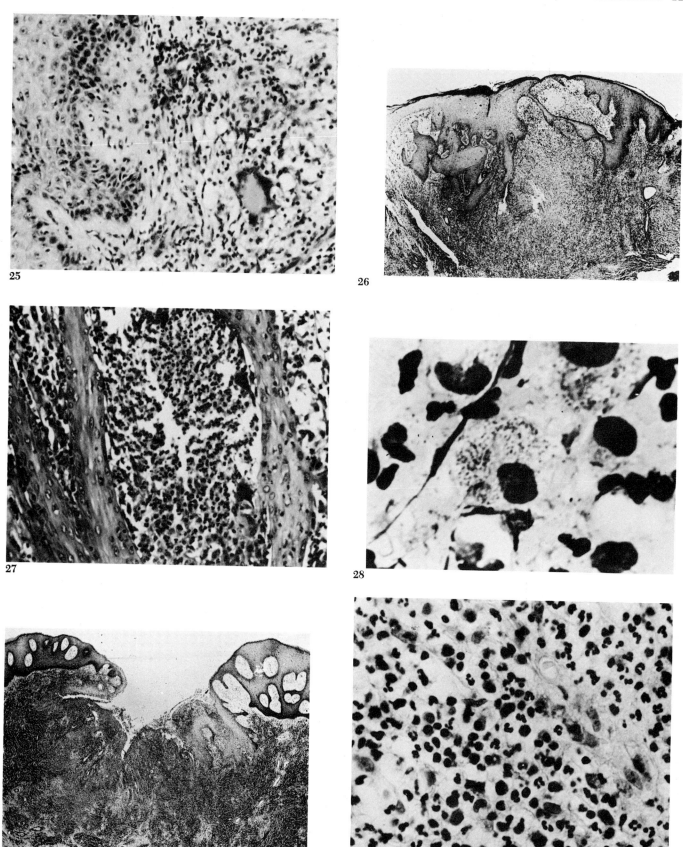

25

26

27

28

29

30

31 Syphilitic chancre (ulcus durum) of the labium majus, primary stage
The margin of an ulcer is shown. There is deep infiltrate composed of lymphocytes and plasma cells. Small foci of necrosis are seen. *Treponema pallidum* can be demonstrated in tissue by application of silver impregnation methods. Perivascular infiltration is seen in deep portions of the dermis. (H&E. ×25)

32 Syphilitic chancre (ulcus durum) of the labium majus, primary stage
High magnification of Fig. 31. The inflammatory exudate is composed of plasma cells, lymphocytes, and occasional polymorphonuclear leukocytes. Capillaries and lymphatics are increased, showing endothelial-cell proliferation. (H&E. ×200)

33 Syphilitic chancre of the labium majus, primary stage
Occlusion of the vascular lumen and formation of perivascular granuloma are observed in the late primary stage. (H&E. ×120)

34 Condyloma latum (secondary syphilis) of the vulva
Marked acanthosis is associated with broadening and elongation of the rete ridges. The dermis shows marked inflammatory infiltration and connective tissue edema. The plasma cells are prominent. (H&E. ×30)

35 Condyloma latum with ecthymalike changes (secondary syphilis) of the vulva—Erosive condyloma latum
Marked inflammatory exudate is seen covering the acanthotic epidermis. The dermal infiltrate is that of secondary syphilis, and shows perivascular infiltrate with numerous plasma cells. There is formation of a pustulelike structure at the epidermodermal junction. (H&E. ×50)

36 Ulceration of nodular tertiary syphilis of the vulva
An extensive ulcer is seen developing from granulomatous inflammation. (H&E. ×30)

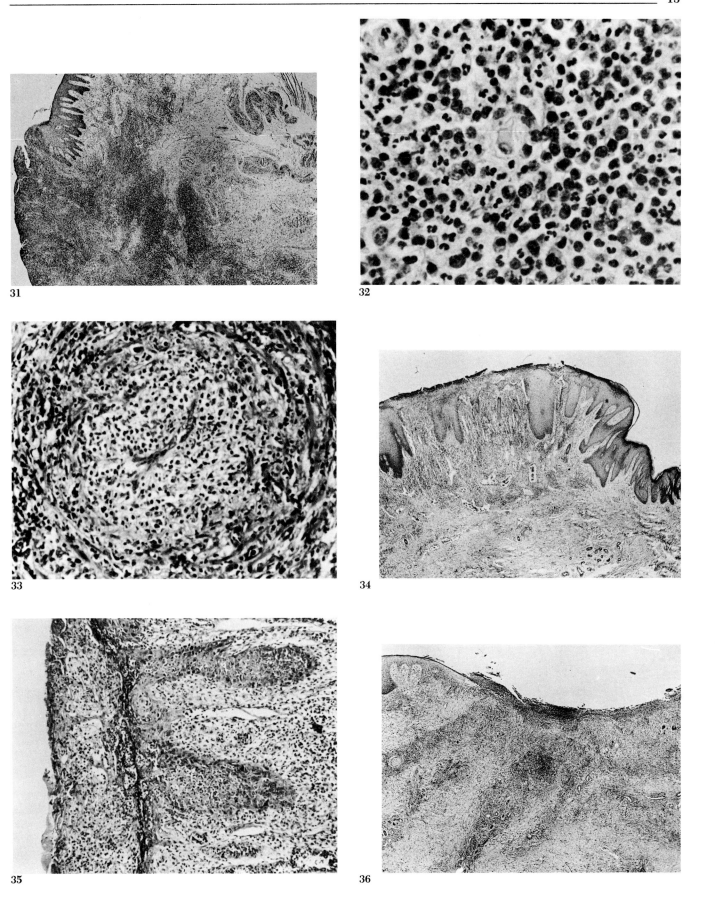

31

32

33

34

35

36

37 Nodular tertiary syphilis of the vulva
High magnification of Fig. 36. The granuloma is composed of giant cells and epithelioid cells. Plasma cells and lymphocytes are scattered throughout. The giant cells are of the foreign-body and/or Langhans type. Verhoeff's elastica stain shows preservation of vascular elastic fibers in otherwise necrotic areas. (H&E. ×200)

38 Gumma (tertiary syphilis) of the vulva
The granulomatous process extends into subcutaneous tissue. Epithelioid cells and giant cells are present. There is extensive obliterative endovasculitis and perivasculitis which may lead to caseation necrosis. Elastica stain demonstrates preservation of vascular elastic fibers in otherwise necrotic areas. (H&E. ×120)

39 Acute suppurative bartholinitis
Deep pyogenic inflammation is seen with extensive destruction of glandular tissue and formation of an abscess. (H&E. ×60)

40 Abscess of Bartholin's gland
Encapsulated abscess of Bartholin's gland is seen with preservation of a few degenerating glandular acini. (H&E. ×50)

41 Inflammatory Bartholin's duct cyst with pseudoabscess formation
Cystic dilated Bartholin's gland duct shows squamous metaplastic changes and contains acute inflammatory exudate. The periductal connective tissue and the glandular acini show diffuse infiltration with acute and chronic inflammatory cells. (H&E. ×50)

42 Inflammatory Bartholin's duct cyst
The large Bartholin's gland duct with stratified columnar epithelium is surrounded by chronic inflammatory exudate leading to obliteration of the excretory pathway and formation of an inflammatory Bartholin's duct cyst. (H&E. ×100)

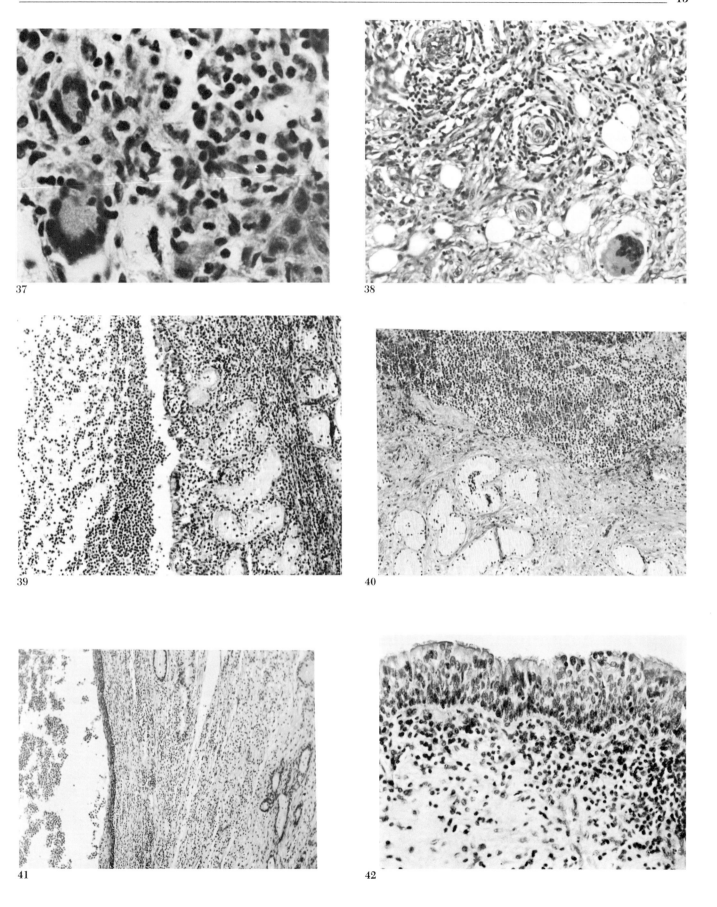

37

38

39

40

41

42

43 Chronic bartholinitis
The marked perilobular fibrosis is associated with a chronic inflammatory process. The individual acini are undergoing destructive changes and replacement by connective tissue. (H&E. ×60)

44 Eosinophilic bartholinitis
Bartholin's gland acini and the periglandular connective tissue are heavily infiltrated with predominantly eosinophilic leukocytes. The reason for their presence is not well known. (H&E. ×50)

45 Ulcus vulvae acutum (Lipschütz ulcer or aphthosis of the vulva)
There is ulceration and necrosis of the epidermis of the vulva. The upper dermis shows a nonspecific inflammatory reaction. The capillaries are dilated, and some are thrombosed. (H&E. ×55)

46 Fasciitis of the vulva (inflammatory pseudotumor of the vulva or pseudosarcomatous fasciitis of the vulva)
A granuloma adherent to the fascia of the vulva is composed of a bizarre proliferation of fibroblasts and variable numbers of inflammatory cells and capillaries. This lesion is frequently misinterpreted as malignant. The pseudotumor in this case developed from fascia of the transversus perinei profundus. If the lesion is inadequately excised, local recurrence is frequent. (H&E. ×125)

47 Molluscum contagiosum of the vulva
Note the marked proliferation of the stratum malpighii. There is formation of small vacuoles and the appearance of granules in the cytoplasm of these cells. The excavated central portion of this structure is filled with cellular detritus and hyalinized molluscum bodies. (H&E. ×120)

48 Molluscum contagiosum of the skin of the vulva
Numerous elementary virus bodies are present within the cytoplasm of the enlarged prickle cells. They fuse to form an oval hyaline body that fills the cell and displaces the nucleus, the so-called molluscum body. (H&E. ×312)

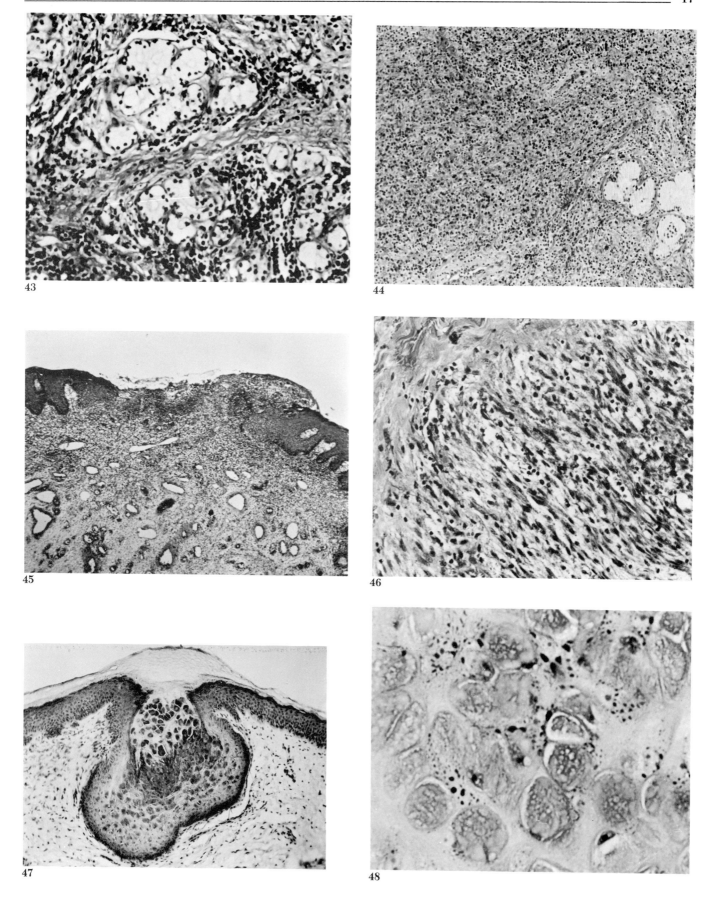

43

44

45

46

47

48

49 Single condyloma acuminatum of the skin of the vulva
Marked branching and elongation of the papillary bodies with pronounced acanthosis of the epidermis is seen. (H&E. ×25)

50 Multiple condylomata acuminata of the skin of the vulva
There is marked papillomatosis and acanthosis with broadening and elongation of the rete ridges. (H&E. ×12)

51 Dysplastic changes occurring in condyloma acuminatum, skin of the vulva
There is parakeratosis and irregular acanthosis associated with moderate cellular atypism and dyskeratosis. Malignant epithelial transformation may also occur in condyloma acuminatum. (H&E. ×100)

52 Verruca vulgaris of the skin of the vulva
There is hyperkeratosis, papillomatosis, and acanthosis. The elongated marginal rete pegs show characteristic inward curvature. The upper stratum malpighii shows the presence of large vacuolated cells. (H&E. ×12)

53 Lymphogranuloma venereum, skin of the labium majus
Granulomatous inflammation of the dermis and subcutis with ulcer formation. The granulomatous infiltrate consists of plasma cells, lymphocytes, epithelioid cells, and occasional polymorphonuclear leukocytes. The epidermis shows hyperkeratosis, acanthosis, and, as a rule, pseudoepitheliomatous hyperplasia. The etiological agent is filtrable virus *Miyagawanella lymphogranulomatosis*. There is possible relationship between lymphogranuloma venereum and cancer. (H&E. ×25)

54 Lymphogranuloma venereum of an inguinal lymph node
The formation of a stellate abscess in an inguinal lymph node is seen. This characteristic lesion is diagnostic of the disease. The stellate abscess is formed by epithelioid cells with central necrosis. (H&E. ×50)

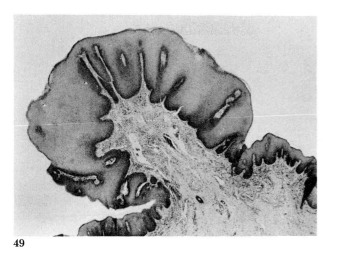

49

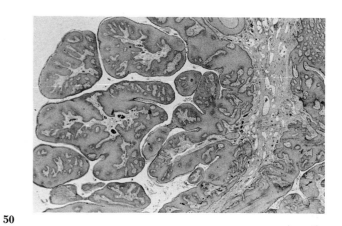

50

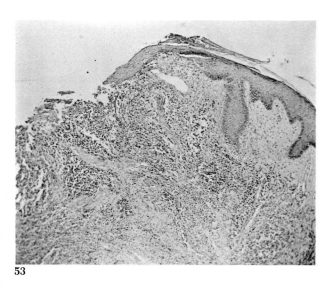

51

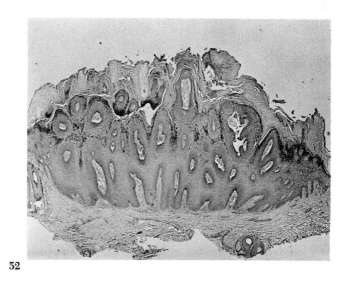

52

53

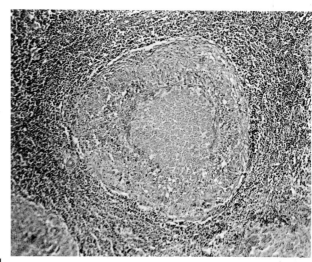

54

55   Varicella of the vulva
The intraepidermal vesicle is the result of ballooning and reticular degeneration of the epidermal cells. (H&E. ×80)

56   Varicella of the vulva
High magnification of Fig. 55. There is advanced reticular degeneration of the epidermal cells. Intranuclear inclusion bodies are seen in varicella, herpes zoster, and herpes simplex. (H&E. ×200)

57   Herpes zoster of the vulva
The unilocular vesicle contains numerous balloon cells. Varicella, herpes zoster, and herpes simplex are indistinguishable histologically. (H&E. ×100)

58   Herpes zoster of the vulva
High magnification of Fig. 57. Degeneration of the epidermal cells (ballooning), with Lipschütz inclusion bodies in the nuclei of cells, is seen. (H&E. ×200)

59   Herpes progenitalis (herpes simplex) of the vulva
There is reticular degeneration at the surface of the vesicle and ballooning degeneration at the floor of the vesicle. The upper dermis shows an inflammatory reaction. (H&E. ×125)

60   Herpes progenitalis (herpes simplex) of the vulva
High magnification of Fig. 59. Intranuclear inclusion bodies are seen in balloon cells. (H&E. ×312)

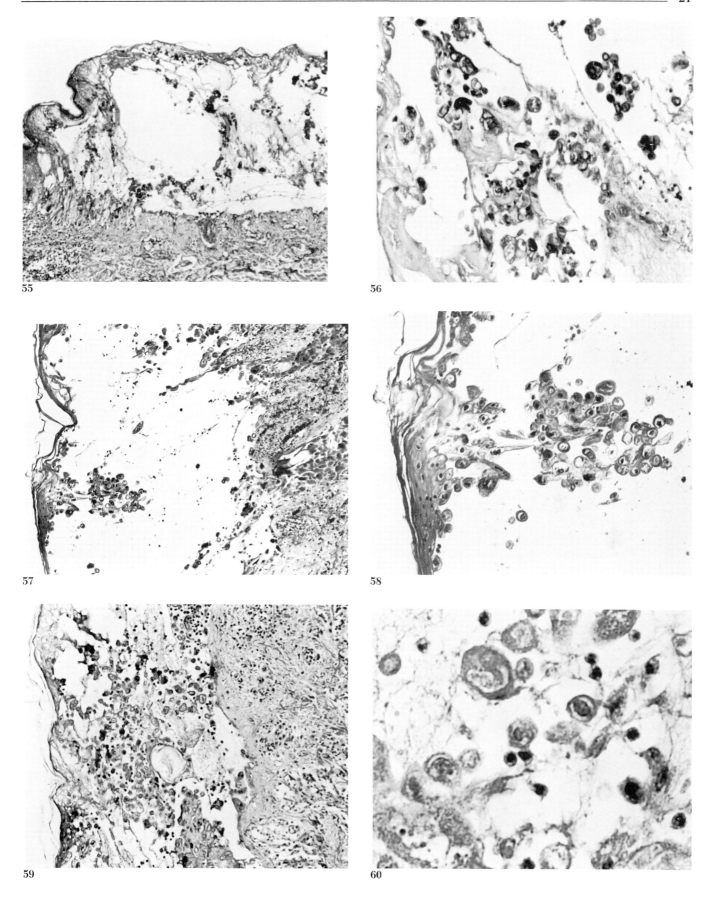

55

56

57

58

59

60

61 Actinomycosis of the skin of the vulva
The actinomycotic granule is surrounded by acute inflammatory exudate forming an abscess. (H&E. ×50)

62 Actinomycosis of the skin of the vulva
High magnification of Fig. 61. The edge of the actinomycotic granule shows a peripheral mycelial fringe with clubs. Polymorphonuclear leukocytes and lipoid macrophages are seen surrounding the granule. (H&E. ×175)

63 Cutaneous blastomycosis, of the skin of the vulva
This section of infected tissue is similar to that seen in South American blastomycosis. There are numerous giant cells, some containing organisms. In some areas, the organisms lie free in the tissue. (H&E. ×120)

64 Cutaneous blastomycosis, of the skin of the vulva
Multiple budding cells and chains of cells are located in the dermal connective tissue. (Gridley fungus stain. ×60)

66 Bancroft's filariasis with lymphoid hyperplasia of the labium majus
An island of mononuclear cell accumulation can be seen. Such islands are scattered in the lower dermis and subcutis. Microfilariae may be found in such lymphoid islands. Isolated lymphatic hyperplasia is characteristic of long-standing infection with *Wuchereria bancrofti*. (H&E. ×50)

65 Dermatophytosis consistent with Tinea cruris, skin of the labium majus
There are fungal mycelia located in keratin layer of the epidermis. (H&E. ×400)

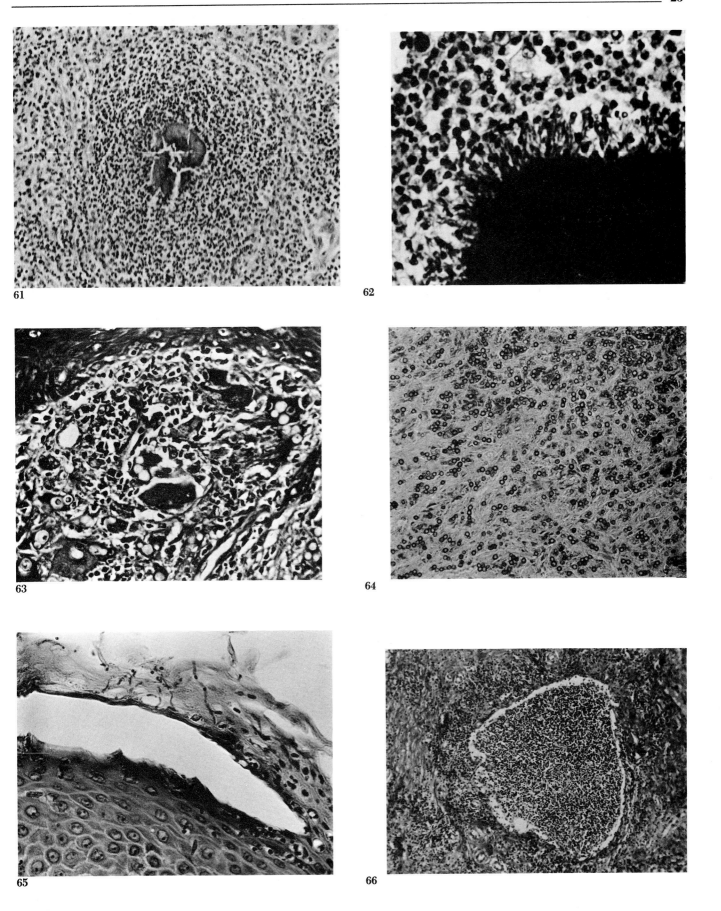

61

62

63

64

65

66

67 Bancroft's filariasis with elephantiasis of the labium majus
There is advanced elephantiasis of the labia majora of the vulva. The proliferation of fibrous connective tissue and chronic edema terminate in marked dermal fibrosis and obliteration of all dermal appendages. (H&E. ×35)

68 Bancroft's filariasis with fibrosis and elephantiasis of the labium majus
High magnification of Fig. 67. Dilated lymphatic channels with marked perivascular fibrosis are seen. These are the result of chronic obstruction of lymphatic drainage. (H&E. ×125)

69 Schistosomiasis (bilharziasis) of the skin of the vulva
Schistosoma mansoni ova are seen surrounded by several foreign-body giant cells. There is marked inflammatory reaction of the dermis with numerous giant cells. (H&E. ×65)

70 Schistosomiasis (bilharziasis) of the skin of the vulva
High magnification of Fig. 69. The nearly spherical ova of the *Schistosoma mansoni* are found in the lower dermis of vulvar skin. The ova are instigating the formation of pseudotubercles. These consist of foreign-body giant cells, epithelioid cells, eosinophils, lymphocytes, and plasma cells. (H&E. ×320)

71 Acute contact dermatitis (eczema) of the vulva
There is formation of intraepidermal vesicles and pronounced intercellular edema. The upper dermis shows marked perivascular infiltrate by eosinophils, lymphocytes, and neutrophilic leukocytes. (H&E. ×120)

72 Chronic dermatitis (eczema) of the vulva
There is slight hyperkeratosis intermingled with areas of parakeratosis. The epidermis shows a slight degree of spongiosis. The perivascular inflammatory exudate consists chiefly of lymphocytes. (H&E. ×120)

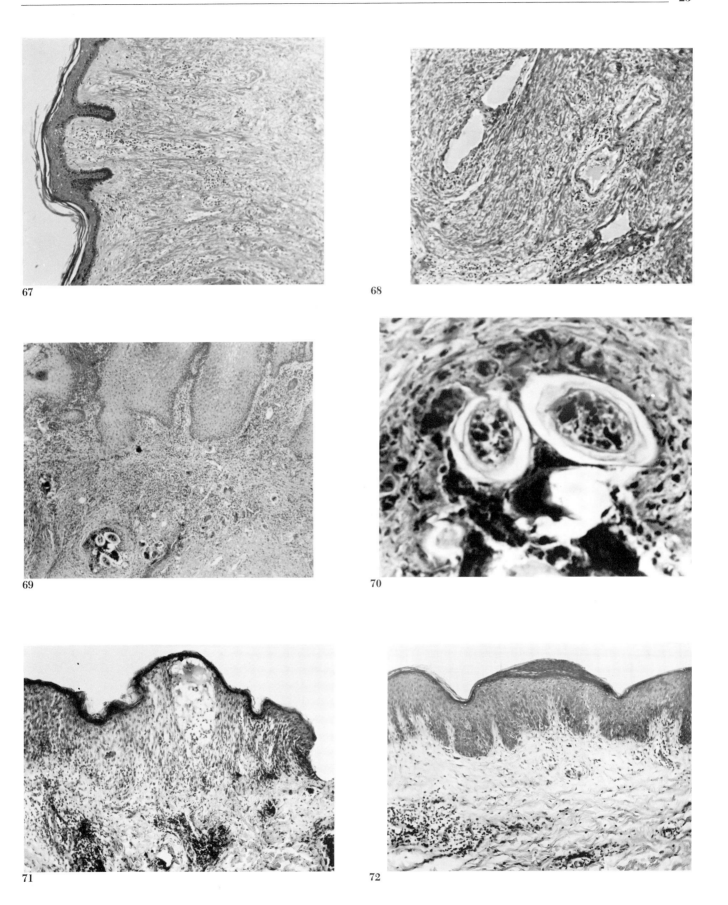

67

68

69

70

71

72

73 Neurodermatitis circumscripta (lichen chronicus simplex) of the vulva
Hyperkeratosis and areas of parakeratosis are prominent. There is acanthosis with regular elongation of rete ridges. The spongiosis is minimal. The upper dermis shows perivascular and diffuse infiltration with chronic inflammatory cells. (H&E. ×50)

74 Psoriasis of the vulva
There is parakeratosis and marked acanthosis. The rete ridges show irregular thickening in their lower portion. There is clubbing and edema of the papillary bodies. The capillaries show tortuosity and dilatation. Lymphatic infiltration is moderate. (H&E. ×180)

75 Lichen planus of the vulva
There is hyperkeratosis and broadening of the stratum granulosum. Some of the epidermal cells show degenerative changes. The inflammatory infiltrate consists entirely of lymphocytes and shows sharp demarcation at its lower border. Acanthosis with irregular elongation of the rete ridges may be present. (H&E. ×100)

76 Lichen planus verrucosus (hypertrophic lichen planus) of the vulva
There is marked papillomatosis, hyperkeratosis, and irregular acanthosis. The characteristic feature is the limitation of the cellular infiltration to a band in the upper dermis. (H&E. ×90)

77 Pemphigus vulgaris of the vulva
Suprabasal intradermal bulla with cavitary acantholytic cells is seen. Little inflammatory reaction is observed in the dermis. (H&E. ×150)

78 Erythema multiforme of the vulva, acute stage
Note the spongiosis and transepidermal infiltration composed mainly of lymphocytes with few polymorphonuclear leukocytes. The basal layer is consequently rendered indistinct. (H&E. ×120)

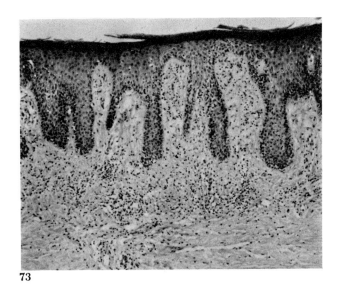

73

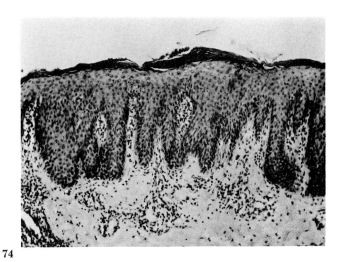

74

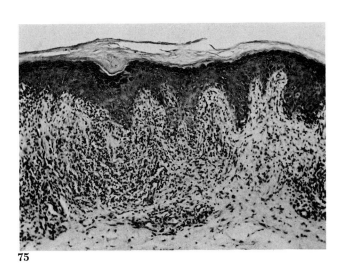

75

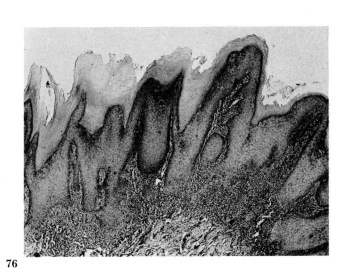

76

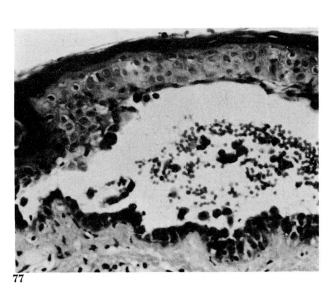

77

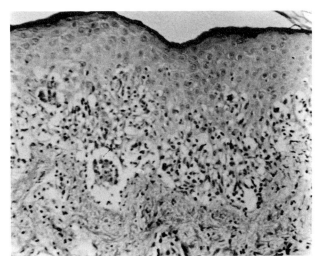

78

79 Erythema multiforme of the vulva, acute stage

The epidermis shows spongiosis, intracellular edema, and formation of an intraepidermal vesicle. Polymorphonuclear cells, particularly eosinophils, are seen in the vesicle. The upper dermis shows edema, dilatation of capillaries, and perivascular infiltration of chronic inflammatory cells and extravasated erythrocytes. (H&E. ×50)

80 Subsiding erythema multiforme of the vulva

Crust formation is seen following the disappearance of intraepidermal vesicles in the healing stage of the disease. (H&E. ×100)

81 Malignant acanthosis nigricans of the vulva

This biopsy was taken from the vulva of a patient with metastasizing endometrial carcinoma. The epidermis shows marked hyperkeratosis, papillomatosis, and areas of acanthosis alternating with areas of epidermal atrophy. There may be increased melanin in the basal layer. The term "malignant" is used to denote that type of acanthosis nigricans which is invariably associated with an internal adenocarcinoma (Curth). H&E. ×80)

82 Pityriasis rubra pilaris of the skin of the vulva

The horny plug in the follicular orifice is associated with diffuse hyperkeratosis and spotty parakeratosis. There is also mild, irregular acanthosis. Occasional chronic inflammatory cells are seen in the upper dermis. Phrynoderma due to vitamin A deficiency takes on a similar histologic appearance. (H&E. ×100)

83 Darier's disease (keratosis follicularis) of the vulva

The characteristic feature is the presence of lacunas in the epidermis which occur above the basal layer. There is hyperkeratosis and moderate acanthosis. Hyperkeratosis and the keratotic plugging are not related to the hair follicles, and the term "keratosis follicularis" is inaccurate. Within the lacunas there is formation of villi due to upward proliferation of the papillary body. (H&E. ×80)

84 Darier's disease (keratosis follicularis) of the vulva

High magnification of Fig. 83. Corps ronds, partially keratinized cells in the process of benign dyskeratosis, are seen within the granular layer. Within the lacunas are degenerating, desquamated, acantholytic cells. Shrunken acantholytic cells and small cells with pyknotic nuclei are called grains. (H&E. ×200)

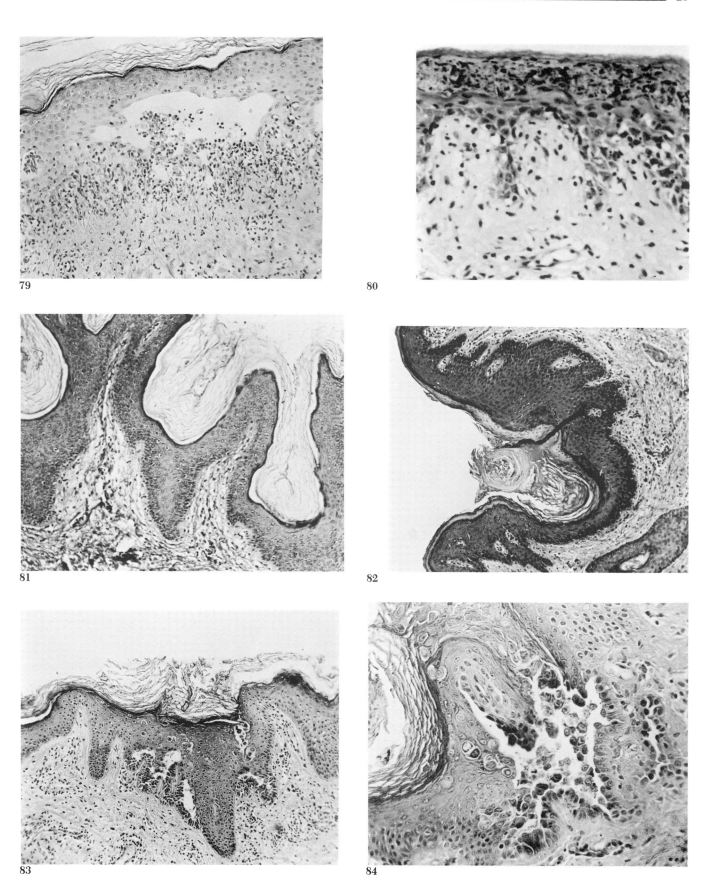

79

80

81

82

83

84

85 Xanthoma diabeticorum (Hyperlipemic xanthoma) of the vulva
There is proliferation of fibroblasts, and numerous foam cells containing lipid droplets are present. Clefts representing cholesterol and fatty acids dissolved by embedding agents are prominent. (H&E. ×120)

86 Localized, nodular amyloidosis of the skin of the vulva
There is marked homogenization affecting almost the entire dermis. The dermal appendages are obliterated. The epidermis is atrophic, and the papillary bodies are obliterated by band-shaped deposition of amyloid. Perivascular distribution of amyloid is also seen. (H&E. ×62)

87 Lichen sclerosus et atrophicus (LSA) of the vulva, early stage
There is hyperkeratosis and atrophy of the epidermis. The upper dermis shows edema and vacuolar degeneration. The mid-dermis shows early homogenization of collagen fibers. (H&E. ×25)

88 Lichen sclerosus et atrophicus (LSA) of the vulva, progressing stage
Marked atrophy of the epidermis and mid-dermal distribution of inflammatory exudate composed mainly of lymphocytes. (H&E. ×25)

89 Lichen sclerosus et atrophicus (LSA) of the vulva, advanced stage
The stage of edema of the upper dermis is followed by homogenization of the collagen fibers. The degree of homogenization may vary from case to case, but this is the pathognomonic feature of LSA. The epidermis is subatrophic. (H&E. ×40)

90 Squamous cell carcinoma developing in a lichen sclerosus et atrophicus of the vulva
There is no statistical relationship between LSA and development of the squamous carcinoma of the epidermis. Here islands of neoplastic squamous cells are invading homogenized collagen tissue. The mid-dermal inflammatory exudate is observed at the right. (H&E. ×50)

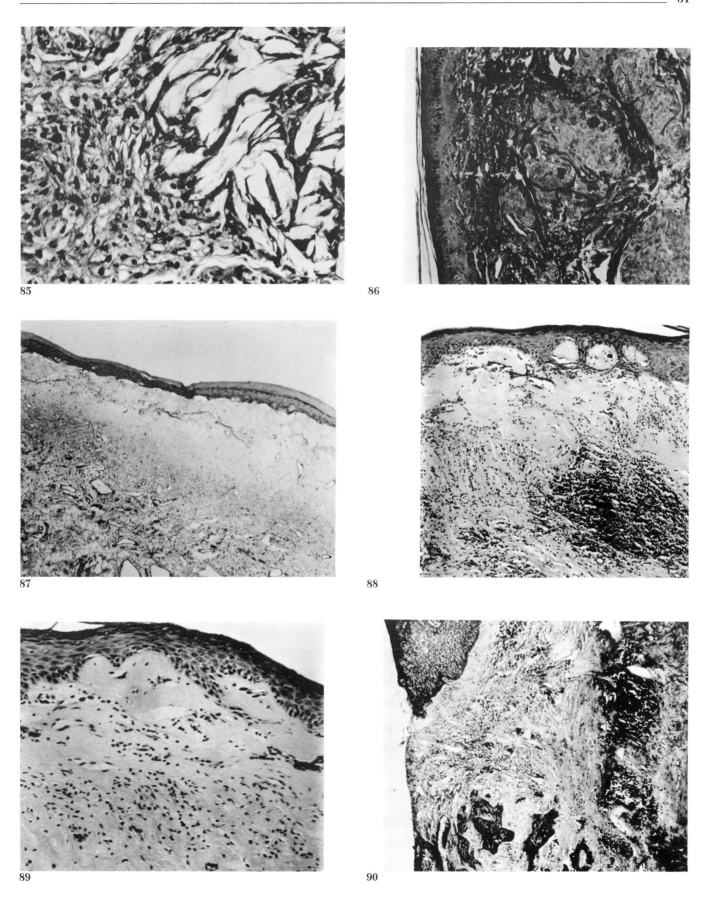

85

86

87

88

89

90

91 Hyperkeratosis with senile atrophy of the skin of the vulva
There is marked production of keratin. The epidermis is atrophic. The upper dermis shows a mild inflammatory reaction. The dermal appendages are partly absent or atrophic. This morphologic alteration of vulvar skin may be found in chronic irritative or traumatic processes of the vulva. (H&E. ×24)

92 Tangential section of the normal vulvar skin
Epidermis is seen simulating pseudoepitheliomatous hyperplasia and frequently is misinterpreted as such. (H&E. ×50)

93 Pseudoepitheliomatous hyperplasia of the skin of the vulva
The downward proliferation of the epidermal cells has some resemblance with squamous cell carcinoma. However the epidermal cells are all well differentiated, and there is absence of cellular and nuclear atypism. This condition is frequently encountered with ulceration and nonspecific inflammation of the skin of the vulva. (H&E. ×25)

94 Hypertrophy of the clitoris
The hypertrophic clitoris is seen in a 2-year-old girl with adrenogenital syndrome. (H&E. ×5)

95 Hypertrophy of the clitoris
High magnification of Fig. 94. There is hypertrophy and hyperplasia of connective tissue elements and an increase of corpus cavernosum spaces and perivascular tissue. (H&E. ×50)

96 Hyperplasia of the apocrine sweat glands of the vulva
Although the cyclic enlargement of the apocrine sweat glands of the vulva in the premenstrual period is well established, the persisting hyperplasia with cystic, dilated glandular structures forming polygonal islands is occasionally observed in Negresses. (H&E. ×20)

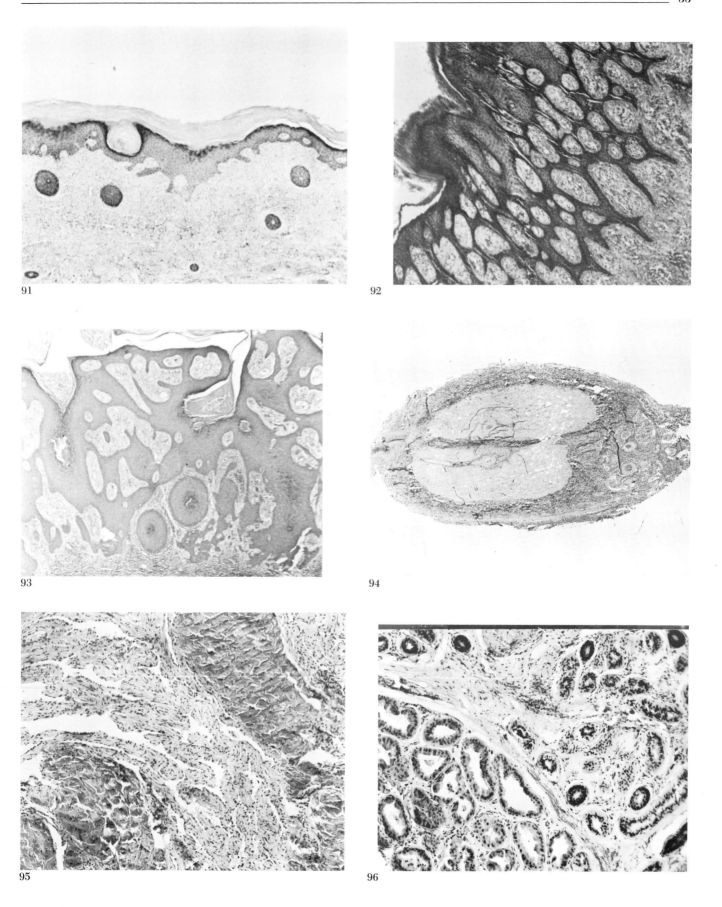

91

92

93

94

95

96

97 Epithelial nevus, skin of the vulva
Marked hyperplasia and irregular acanthosis of the epidermis. There is increased pigment content of basal cells. Melanin pigment is also seen in upper dermis. There is absence of nevus cells. Occurring in 22-year-old patient and presenting as multiple, small, brownish nodular structures of the skin of the vulva. This lesion may be congenital or acquired. (H&E. ×30)

98 Hyperplasia of the sebaceous gland of the labium minus
Hyperplasia of the sebaceous glands associated with chronic inflammatory infiltration of the connective tissue stroma and increased vascularity denote mechanical irritation of the labia. These morphologic findings are consistent with masturbation hypertrophy of the labia. (H&E. ×45)

99 Keloid of the vulva
There is absence of dermal appendages and formation of coarse collagen bundles with interspersed fibroblasts. The hypertrophic scar on the mons veneris was present for 2 years. (H&E. ×17)

100 Keloid of the vulva
High magnification of Fig. 99. Irregularly arranged collagen bundles which are partly hyalinized indicate the aging process. The fibroblasts are inconspicuous. (H&E. ×100)

101 Traumatic lipogranuloma of the mons veneris and vulva
There is replacement of adipose tissue by phagocytic cells and multinucleated giant cells. Some of these contain phagocytized lipid. Focal necrosis and scattered chronic inflammatory cells are present. A similar histologic picture is observed in patients receiving steroid injections in the vulvar area for vulvar pruritus, so-called poststeroid panniculitis. (H&E. ×100)

102 Cystic dilatation of Bartholin's acini in association with a large cyst
The cyst on the left is lined by cuboidal mucus-secreting epithelium. The fibrous wall contains cystic dilated glands with inspissations. (H&E. ×50)

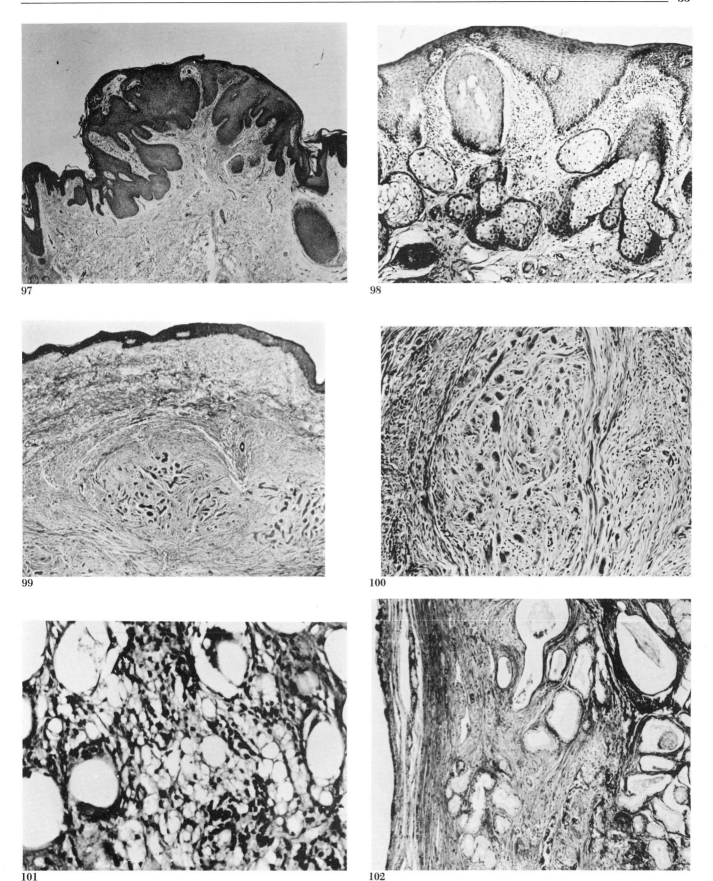

97

98

99

100

101

102

103 Bartholin's gland with ductal ectasia
Ductal ectasia of Bartholin's gland occurs following an obstruction within the main excretory ductal system. It is the first step in the development of a Bartholin's duct cyst. (H&E. ×150)

104 Bartholin's gland cyst
The typical cyst is lined by a single row of tall columnar mucin-producing epithelial cells with basally placed uniform nuclei. The wall of the cyst is fibrous and contains an isolated compressed small gland. (H&E. ×70)

105 Bartholin's duct cyst
The duct of the Bartholin's gland is cystic, dilated, and lined by several layers of transitional epithelium. (H&E. ×10)

106 Squamous metaplasia of a Bartholin's gland duct
(H&E. ×150)

107 Peritoneal cyst of the canal of Nuck vulva
The unilocular cyst shows fibrous tissue wall and is lined by flattened mesothelial cells. (H&E. ×100)

108 Cyst of the vulva caused by ectopic lactating breast tissue
A cystic, dilated duct of lactating ectopic breast tissue is seen. The acini are dilated, showing secretory activity. (H&E. ×12)

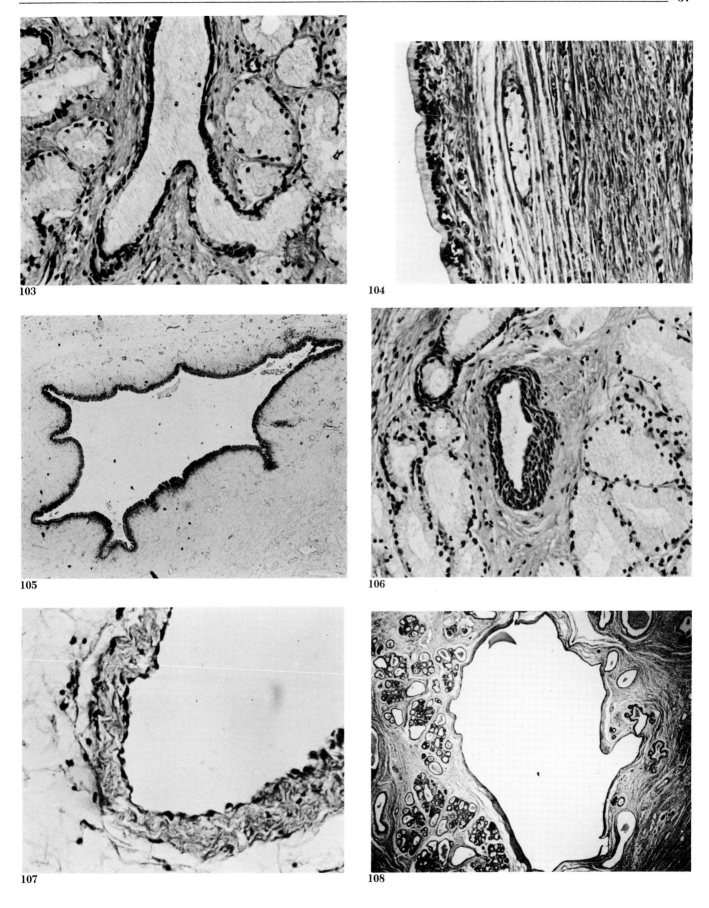

103

104

105

106

107

108

109 Cyst of an eccrine sweat gland duct of the labium majus
The cystic, dilated eccrine sweat gland duct shows a fibrous wall. (H&E. ×30)

110 Epidermal inclusion cyst of the labium majus
The cyst is lined with attenuated squamous epithelium and contains keratinized material. (H&E. ×10)

111 Traumatic epidermal inclusion cyst developing in an episiotomy scar of the vulva
The cyst is lined with squamous epithelium. The wall shows dense fibrous tissue consistent with cicatrization. (H&E. ×60)

112 Sebaceous duct cyst of the labium majus
The cyst is lined in places with several rows of cuboidal cells with round nuclei. In other areas it is lined by stratified squamous epithelium continuous with the ducts of neighboring sebaceous glands. (H&E. ×50)

113 Dysontogenetic (Müllerian) cyst of the labium minus
The cross section of the labium minus shows the centrally located cyst. Note the considerable stromal edema and pronounced vascularity. (H&E. ×5)

114 Dysontogenetic (Müllerian) cyst of the labium minus
High magnification of Fig. 113. The lining epithelium has a striking resemblance to tubal type of epithelium. (Wilder's reticulum stain. ×250)

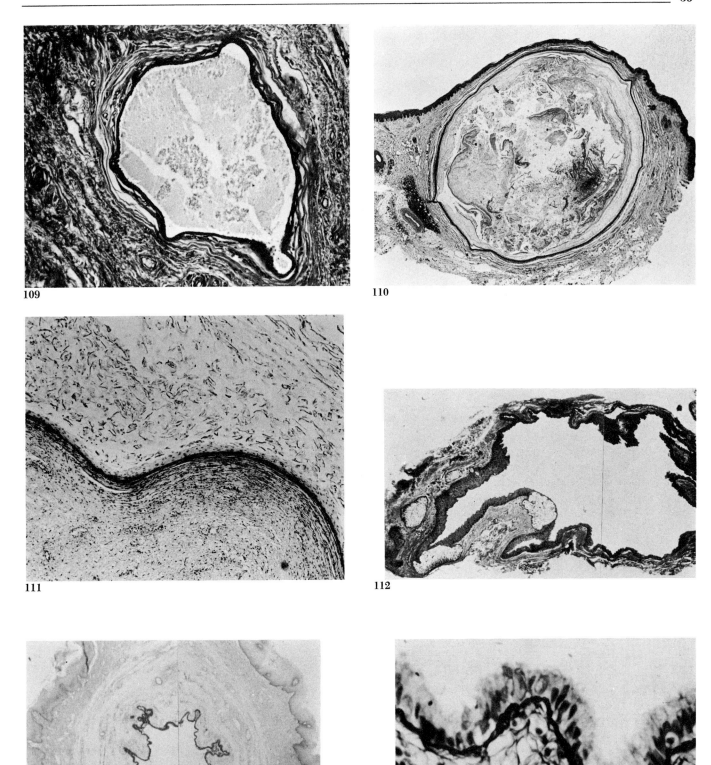

109

110

111

112

113

114

115 Fibroepithelial papilloma of the skin of the vulva
Multiple cores of connective tissue are covered by epidermis. Moderate keratosis and/or parakeratosis may be present. (H&E. ×15)

116 Congenital fibroepithelial papilloma of the skin of the vulva
The tumor has a broad stalk. The epidermis shows papillomatosis, hyperkeratosis, and irregular acanthosis. The connective tissue core is vascular and infiltrated with chronic inflammatory cells. The patient with this congenital vulvar lesion is 13 years old. (H&E. ×24)

117 Seborrheic keratosis of the skin of the vulva
There is hyperkeratosis, acanthosis, and papillomatosis. Because of invagination of the stratum corneum, there are frequent cystic inclusions of horny material known as pseudohorn cysts. The tumor is made up of small cells resembling cells of the stratum germinativum. Increased pigmentation is noted in epidermal cells, and there are numerous melanophages in the upper dermis. (H&E. ×60)

118 Inverted follicular keratosis of the vulva
The tumor consists of islands of keratinizing squamous epithelium which has become inverted into itself. The margins and the base of the tumor exhibit normal epidermis. This lesion is occasionally misinterpreted as being an invasive squamous cell carcinoma. (H&E. ×10)

119 Inverted papilloma (pseudoepitheliomatous hyperplasia) following simple vulvectomy
At the surgical mucocutaneous margin of the vulva, 1 year after simple vulvectomy, a tumor developed which has been variously interpreted as squamous carcinoma, papilloma, verruca, etc. There is irregular invasion of the dermis by epidermal cells with horn pearls and cyst formations. The lesion resembles an inverted papilloma. The squamous cells are well differentiated, and there is no evidence of atypism. (H&E. ×20)

120 Keratoacanthoma of the vulva
The marked epithelial hyperplasia suggests either a pseudoepitheliomatous or a highly differentiated squamous cell carcinoma. The central crater of the tumor is filled with keratin. At the base there is marked proliferation of the epidermal cells with formation of keratin pearls and cysts. The margins of the tumor consist of normal epidermis and are characteristically "pulled up" over the tumor. Dense inflammatory infiltrate is found in the surrounding connective tissue. This tumor is often misdiagnosed as squamous cell carcinoma. (H&E. ×8)

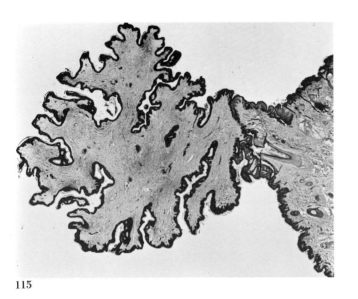

115

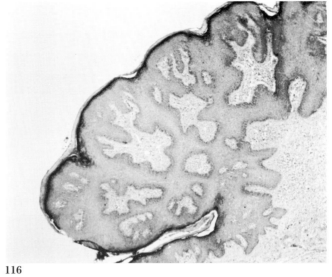

116

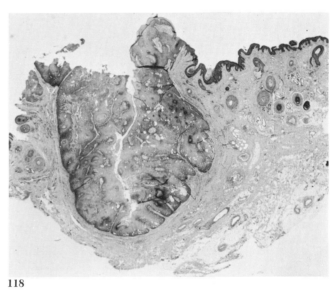

117

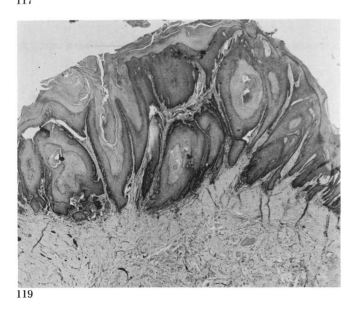

118

119

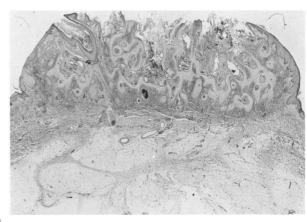

120

121 Keratoacanthoma of the skin of the vulva
High magnification of Fig. 120. The base of the keratoacanthoma shows marked acanthotic changes, associated with epidermal cell hyperplasia, formation of keratin pearls and cysts. The connective tissue shows a dense inflammatory reaction. The resemblance to squamous cell carcinoma is striking. However, if the lesion is excised in its entirety, the general architecture is pathognomonic for this tumor. (H&E. ×80)

122 Hidradenoma papilliferum of the labium majus
This is usually a small benign tumor of apocrine sweat glands. It is well encapsulated, exhibiting both a papillary and glandular pattern. (H&E. ×8)

123 Hidradenoma papilliferum of the labium majus
High magnification of Fig. 122. The glandular structures vary in size showing occasional typical apocrine metaplasia consisting of a double layer of eosinophilic epithelial cells. (H&E. ×120)

124 Hidradenoma papilliferum of the labium majus
High magnification of Fig. 122. The papillary structures are slender and covered by a single or double layer of tall columnar cells. In places these columnar cells are seen resting on a second layer of small cuboidal cells with round nuclei and clear cytoplasm. (H&E. ×120)

125 Syringoma of the labium majus
Numerous cystic structures are located in the dermis. Colloidal material is seen in the same cysts. This is a benign tumor of sweat gland origin. (H&E. ×50)

126 Syringoma of the labium majus
High magnification of Fig. 125. The cyst is lined by two layers of cells. There are several solid strands of epithelial cells. Colloid material is within the cyst. (H&E. ×312)

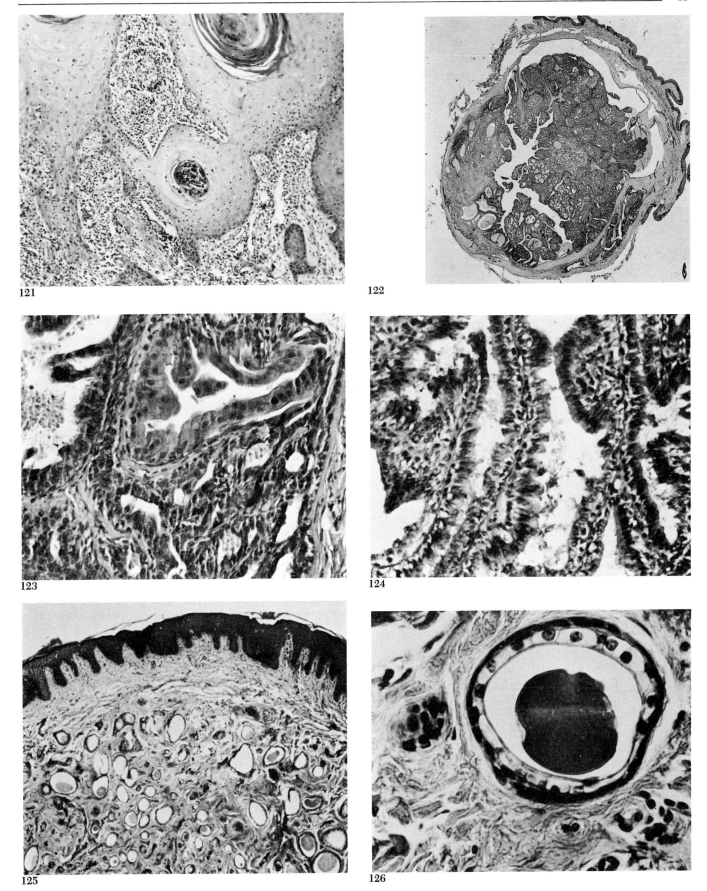

121

122

123

124

125

126

127   Adenoma of Bartholin's gland
The normal architecture is replaced by neoplastic glandular structures showing considerable variation in size. The ducts are well preserved. (H&E. ×50)

128   Adenoma of Bartholin's gland
High magnification of Fig. 127. Masses of epithelial acini, tubules, and buds have replaced normal glandular structures. The intervening connective tissue is sparse. The neoplastic epithelium is cuboidal with round prominent nuclei. There is absence of mitotic activity. Some glandular lumens contain mucinous secretions. (H&E. ×120)

129   Adnexal papilloma (papillary adenoma) of the labium minus
The small, poorly developed fibrovascular papillomatous processes are covered by uniform stratified epithelium. The tumor is benign. The origin is not clear. (H&E. ×62)

130   Adnexal papilloma (papillary adenoma) of the labium minus
High magnification of Fig. 129. The cells lining the free surface of the papillary projections are flattened and have dark nuclei. The cells of the basal layer are slightly basophilic, orderly, and contain no mitotic figures. (H&E. ×125)

131   Dermatofibroma of the skin of the vulva
There is disorderly arrangement of collagen fibers. Individual fibers are prominent. The pale stained areas represent young collagen. Fibroblasts are increased in number. The overlying epidermis is attenuated. (H&E. ×50)

132   Fibroepithelial polyp (skin tag, fibroma molle) of the labium majus
Attenuated squamous epithelium covers edematous and well-vascularized connective tissue core. The polyp is attached by a stalk to the vulvar skin. (H&E. ×5)

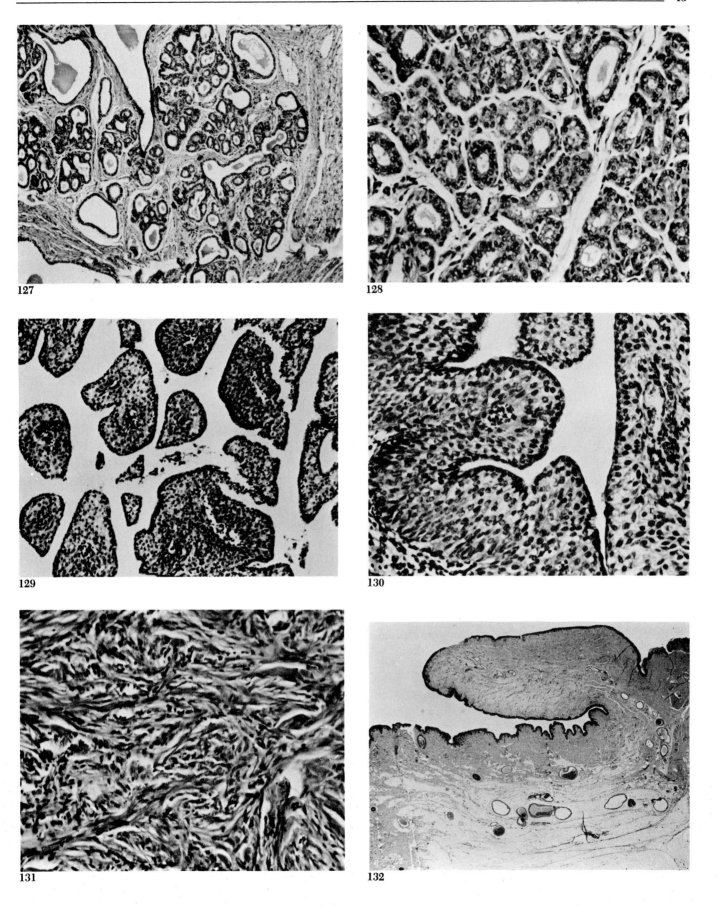

127

128

129

130

131

132

133   Histiocytoma of the skin of the vulva
The tumor is composed of whorls of fibrous connective tissue. Hemosiderin, foam cells, and an increased number of vessels are constant components of the tumor. Special stains for fat or lipid are useful for demonstration of lipid phagocytizing histiocytes. (H&E. ×50)

134   Histiocytoma of the skin of the vulva
High magnification of Fig. 133. There is marked proliferation of fibroblasts and histiocytes with large nuclei rich in chromatin and cytoplasm containing lipid or phagocitized hemosiderin. Multinuclear giant cells are frequent. (H&E. ×312)

135   Fibroma of the vulva, with myxomatous changes
To the right is a fibroma. To the left one sees marked myxomatous changes of the tumor. (H&E. ×125)

136   Myxoma of the vulva
The tumor is made up of elongated and stellated well-differentiated fibroblastic cells. They are producing mucoid material (hyaluronic acid). This tumor has a tendency to recur but does not metastasize. (H&E. ×125)

137   Angiolipoma of the labium majus
The tumor may or may not be encapsulated. It consists of mature fat cells and proliferated capillaries. The connective tissue framework may be more or less developed, depending on the tumor. (H&E. ×80)

138   Hibernoma of the mons veneris and vulva
The tumor is formed by oval cells with centrally located nuclei. The cytoplasm contains fine granules and vacuoles which stain with fat stains. Several normal, mature fat cells are seen. (H&E. ×200)

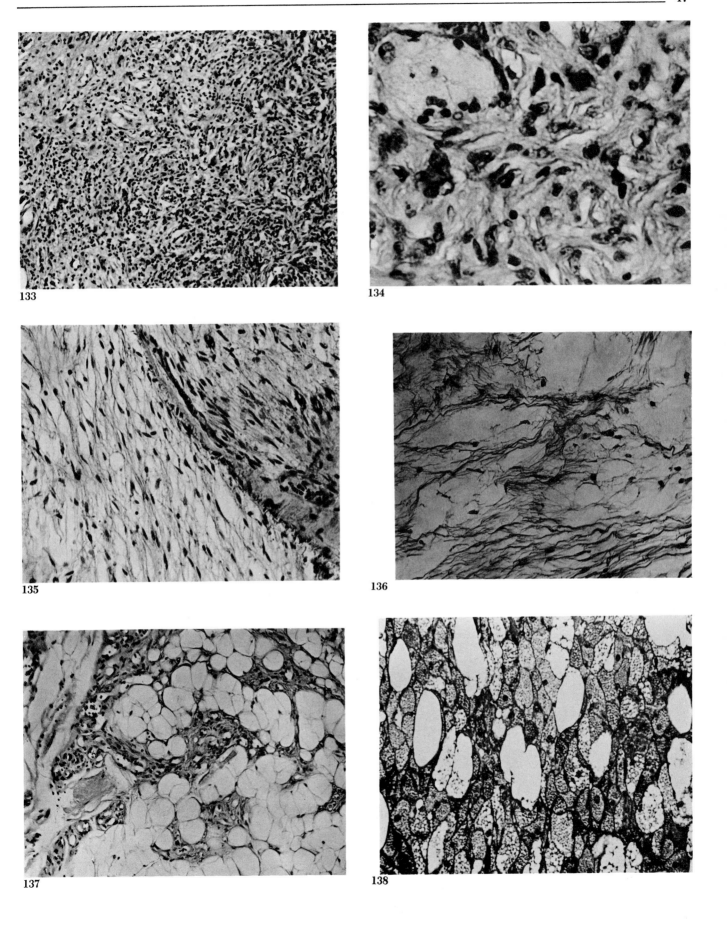

133

134

135

136

137

138

139   Leiomyoma of the vulva
The tumor consists of interlacing bundles of smooth muscle fibers. Special stains are indicated in order to differentiate muscle from collagen. (Masson's trichrome stain. ×50)

140   Granular cell myoblastoma of the vulva
Large polygonal cells are seen with small deeply stained nuclei and cytoplasm containing many fine acidophilic granules. The cells may be arranged in cords, sheets, or alveolar structures. A special stain for lipid will differentiate these cells from xanthomatous histiocytes. (H&E. ×312)

141   Neuroma of the vulva following episiotomy
The tumor consists of numerous bundles of medullated nerves. Each nerve bundle is surrounded by fibrous tissue. The diagnostic features of the tumor are best represented on transverse section, as in this picture. The demonstration of myelin sheaths will definitely identify the tumor. (H&E. ×125)

142   Neurilemmoma of the vulva
The tumor is formed by interlacing bundles of fibrillary tissue. The dark nuclei are arranged in palisading form with intervening spaces without nuclei. This organoid arrangement of cells, nuclei, and fibers is known as a Verocay body. (H&E. ×120)

143   Neurofibroma of the vulva
The tumor is formed of fine, wavy fibers with spindle-shaped somewhat angulated dark nuclei. There is a tendency toward whorl formations. (H&E. ×120)

144   Multiple neurofibromatosis (von Recklinghausen's disease) of the vulva
There is proliferation of Schwann cells in a diffuse and haphazard fashion. (H&E. ×150)

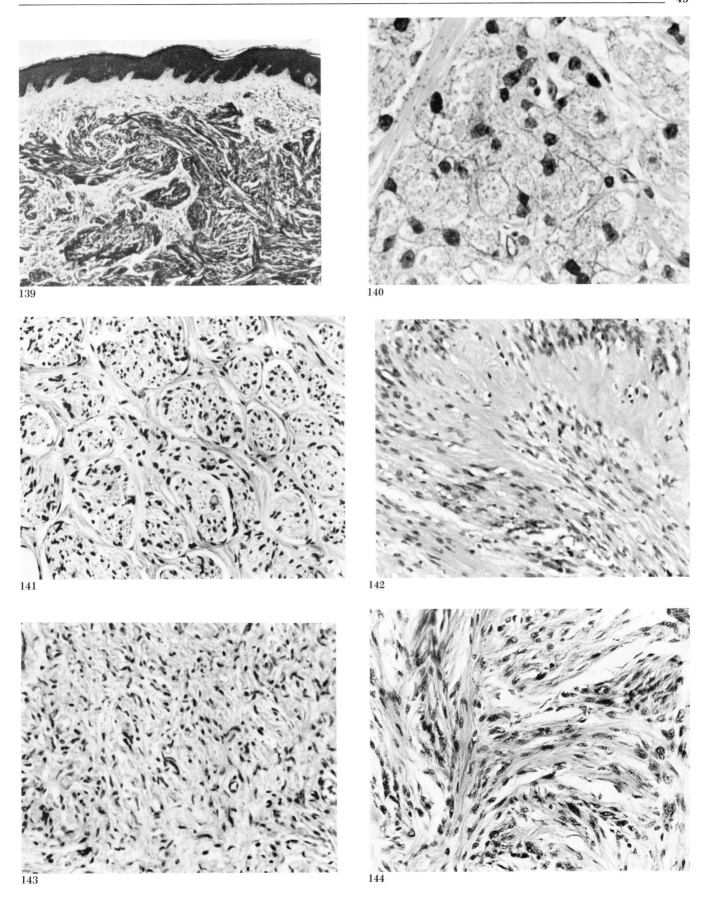

139

140

141

142

143

144

145 Café-au-lait spot in multiple neurofibromatosis (von Recklinghausen's disease) of the skin of the vulva

There is deposition of melanin pigment in the basal layer of the epidermis and in melanophages of the upper dermis. There is marked telangiectasis. The dermis shows fibrosis. (H&E. ×60)

146 Capillary hemangioma of the labium majus

The tumor is formed of a solid mass of capillaries with prominent endothelial lining cells. (H&E. ×150)

147 Lymphangioma of the labium majus

This tumor, 2 cm in diameter, removed from labium majus, is formed by various sized lymphatic channels. The intervening connective tissue is focally infiltrated with lymphocytes. (H&E. ×160)

148 Angiokeratoma of Mibelli of the skin of the labium majus

There is acanthosis with irregular proliferation of rete ridges. Greatly dilated capillaries are completely surrounded by the hypertrophic stratum malpighii. (H&E. ×50)

149 Glomus tumor of the clitoris

Islands of glomus cells with faintly eosinophilic cytoplasm and large nuclei are seen. Glomus cells surround the vascular channels. (H&E. ×80)

150 Lentigo of the vulva

There is elongation and clubbing of the rete ridges. An increase of melanin pigment is seen in the stratum germinativum. The epidermodermal junction is normal. There may be an increase of melanocytes (clear cells). The upper dermis contains melanophores and mild lymphocytic infiltrate. (H&E. ×180)

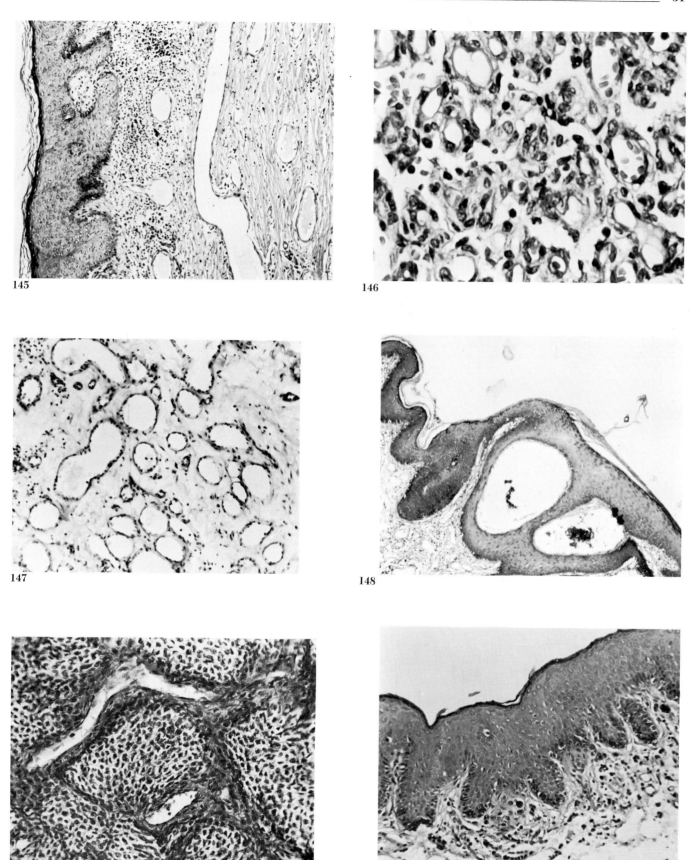

145

146

147

148

149

150

151   Junctional nevus of the labium majus
There are nevus cells at the lower epidermis
and/or at the epidermodermal junction. Melanophores are present in the dermis. The junctional
nevus, also called "active nevus," has malignant
potentiality. (H&E. ×100)

152   Intradermal nevus of the skin of the vulva
Cords of nevus cells are located in the upper and
mid-dermis. They may contain melanin. (H&E.
×50)

154   Blue nevus of the vulva
There is attenuated epidermis. The mid-dermis
and lower dermis are replaced by a tumor composed of elongated and spindle-forming melanocytes rich in dopa-positive melanin. In between
are scattered dopa-negative ovoid melanophores.
Considerable fibrosis is seen. (H&E. ×50)

153   Compound nevus of the skin of the vulva
The features of the intradermal and junctional
nevus are present in compound nevi. The nevus
cells are oval or cuboidal and the nuclei large
and round. (H&E. ×120)

**156   Benign mixed mesodermal tumor of the
         vulva**
High magnification of Fig. 155. Large groups of
cartilaginous cells are haphazardly arranged.
There is preponderance of matrix. Chondroma-
tous changes in vulvar tumors appear mostly in
association with fibroma or myxoma. In such
tumors these changes may represent chondroma-
tous metaplasia of fibrous connective tissue.
(H&E. ×125)

**155   Benign mixed mesodermal tumor of the
         vulva**
To the right, the tumor consists of scattered
fibroblasts in a mucoid matrix. To the left, the
tumor shows a cartilaginous island formed of
mature chondrocytes. (H&E. ×50)

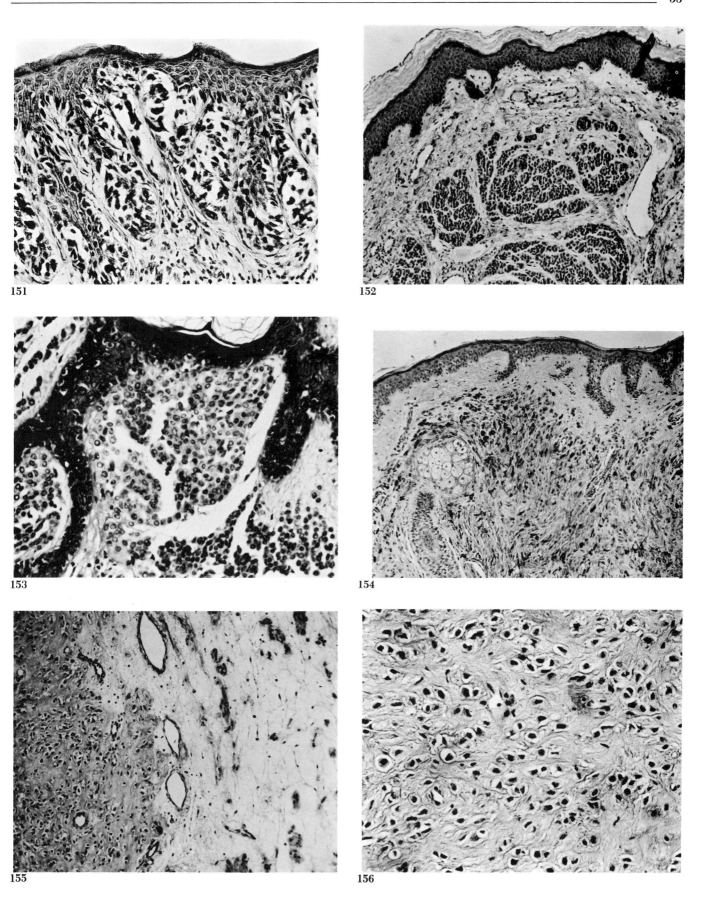

151

152

153

154

155

156

157 Mixed tumor of Bartholin's gland
The glands are distorted and compressed by a marked increase of connective tissue stroma showing cartilaginous metaplasia. Glandular spaces show marked variation in size and shape. A variegated and haphazard tissue pattern is seen in this tumor. A high percentage of local recurrence of this tumor is probably due to persistence of a previously inadequately excised tumor tissue. (H&E. ×50)

158 Mixed tumor of Bartholin's gland
High magnification of Fig. 157, right portion. As a rule there is marked cellularity of the tumor in association with capsular invasion. The stromal cells are hyperplastic and show pathognomonic mucoid or myxomatous changes. (H&E. ×100)

159 Early dyskeratosis of the outer aspect of the labium majus
Severe hyperkeratosis is seen. The stratum granulosum is somewhat enlarged. There is slight variation in the appearance of the epidermal cells. Some of the nuclei show slight hyperchromatism and dyskeratosis. Hyperkeratosis is usually observed in connection with traumatic, irritative, and inflammatory affections of the vulva. Hyperkeratosis, without displastic alteration of the epidermis, has no malignant potentiality. (H&E. ×120)

160 Dyskeratosis with epidermal dysplasia of the inner aspect of the labium majus
An advanced form of dyskeratotic changes is seen. The occurrence of malignant tumors in such epidermal alterations is 10 to 20 per cent. (H&E. ×200)

161 Epidermal dysplasia of the inner aspect of the labium majus
There is hyperkeratosis, acanthosis, and moderate epithelial dysplasia. The prickle cells are relatively young and show an increased number of mitotic figures. The upper dermis shows an inflammatory reaction. The changes observed in Figs. 159 to 161 are usually referred to by pathologists as leukoplakia. The term "leukoplakia" denotes the gross appearance of a "white lesion" of the vulva and is a common finding in numerous vulvar affections. The histomorphologic alteration of the vulvar epidermis as shown here should be referred to as dyskeratosis or dysplasia, rather than leukoplakia. (H&E. ×150)

162 Intraepidermal carcinoma of the inner aspect of the labium majus
There is marked parakeratosis. Atypical cells are seen in the stratum malpighii. There is proliferation of basal cells with loss of cellular polarity. Mitoses are frequent. Dyskeratotic changes are not remarkable. (H&E. ×170)

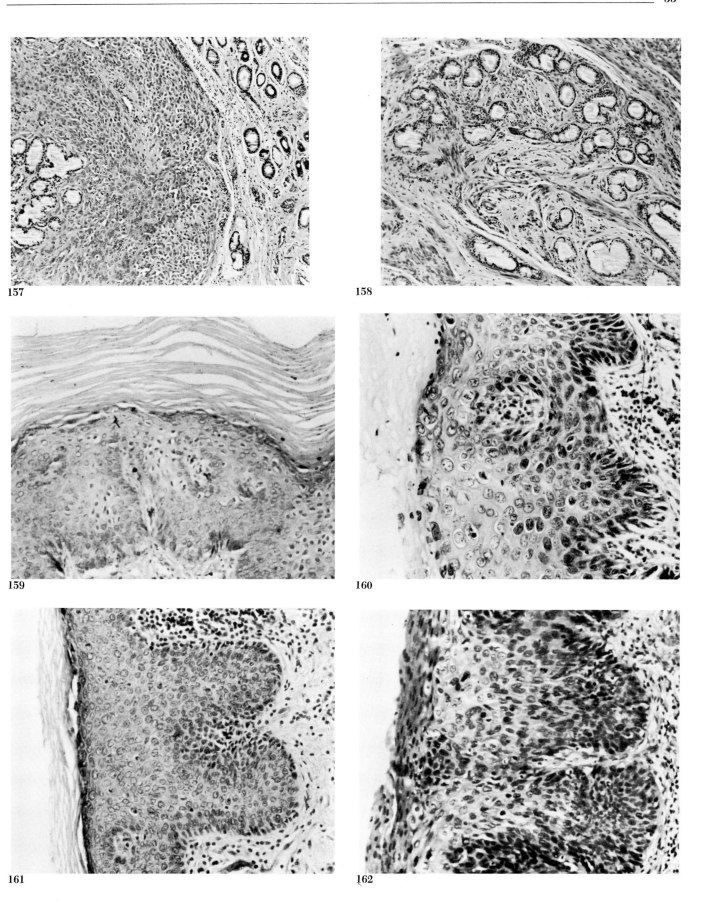

157

158

159

160

161

162

163 Intraepidermal carcinoma (Bowenoid type) of the outer aspect of the labium majus
There is hyperkeratosis and acanthosis. Disarrangement of the epidermal layers is pronounced. The atypical cells are predominately in the stratum malpighi. Multinuclear cells are occasionally seen and mitotic figures are infrequent. The dyskeratosis is not striking. The architecture of the stratum germinativum is relatively preserved. The basal membrane is intact. (H&E. ×140)

164 Intraepidermal carcinoma (Bowen's disease) of the skin of the vulva
There is hyperkeratosis, parakeratosis, and acanthosis. There is complete disarrangement of the cells throughout the entire thickness of the involved epidermis. Cellular atypism and nuclear hyperchromasia are striking. Numerous multinuclear cells are seen. Atypical mitotic figures are frequent. Dyskeratosis dominates the histological picture. The basal membrane is intact. (H&E. ×150)

165 Intraepidermal carcinoma (erythroplasia of Queyrat) of the inner aspect of the labium majus
There is slight parakeratosis and minimal hyperkeratosis. The remaining changes are identical with those seen in Figs. 163 and 164. The absence of hyperkeratosis is responsible for the pink-red appearance of the lesion. In addition, the lesion is more frequent on the mucosal surface than on the skin. It is actually Bowen's disease of the mucosa. (H&E. ×140)

166 Extramammary Paget's disease of the vulva
View of general distribution of Paget's cells within the epidermis and involvement of the hair follicles. The dermis shows a varied degree of inflammatory infiltration with lymphocytes, mast cells, and plasma cells. (H&E. ×50)

167 Extramammary Paget's disease of the vulva
Note the downward growth of Paget's cells from the epidermis along the duct of the sweat gland. (Alcian blue. ×120)

168 Extramammary Paget's disease of the vulva
There is elongation of the rete ridges and infiltration of the lower epidermis with Paget's cells. Extramammary Paget's disease of the vulva begins in the epidermis and advances downward along the epidermal appendages, hair follicles, and sebaceous and sweat glands. (H&E. ×120)

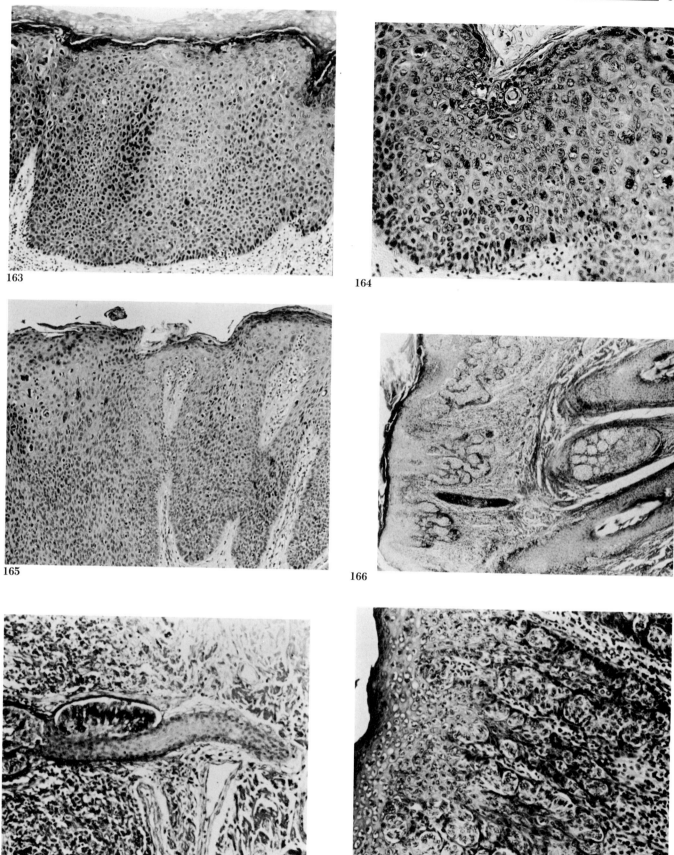

163

164

165

166

167

168

169 Extramammary Paget's disease of the vulva
There is diffuse infiltration of the epidermis with
Paget's cells. The Paget's cells are being ex-
foliated, giving an eczemalike clinical picture.
Paget's disease is probably multicentric in origin.
(H&E. ×200)

170 Extramammary Paget's disease of the vulva
Typical distribution of Paget's cells is seen in the
epidermis. This picture is frequently misdiagnosed as malignant melanoma or as the so-
called "superficial malignant melanoma." (H&E.
×125)

171 Extramammary Paget's disease of the vulva
Massive involvement of the epidermis by Paget's
cells is present. There is early invasion of the
upper dermis. Following massive invasion of the
dermis, distant metastases are possible. (H&E.
×80)

172 Basal cell carcinoma of the vulva
Several groups of neoplastic basal cells are growing from the stratum germinativum into the dermis. In the lower dermis, the tumor is widely
scattered as bands and columns. (H&E. ×50)

173 Basal cell carcinoma of the skin of the vulva
High magnification of Fig. 172. There is variation in the appearance of the neoplastic basal
cells. The basal cell nests are rimmed by layers
of dark-staining palisading cells. The neoplastic
cells have elongated deeply basophilic nuclei
with little cytoplasm. Intercellular bridges are
absent. (H&E. ×150)

174 Basal cell carcinoma of the skin of the vulva
There are branching nests of relatively small
basal cells with dark nuclei infiltrating the upper
dermis. (H&E. ×120)

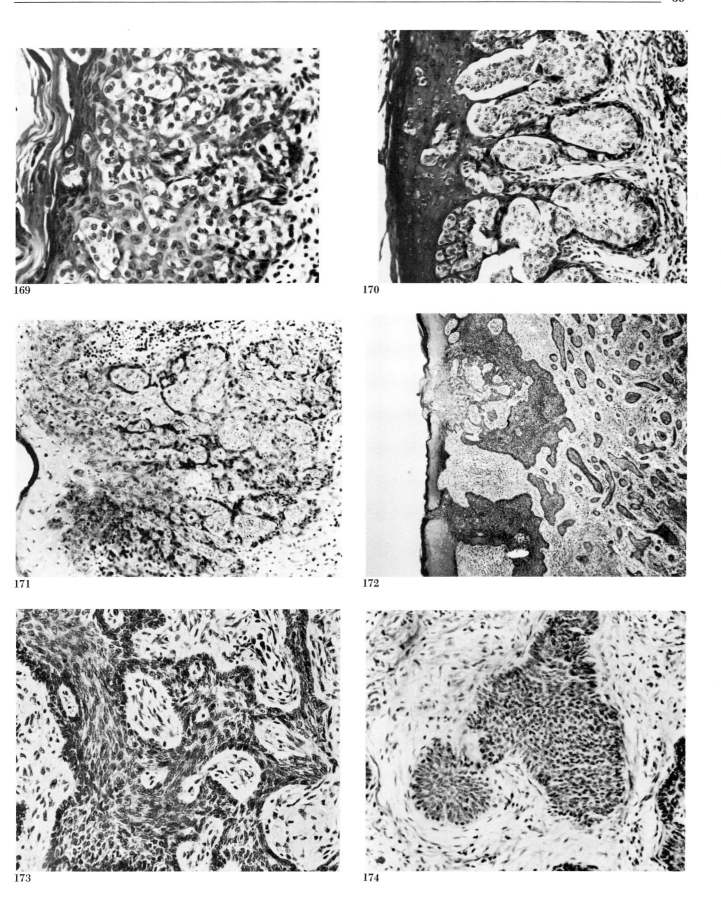

169

170

171

172

173

174

175 Adenoma (dermal eccrine cylindroma) of the adnexal gland of the labium majus
The collections of hyaline material are surrounded by basophilic cells which form rosettes. There is a tendency for hyaline material to coalesce. The tumor is located in the upper dermis. It is benign, slow growing, and is derived from eccrine sweat apparatus. There is recurrence in one-third of cases. (H&E. ×100)

176 Adnexal carcinoma of the skin of the vulva
The mid-dermis is replaced by multilocular nodules of tumor tissue. Numerous cystic spaces are seen within the tumor mass. The degree of malignancy is difficult to ascertain in adnexal carcinomas. Some are of low degree and warrant wide local excision. Some, however, are prone to metastasize. (H&E. ×60)

177 Adnexal carcinoma associated with "leukoplakia" of the labium majus
Biopsy was performed for vulvar "leukoplakia," and a coincidental adnexal tumor located in the mid-dermis was detected. *Adnexal tumors* or *appendage tumors* develop from skin appendages. They can be benign or malignant. The skin of the vulva shows a predilection for such tumors. They belong to a broad group of basal cell tumors. However, their precise origin is at times difficult to determine. See Fig. 161. (H&E. ×15)

178 Adnexal carcinoma of the labium majus
High magnification of Fig. 177. The islands of neoplastic cells surround several eccrine glands. The neoplastic cells are small, basophilic, and the nuclei are dark and ovoid. There is tendency toward cyst formation and hyaline deposition in such tumor islands. (H&E. ×100)

180 Adnexal carcinoma (adenoid cystic carcinoma) of the labium majus
High magnification of Fig. 179. The neoplastic cells are small and basophilic. The nuclei are uniform in size, ovoid, and have clearly discernible nucleoli. Microcyst formation is characteristic of this tumor. The cystic lumens contain mucoid material. There is also deposition of homogenous eosinophilic material between the tumor cells. Mitotic figures are uncommon. (H&E. ×200)

179 Adnexal carcinoma (adenoid cystic carcinoma) of the labium majus
There are cords, ductlike and glandlike arrangement of the neoplastic cells. Perineural and intraneural propagation of such a tumor is occasionally observed. Intervening connective tissue shows inflammatory reaction and edema. (H&E. ×24)

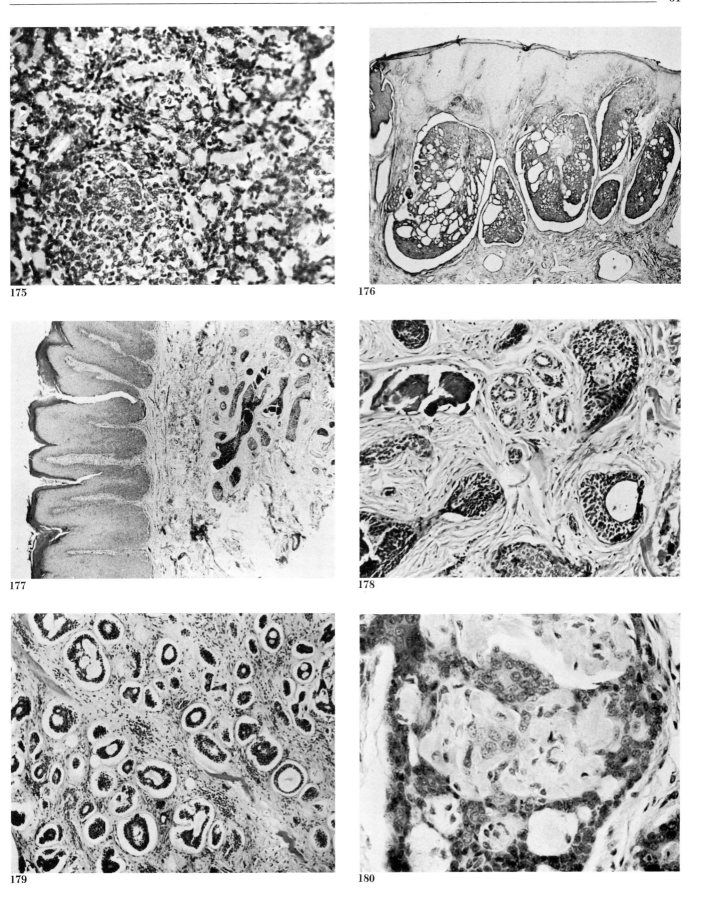

175

176

177

178

179

180

181 Mucus-secreting adnexal carcinoma of the skin of the vulva
There are ovoid islands of neoplastic tissue associated with cystic dilated ductal structures. Within the neoplastic islands are numerous microcysts containing mucoid material. (H&E. ×24)

182 Mucus-secreting adnexal carcinoma of the skin of the vulva
High magnification of Fig. 181. The neoplastic cells vary in size and appearance. Some are small and basophilic, and others are vesicular with clear cytoplasm. Mucinous material is detected in the latter. Microcyst formation is noted. There is absence of hyaline deposition. This tumor is a mucus-secreting variant of an adnexal carcinoma. (H&E. ×180)

183 Invasive squamous cell carcinoma of the vulva
There is invasion of the dermis by an island of neoplastic epidermal cells showing moderate atypism. There is marked inflammatory reaction of the dermis. (H&E. ×60)

184 Invasive squamous cell carcinoma of the vulva
High magnification of Fig. 183. The neoplastic islands and cords consist of moderately well-differentiated squamous cells. There are several keratin pearls and incompletely keratinized centers. Note the marked vascularity of the dermis. Some of the neoplastic islands are in lymphatic channels. (H&E. ×90)

185 Squamous carcinoma of Bartholin's gland
The tumor consists of poorly differentiated squamous epithelial cells forming alveolar structures. There is marked inflammatory reaction. (H&E. ×120)

186 Adenocarcinoma of Bartholin's gland
The tumor consists of irregular neoplastic glands. The glands are lined by atypical cells with large, dark pleomorphic nuclei. The secretion is inconspicuous. There is increase in connective tissue stroma and infiltration with mononuclear cells. (H&E. ×80)

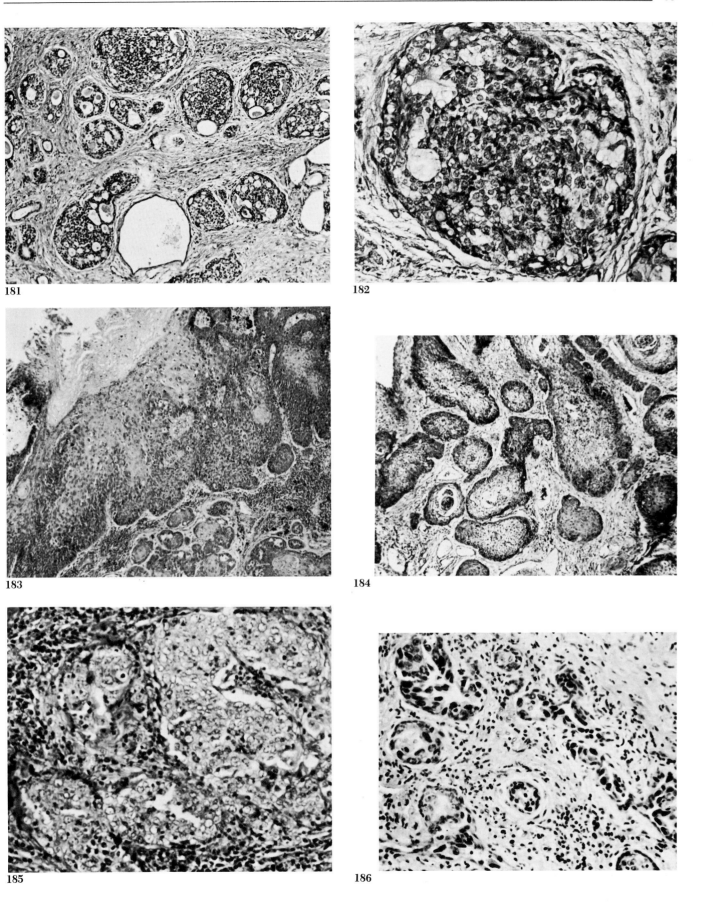

181

182

183

184

185

186

187 Adenoid cystic carcinoma of Bartholin's gland
There is rosette formation by neoplastic cells with central accumulation of microcysts containing mucoid material. (H&E. ×200)

188 Adenoid cystic carcinoma of Bartholin's gland
The tumor is formed by relatively uniform small basophilic cells with round to ovoid dark nuclei. Intervening microcystic structures are present. This is a different area of the tumor shown in Fig. 187. (H&E. ×200)

189 Mucus-secreting adenocarcinoma of Bartholin's gland
The tumor consists of neoplastic glands of various size which contain mucoid material. The tumor shows infiltrative growth with no demarcation. Interspersed are connective tissue strands. (H&E. ×24)

190 Mucus-secreting adenocarcinoma of Bartholin's gland
High magnification of Fig. 189. The glands are lined by flattened cells with prominent dark ovoid nuclei. Mucoid material fills the lumens. In addition, there are solid strands of neoplastic epithelial cells independent of the glands. (H&E. ×80)

191 Adenoacanthoma of Bartholin's gland
Cords and island of infiltrating neoplastic tissue are formed by squamous epithelial cells. There is variation in size and shape of the cells, and the nuclei are large, hyperchromatic, and atypical. The surrounding tissue is infiltrated with inflammatory cells. In addition, islands formed by neoplastic glandular and papillary structures are seen. (H&E. ×125)

192 Sebaceous gland carcinoma of the vulva
The lobulated tumor is formed by poorly differentiated sebaceous cells. The central area shows necrosis and accumulation of lipid material. (H&E. ×50)

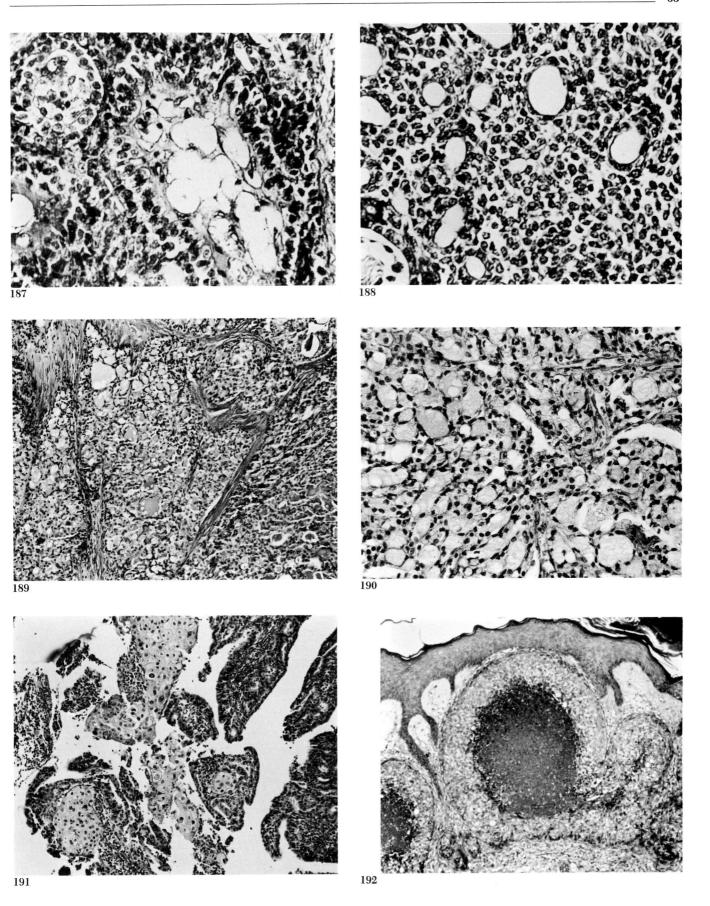

187

188

189

190

191

192

193 Well-differentiated sebaceous gland carcinoma of the vulva
The tumor consists of well-differentiated sebaceous cells. For demonstration of lipid material, special stains are useful. (H&E. ×80)

194 Highly anaplastic sebaceous gland carcinoma of the vulva
The tumor is formed by undifferentiated cells with extreme cellular atypism. Lipid material is seen in most of these cells. (H&E. ×200)

195 Apocrine carcinoma of the vulva
The dermis is infiltrated by neoplastic cells forming irregular tumor islands. The tumor consists of atypical glandular cells with eosinophilic cytoplasm and active "decapitation" secretion. (H&E. ×100)

196 Fibrosarcoma of the vulva
The tumor is characterized by marked cellularity and young appearing fibroblasts. Hyperchromatic nuclei and mitotic figures are frequent. (H&E. ×120)

198 Rhabdomyosarcoma of the vulva
The tumor is composed of large spindle cells which show variation in size and shape. Most of the tumor cells are bipolar. Their lateral cell margins are invariably distinct, but their poles are quite indistinct, suggesting syncytium formation. Many irregular multinucleated tumor giant cells are seen. Bizarre "strap" cells with abundant eosinophilic cytoplasm are frequent. (H&E. ×200)

197 Leiomyosarcoma of the vulva
The tumor consists of solid sheets of anaplastic cells. There is marked pleomorphism and hyperchromatism of the nuclei. The blunt ends of the nuclei favor the diagnosis of leiomyosarcoma. (H&E. ×180)

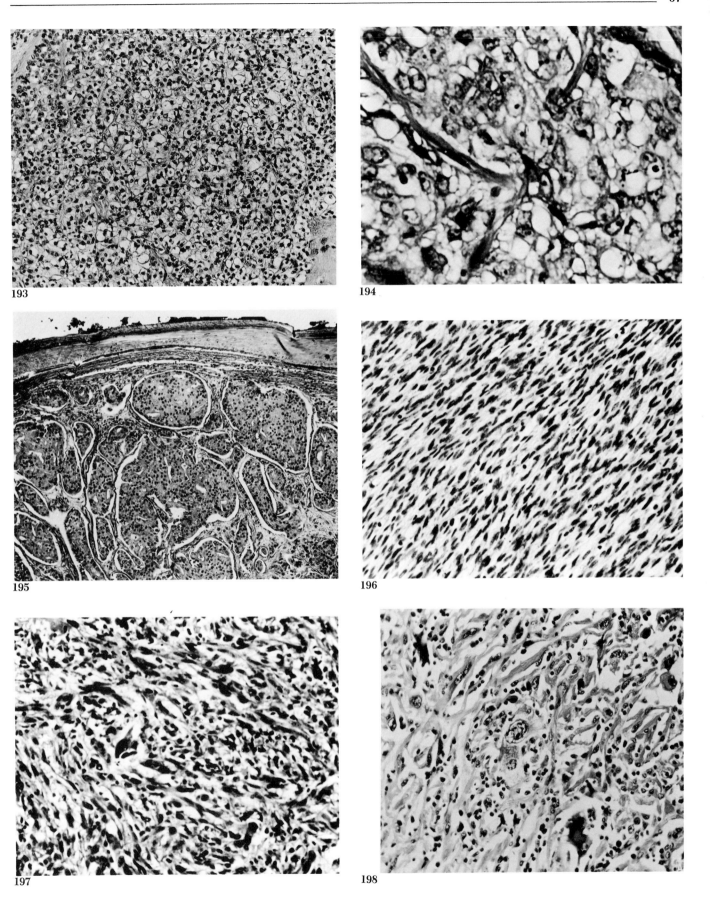

193

194

195

196

197

198

199   Liposarcoma of the vulva
The tumor is composed of poorly differentiated cells containing numerous lipid vacuoles. Tumor giant cells and pleomorphic cells are present. Special stains for lipid are helpful diagnostic aids. (H&E. ×312)

200   Dermatofibrosarcoma protuberans of the vulva
The tumor is formed by relatively uniform spindle-shaped connective tissue cells. The characteristic cartwheel pattern of proliferating fibroblasts is pathognomonic for this tumor. Mitotic figures are infrequent. (H&E. ×80)

201   Malignant lymphoma (lymphoblastic lymphosarcoma) of the vulva
Note the massive infiltration of the entire dermis by lymphoma cells. (H&E. ×70)

202   Malignant lymphoma (lymphoblastic lymphosarcoma) of the skin of the vulva
High magnification of Fig. 201. The tumor is formed by relatively uniform cells with nuclei larger than those of lymphocytes. (H&E. ×300)

203   Hodgkin's disease of the vulva
The polymorphous infiltrate consists of atypical reticulum cells, mononuclear cells, and multi-nucleated Reed-Sternberg cells. (H&E. ×250)

204   Malignant melanoma of the clitoris
There is marked junctional activity. The tumor cells show downward and upward infiltration. The tumor cells contain melanin. They are large and disorganized. The upper dermis shows a bandlike inflammatory reaction. (H&E. ×50)

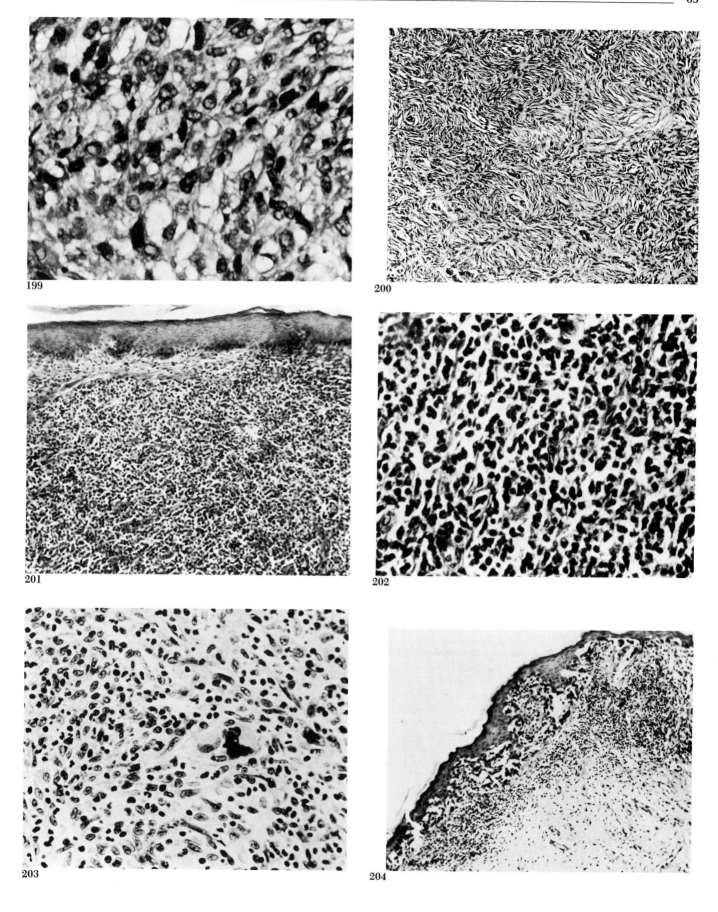

199

200

201

202

203

204

205   Malignant melanoma of the clitoris
At the dermoepidermal junction and throughout the entire dermis, there are densely packed cells with pleomorphic and hyperchromatic nuclei. Some of the cells contain fine melanine granules. (H&E. ×180)

206   Ulcerated malignant melanoma of the labium minus
The ulcer shows a base of necrotic tissue, cellular debris, and tumor cells. The neoplastic cells are cuboidal with large, irregular dark nuclei. The tumor cells are engulfing the capillaries. (H&E. ×180)

207   Malignant melanoma of the labium minus
The tumor cells exhibit an alveolar arrangement. Mitoses are rare. There are occasional fine intracytoplasmic melanin granules. (Masson's trichrome stain. ×180)

208   Carcinoma of the breast metastatic to the labium majus
The metastatic tumor is made up of cuboidal cells with prominent nuclei, suggesting ductal carcinoma of the breast. The patient, age 52, had a large tender mass in her right breast for several years. (H&E. ×120)

209   Adenocarcinoma of the endometrium metastatic to the mons pubis
Glands with papillary projections are lined by stratified neoplastic epithelium. The tumor developed 1 year after hysterectomy for endometrial carcinoma. (H&E. ×120)

210   Adenocarcinoma of the large intestine metastatic to the skin of the vulva
Moderately anaplastic glands show marked inflammatory reaction of the dermis and subcutis. This woman, age 62, had a history of progressive weight loss and abdominal pain for 8 months. (H&E. ×100)

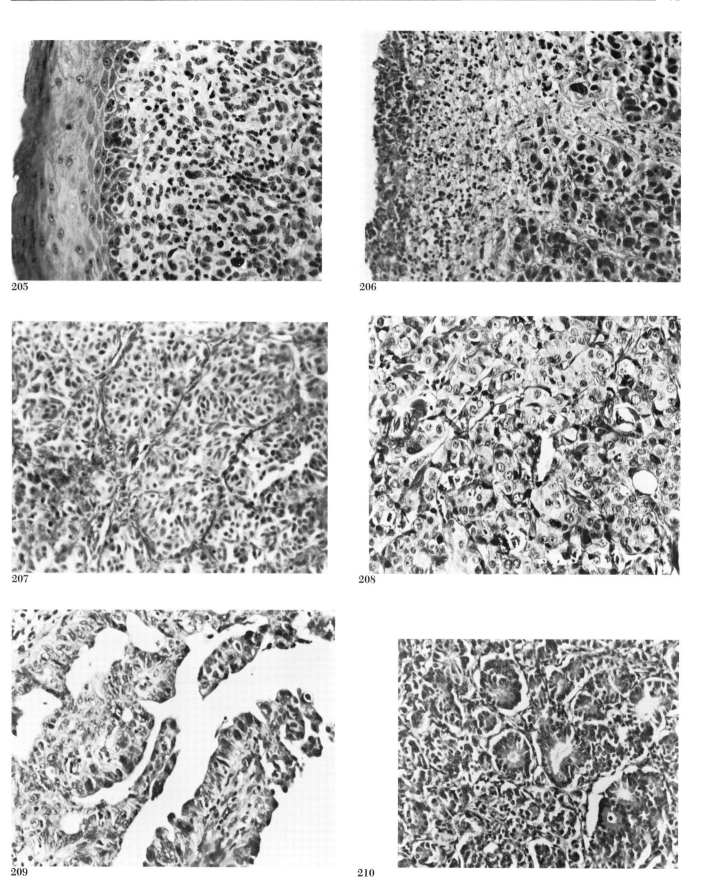

205

206

207

208

209

210

211 Ectopic or accessory breast tissue (mamma accessoria pendulans) of the labium majus
There is marked fibrosis of the connective tissue stroma and moderate cystic dilatation of the glandular ducts. The acini are sparse. (H&E. ×60)

212 Ectopic or accessory lactating breast tissue of the vulva
There is lobular hyperplasia. The acini are lined by cuboidal epithelium. Distended ducts contain inspissated material. The vestigial remnants of breast tissue located in the vulva show hyperplasia of pregnancy. (H&E. ×50)

213 Endometriosis of the labium majus
Several glandular structures lined by cuboidal to columnar epithelium are seen in connective tissue stroma and at the epidermodermal junction. They are surrounded by endometrial stromal cells, hemosiderin, and chronic inflammatory cells. (H&E. ×50)

214 Early acute radiodermatitis of the labium majus
There is considerable hyperkeratosis. The cells of the stratum malpighii show hydropic degeneration, and the nuclei are pyknotic. There is edema of the dermis. The vessels are dilated and show perivascular infiltrates. (H&E. ×50)

216 Postirradiation, metastasizing intermediary cell carcinoma of the vulva
The patient received local x-ray therapy applied to the vulva for an otherwise benign condition. Three years thereafter an ulcerating tumor developed and inguinal lymph nodes revealed metastatic foci. This ulcerating tumor simulates a basal cell carcinoma and is difficult to classify. Similar tumors have been reported as "metastasizing basal cell carcinoma." However there is transepidermal involvement by the neoplastic cells, suggesting an intermediary cell carcinoma. (H&E. ×24)

215 Edge of radiation ulcer of the vulva
The changes are those seen in late chronic radiodermatitis. There is hyperkeratosis and acanthosis. The vessels show marked ectasia, and the dermis is sclerotic. Perivascular fibrosis is also prominent. Dermal appendages are absent. The ulcerative area is located to the left. (H&E. ×50)

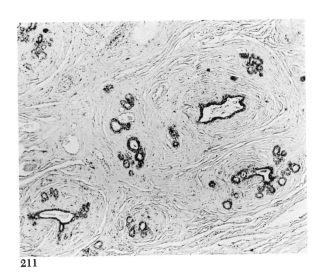

211

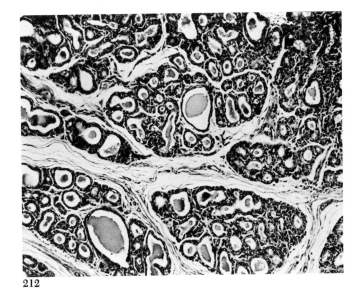

212

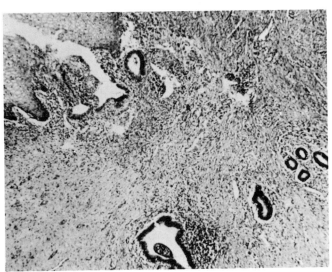

213

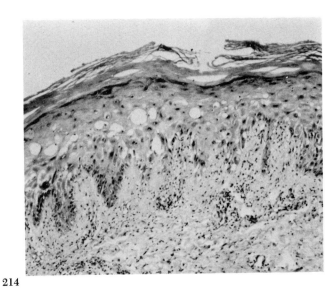

214

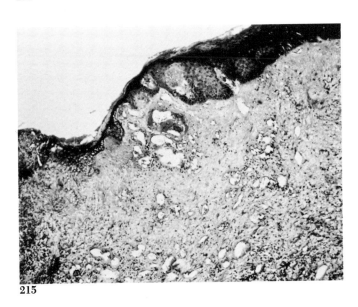

215

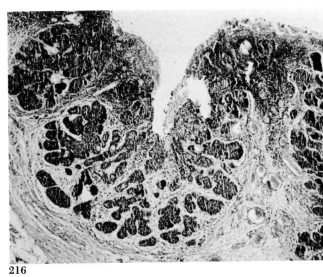

216

217 Postirradiation, metastasizing intermediary cell carcinoma of the vulva

High magnification of Fig. 216. Although the tumor appears to be attached to the undersurface of the epidermis, the transepidermal neoplastic alteration is evident. The neoplastic cells are somewhat larger than the basal cells, but they lack any resemblance to the prickle cell. The neoplastic cells of this tumor are neither typically basal nor typically prickle cells. (H&E. ×150)

218 Chronic skenitis of the urethral meatus (chronic paraurethritis)

There is periglandular infiltration with chronic inflammatory cells. (H&E. ×50)

219 Chronic skenitis of the urethral meatus, undergoing transitional cell metaplasia

Transitional cell metaplasia is seen in Skene's gland. The periglandular connective tissue is heavily infiltrated with chronic inflammatory cells. (H&E. ×125)

220 Suburethral diverticulum

The diverticulum is lined by transitional epithelium. The submucosa is thickened and infiltrated with acute and chronic inflammatory cells. (H&E. ×24)

221 Urethral diverticulum with pseudoxanthomatous inflammation

The lining epithelium of the diverticulum is destroyed and replaced by inflammatory tissue. It consists of numerous large lipid macrophages intermingled with lymphocytes, plasma cells, and occasional polymorphonuclear leukocytes. (H&E. ×50)

222 Papillomatous caruncle of the urethral meatus

The papillomatous growth is composed of stratified squamous epithelium. The connective tissue core shows a mild inflammatory reaction. (H&E. ×15)

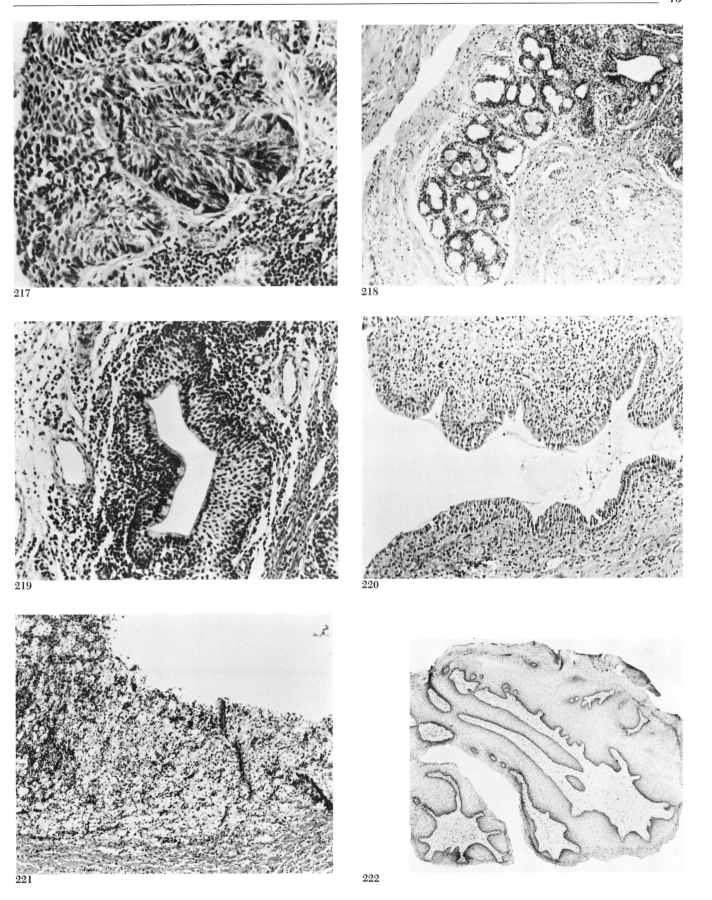

217

218

219

220

221

222

223 Granulomatous caruncle of the urethral meatus
The overlying squamous epithelium is eroded. The submucosa is heavily infiltrated with inflammatory cells. The connective tissue shows dilated vessels, proliferation of fibroblasts, infiltration with acute and chronic inflammatory cells, and focal erythrocytic extravasation. The inflammatory process has resulted in a very cellular and vascular granulation tissue. (H&E. ×15)

224 Caruncle with isolated ectasia of a vein of the urethral meatus
The covering epithelium is intact and of transitional cell type. The underlying connective tissue contains a large single dilated vein filled with blood. Several small vascular spaces are present; to the left metaplasia of Skene's glands is seen. (H&E. ×50)

225 Telangiectatic or angiomatous caruncle of the urethral meatus
The growth consists of edematous connective tissue stroma with many dilated vessels. The overlaying epithelium is of either squamous or transitional cell type. (H&E. ×80)

226 Caruncle of the urethral meatus simulating carcinoma
Multiple epithelial invaginations and metaplastic changes frequently occurring in the caruncle of the urethral meatus may be misinterpreted as being malignant changes. (H&E. ×80)

227 Condyloma acuminatum of the urethral meatus
Papillary projections are formed by nonkeratinizing epithelium with well-vascularized connective tissue core and show moderate inflammatory infiltration. (H&E. ×24)

228 Squamous papilloma of the urethral meatus
The pedunculated, branching tumor is covered with keratinizing squamous epithelium and shows a markedly vascularized connective tissue core. (H&E. ×50)

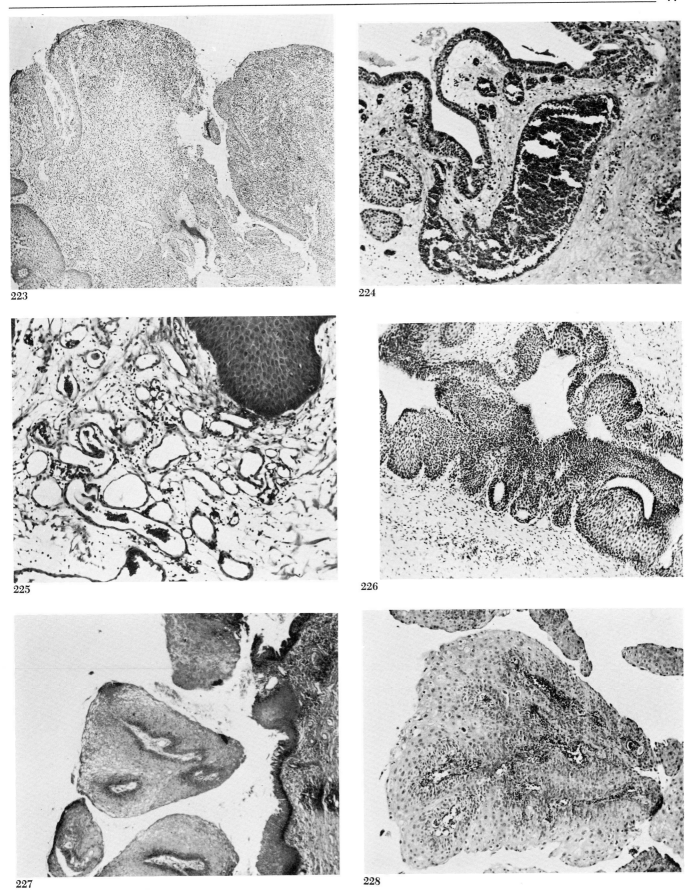

223

224

225

226

227

228

229 Adenoma of Skene's paraurethral glands
The tumor consists of small dilated glandular structures. They are lined by cuboidal epithelium with relatively large, dark ovoid nuclei. Fusion of the glandular epithelium and production of more solid cords are seen occasionally. Mitoses are absent. Sparse connective tissue is infiltrated with chronic inflammatory cells. (H&E. ×120)

230 Caruncle with cellular atypism (dysplasia) of the urethral meatus
The squamous epithelium covering the caruncle shows marked proliferation of basal cells and the presence of atypical cells with hyperchromatic nuclei. At the surface of the epithelium, there appears to be normal maturation. (H&E. ×80)

231 Caruncle with cellular atypism (dysplasia) of the urethral meatus
The squamous epithelium covering a granulomatous caruncle is replaced by relatively large cells with large hyperchromatic nuclei. The polarity of the cells is preserved. There appears to be progressive maturation with absence of mitotic activity. (H&E. ×125)

232 Intraepidermal carcinoma of the urethral meatus
There is marked epidermal hyperplasia with disorderly arrangement of cells. Loss of cellular polarity, the presence of dyskeratotic cells, and large pleomorphic and hyperchromatic nuclei are indicative of malignant changes. (H&E. ×60)

234 Cloacogenic carcinoma of the vulva
The tumor is formed by islands of poorly differentiated neoplastic cells. The tumor islands infiltrate the connective tissue stroma and the muscle fibers of the lower third of the rectovaginal septum and perineum. Rectal and vaginal mucosa were not involved by tumor. Histogenetically this tumor developed from the epithelial rests of the cloaca. (H&E. ×50)

233 Invasive squamous cell carcinoma of the urethral meatus
The connective tissue shows nests of infiltrating neoplastic squamous cells with some keratinization. (H&E. ×15)

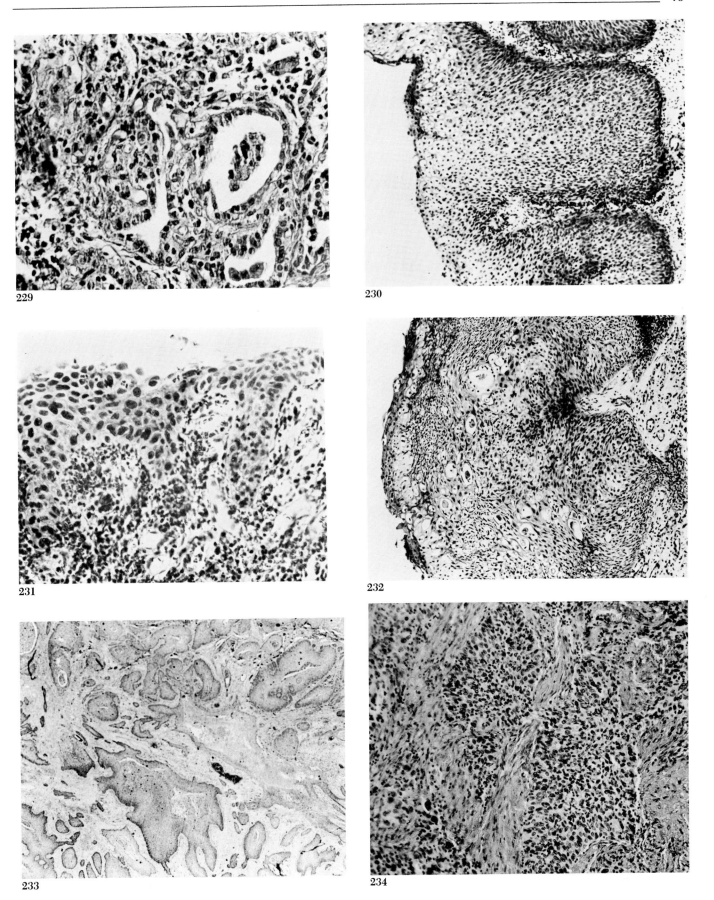

229

230

231

232

233

234

235 Malignant melanoma of the clitoris, metastatic to the urethral meatus
One year following vulvectomy for malignant melanoma of the clitoris, a nodule appeared at the urethral meatus which was biopsied. The metastatic tumor is made up of large pleomorphic cells, some containing melanin granules, which are diffusely invading the connective tissue of the urethral meatus. (H&E. ×120)

236 Caruncle of the hymen (caruncula hymenalis)
The broad-based, papillomalike structure is covered by squamous epithelium and represents relics of the ruptured hymen. (H&E. ×50)

237 Fibrosis of the hymen (hymenal band)
Fibrosis of the connective tissue core of the hymen produces lack of distensibility and dyspareunia. (H&E. ×6)

238 Imperforate hymen associated with hematocolpos, anterior aspect
The introital surface of the imperforate hymen is lined by squamous epithelium. There is increase of the connective tissue core. (PAS. ×50)

239 Imperforate hymen associated with hematocolpos, posterior surface
Same specimen as Fig. 238. The vaginal surface of the imperforate hymen is lined by cuboidal, Müllerian, mucin-producing epithelium. This epithelium is responsible for the occasional formation of a hymenal cyst. Apparently the nonperforation of some hymens is conditioned by the presence of displaced paramesonephric epithelium. (PAS. ×50)

240 Subhymenal annular sclerosis, Halban
Note the marked circumferential increase of the dense fibrous connective tissue of the base of the hymen. (H&E. ×60)

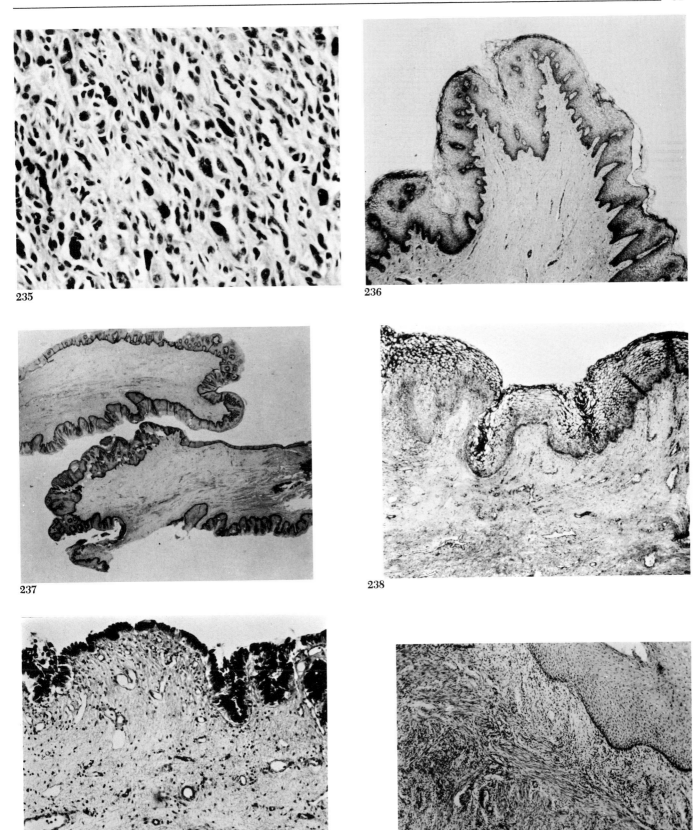

235

236

237

238

239

240

COLOR PLATES

Chapter 1

Diseases of the Vulva

Plates 1, 2, and 3

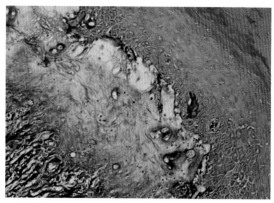

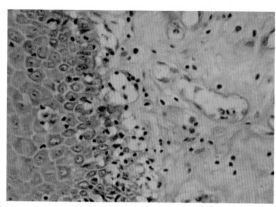

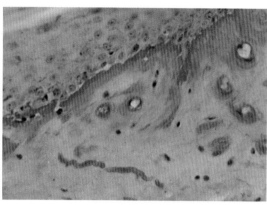

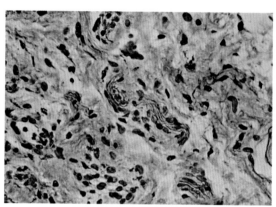

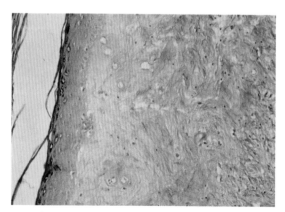

1 Lichen sclerosus et atrophicus (LSA) of the vulva Edema and vacuolar degeneration of the upper dermis are seen. (Masson's trichrome stain. ×100)

2 Lichen sclerosus et atrophicus (LSA) of the vulva There is spongiosis of the basal cells and ectasia of the dermal capillaries. (PAS. ×100)

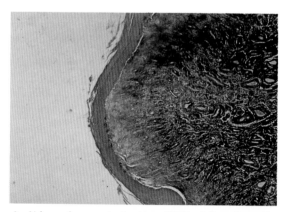

3 Lichen sclerosus et atrophicus (LSA) of the vulva Homogenization of the upper dermis and obliteration of the capillaries can be seen. (PAS. ×150)

4 Lichen sclerosus et atrophicus (LSA) of the vulva Note the degenerative changes of the terminal nerve fibers. (Bodian stain. ×100)

5 Lichen sclerosus et atrophicus (LSA) of the vulva Note the disappearance of elastic fibers in the upper dermis. (Verhoeff's elastica stain. ×50)

6 Lichen sclerosus et atrophicus (LSA) of the vulva The terminal stage of LSA consists of massive homogenization and sclerosis of the upper dermis. (Masson's trichrome stain. ×50)

Plate 1

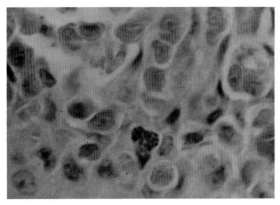

7 Extramammary Paget's disease of the vulva Mucin is present within the Paget's cells. Note the accumulation of melanin granules within the cytoplasm of occasional Paget's cells. (Mayer's mucicarmine stain. ×250)

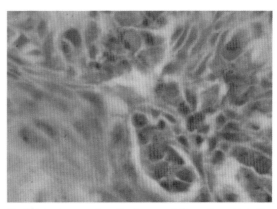

8 Extramammary Paget's disease of the vulva Note the presence of diastase-resistant PAS material within Paget's cells. (PAS stain. ×250)

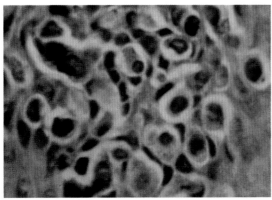

9 Extramammary Paget's disease of the vulva There is an accumulation of acid mucopolysaccharides in Paget's cells. (Alcian blue. ×250)

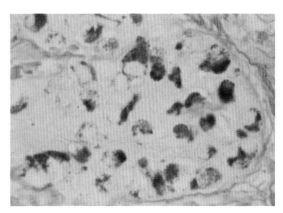

10 Extramammary Paget's disease of the vulva An accumulation of hyaluronidase-resistant acid mucopolysaccharides is seen in the cytoplasm of Paget's cells. (AMP stain. ×250).

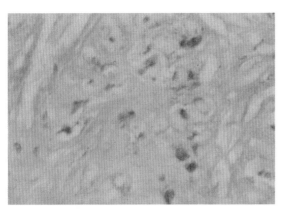

11 Extramammary Paget's disease of the vulva A distinct accumulation of sulfomucopolysaccharides is visible in the cytoplasm of Paget's cell. (Aldehyde fuchsin. ×250)

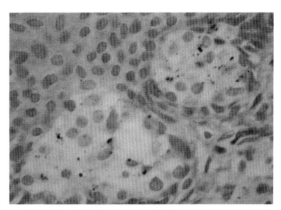

12 Extramammary Paget's disease of the vulva Fine and coarse distribution of melanin pigment is seen within the cytoplasm of Paget's cells. (Fontana-Masson reaction. ×250)

Plate 2

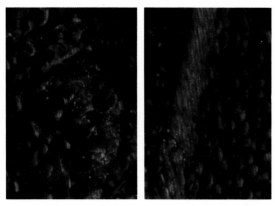

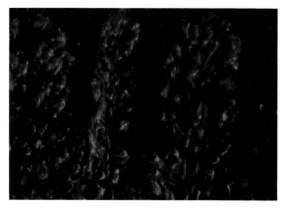

13 Extramammary Paget's disease of the vulva To the right is normal stratum granulosum and stratum germinativum; to the left, Paget's cells exhibit marked fluorescence of mucopolysaccharides. This technique is very sensitive. (Fluorescent PAS technique. ×300)

14 Extramammary Paget's disease of the vulva There is marked fluorescence of Paget's cells. The fluorescent droplets and granules are more evident by application of this technique than when using the standard technique for demonstration of mucopolysaccharides. (Fluorescent Feulgen technique. ×300)

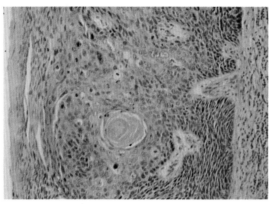

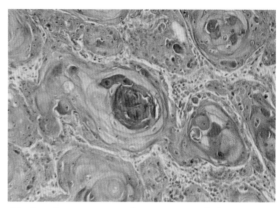

15 Intraepidermal carcinoma (Bowen's disease) of the skin of the labium majus The epidermis is thickened. There is hyperkeratosis and parakeratosis. The cells of the stratum malpighii are atypical, showing large hyperchromatic nuclei and horn-pearl formation. (H&E. ×80)

16 Invasive squamous cell carcinoma, with keratin pearl formations of the skin of the vulva (H&E. ×150)

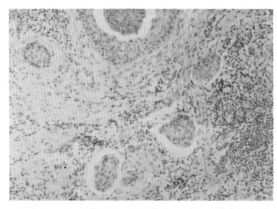

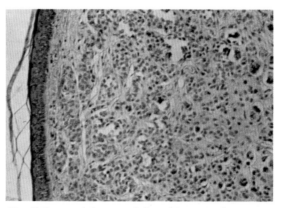

17 Squamous cell carcinoma of the vulva with lymphatic spread (H&E. ×120)

18 Malignant melanoma of the vulva Note the presence of melanin granules in neoplastic cells. (H&E. ×120)

Plate 3

2

Diseases of the Vagina

241   Acute, nonspecific vaginitis
The stratified squamous epithelium of the vagina is destroyed. The submucosal connective tissue is infiltrated with predominantly acute and some chronic inflammatory cells. (H&E. ×120)

242   Candidiasis of the vagina
The desquamated superficial squamous epithelial cells of the vaginal wall are invaded by typical fungal elements—mycelial threads and round blastospores. (H&E. ×350)

243   Trichomoniasis of the vagina
This flagellate protozoon is approximately the size of a polymorphonuclear leukocyte. Quick fixation with osmic acid is useful in demonstrating flagella. (H&E. ×600)

244   Ulcer of the vagina due to potassium permanganate
There is deep coagulation necrosis with exposure and damage of the vaginal wall vessels. This is frequently a cause of massive vaginal hemorrhage. (H&E. ×50)

245   Inflammatory pseudotumor of the vagina
The stratified squamous epithelium lining the vagina is attenuated and atrophic. The submucous connective tissue and the muscular coats are infiltrated by dense inflammatory exudate, the picture simulating a lymphoma. (H&E. ×25)

246   Inflammatory pseudotumor of the vagina
High magnification of Fig. 245. The "pseudotumor" consists of proliferating, dilated vessels, inflammatory exudate, and an occasional proliferating fibroblast. The mononuclear inflammatory exudate consists of plasma cells, mast cells, and lymphocytes. (H&E. ×220)

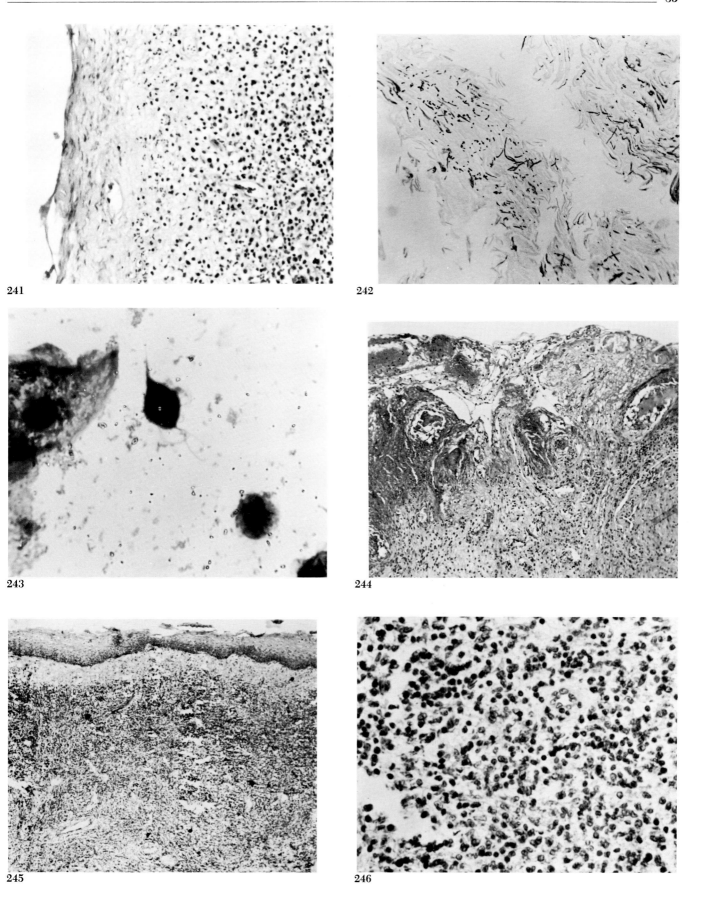

241

242

243

244

245

246

247 Vaginitis emphysematosa
Gas-containing cysts are located within the submucosa. They are surrounded by foreign-body-type giant cells. There is a mild inflammatory reaction of the connective tissue. (H&E. ×50)

248 Granulation tissue of the vaginal vault
Granulation tissue following hysterectomy is composed of fibroblasts, newly formed capillaries, histiocytes, and acute and chronic inflammatory cells. (H&E. ×125)

249 Surgical granuloma of the vaginal vault
An accumulation of foreign-body giant cells is seen. The nuclei are numerous, and scattered through the cytoplasm are fragments of phagocytized material. (H&E. ×120)

250 Condyloma acuminatum of the vagina
A papilloma with a central core of connective tissue is covered by a thick layer of squamous epithelium. It is caused by virus and is infectious and autoinoculable. (H&E. ×50)

251 Varicose vein of the vagina
The enlarged and tortuous vein shows an irregular lumen and an asymmetric thickening and thinning of the vessel wall. (H&E. ×50)

252 Epidermal inclusion cyst of the vagina
The cyst is lined by stratified squamous epithelium and is located within the vaginal wall. It is probably traumatic in origin. (H&E. ×15)

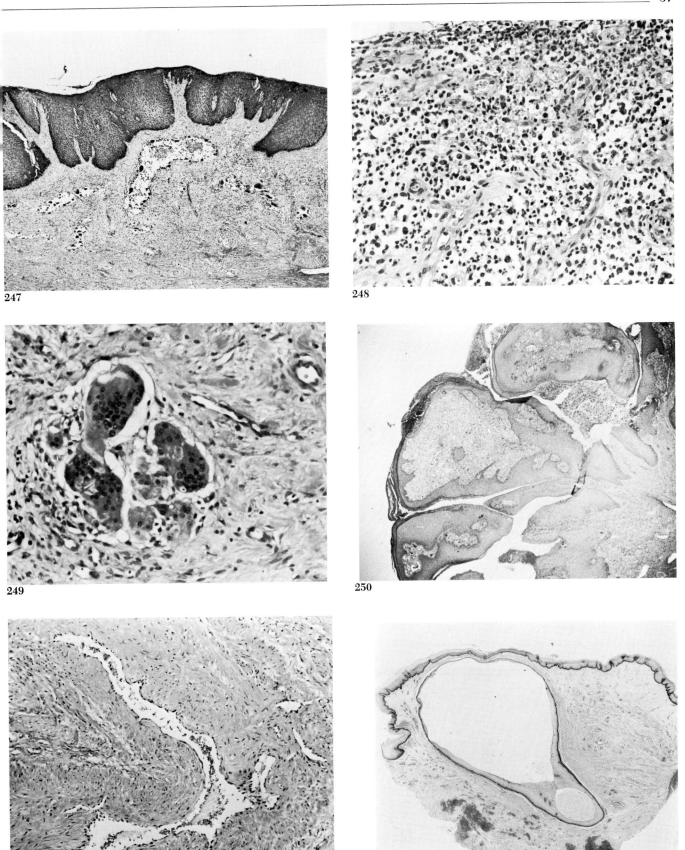

247

248

249

250

251

252

253 Dysontogenetic, paramesonephric cyst of the vagina
The cyst is lined by cuboidal mucus-producing epithelium of Müllerian-paramesonephric origin. The wall of the cyst shows fibrosis. (H&E. ×125)

254 Dysontogenetic cyst of the vagina, with squamous metaplasia
To the left, the cyst is lined by squamous epithelium; the Müllerian, tall columnar mucin-producing epithelium is to the right. (H&E. ×150)

255 Endometriosis of the vagina
The superficial ulceration of the vaginal wall is due to an island of endometrial glands and a chronic inflammatory exudate located in the submucosa. (H&E. ×50)

256 Endometriosis of the vagina
This island consists of endometrial glands, cytogenic endometrial stroma, and mononuclear inflammatory cells located deep in the muscle layers of the vaginal wall. (H&E. ×80)

257 Leukoparakeratosis of the vagina
The lining stratified squamous epithelium exhibits parakeratosis: a retention of pyknotic nuclei in keratinized superficial cells. It represents an imperfect keratinization process. (H&E. ×220)

258 Papillomatosis of the vagina
The vaginal mucosa shows papillomatosis. The squamous epithelium is thickened and shows focal areas of hyperkeratosis. Although benign, the lesion is resistant to therapy, and recurrence after excision is frequent. (H&E. ×50)

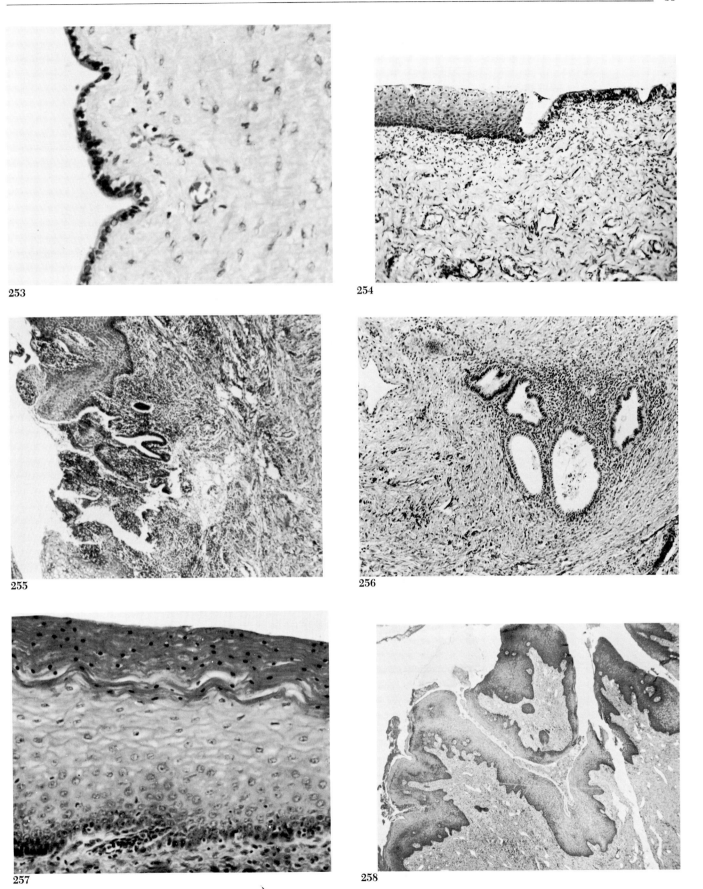

253

254

255

256

257

258

259   Papillomatosis of the vagina

In addition to excessive papilloma formation, there is also marked pseudoepitheliomatous hyperplasia. The cause is unknown. (H&E. ×24)

260   Pseudoepitheliomatous hyperplasia of the vagina

High magnification of Fig. 259. There is downward proliferation of stratified squamous epithelium associated with a mild inflammatory reaction. (H&E. ×120)

261   Mesonephric papilloma of the vagina

The lesion is polypoid in appearance and shows variation in the size and shape of the papillary structures. (H&E. ×70)

262   Mesonephric papilloma of the vagina

High magnification of Fig. 261. The papillary structures are covered by uniform cuboidal epithelial cells with prominent hyperchromatic nuclei. The connective tissue stroma is infiltrated with mononuclear inflammatory cells. The tumor, if not adequately excised, will recur. Such tumors are mostly observed in childhood. (H&E. ×180)

263   Polyp of the vagina

Low magnification shows a polypoid structure covered with normal stratified squamous vaginal epithelium. The connective tissue stroma is edematous and vascular. High magnification (right enclosure) of the connective tissue stroma shows fibroblasts with nuclear pyknosis, nuclear degeneration, and clumping. The bizarre hyperchromatic nuclei are degenerative changes frequently misinterpreted as sarcomatous. Note the absence of mitoses. (H&E. ×25, and ×160)

264   Benign mixed tumor of the vagina

The vaginal wall shows a tumor composed of solid islands of tumor cells and several cystic structures lined by neoplastic squamous epithelium. (H&E. ×50)

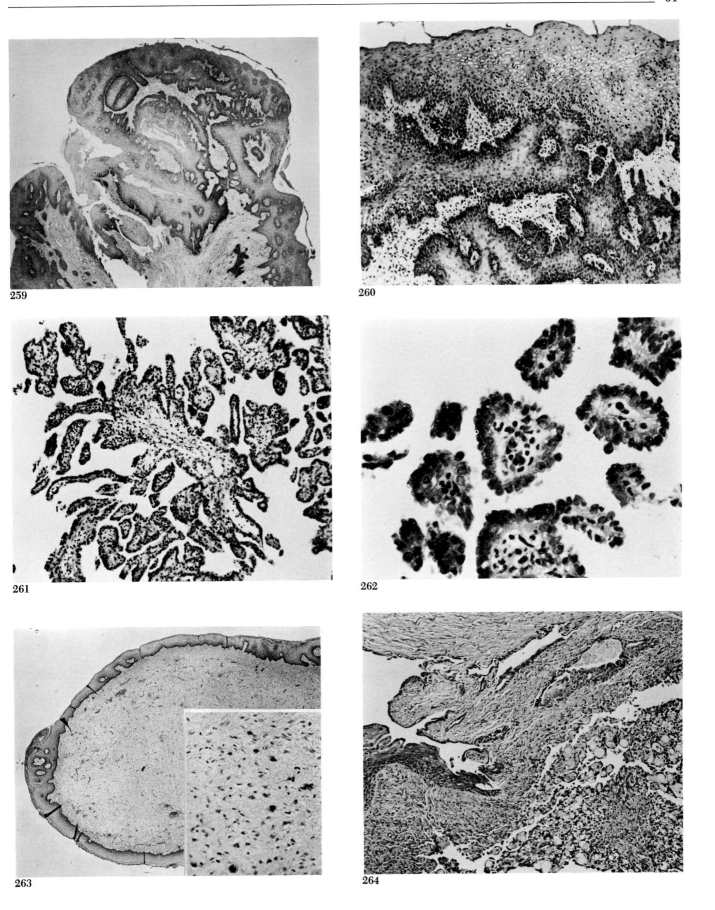

259

260

261

262

263

264

265　Benign mixed tumor of the vagina
High magnification of Fig. 264. The island of keratinized squamous cells is surrounded by poorly defined ovoid cells with prominent round hyperchromatic nuclei. The cytoplasm of these cells contains mucin. (H&E. ×120)

266　Fibroma of the vagina
The tumor consists of edematous fibrous connective tissue, rather diffuse in arrangement, with prominent vessels. (H&E. ×15)

267　Fibroma of the vagina
High magnification of Fig. 266. The tumor consists of elongated fibrous connective tissue cells with prominent nuclei. They are relatively uniform in size and shape. No mitoses are observed. (H&E. ×100)

268　Leiomyoma of the vagina
The tumor consists of smooth muscle fibers forming bundles and whorls. It is moderately vascular, with focal areas of necrosis. (H&E. ×50)

269　Hemangioma of the vagina
The numerous, well-developed vascular spaces are surrounded by loose connective tissue. (H&E. ×150)

270　Neurilemmoma of the vagina
Interlacing bundles of fibrillary tissue are seen with slender elongated nuclei in a palisading arrangement. (H&E. ×50)

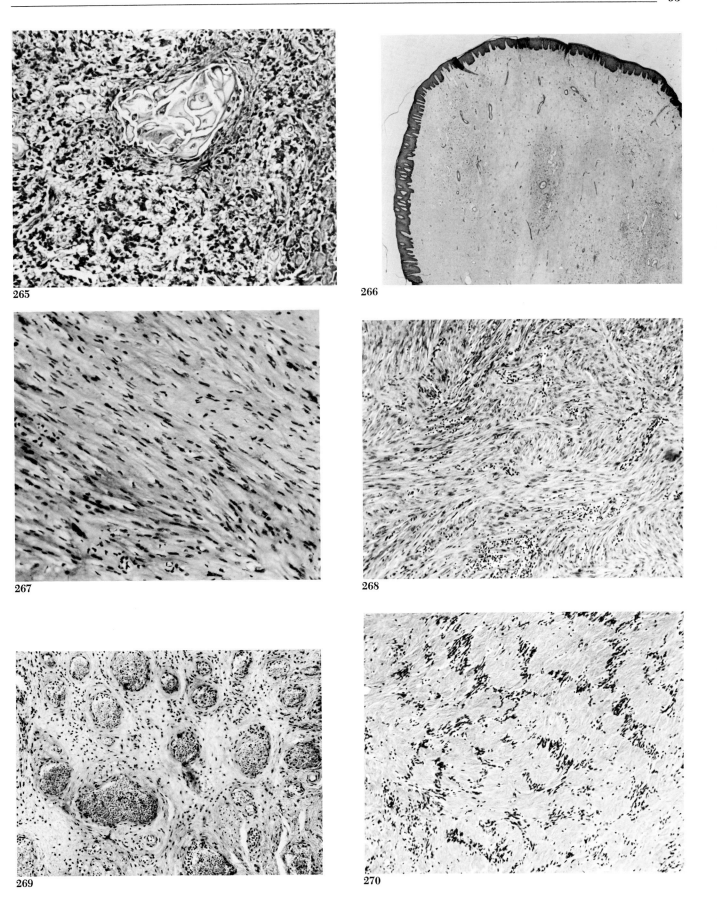

265

266

267

268

269

270

271 Lentigo of the vagina
The stratum germinativum shows hyperpigmentation. Several melanophores are seen in the submucosa. (H&E. ×200)

272 Dysplasia of the vaginal mucosa
The squamous epithelium is thickened because of uniform proliferation of basal cells. The normal maturation is preserved. Mitoses are frequent. The submucosa shows inflammatory reaction. (H&E. ×150)

273 Intraepithelial carcinoma (carcinoma in situ) of the vagina
There is loss of cellular polarity, and pleomorphic neoplastic cells are present with large atypical hyperchromatic nuclei. The basement membrane is intact and relatively straight. (H&E. ×150)

274 Intraepithelial carcinoma (carcinoma in situ) of the vagina
The changes encountered in the squamous epithelium are identical with those seen in Bowen's disease of the skin or erythroplasia of Queyrat of the mucosa. Progression into invasive squamous cell carcinoma occurs sooner in the vagina than with Bowen's disease of the vulva. (H&E. ×100)

275 Squamous cell carcinoma of the vagina
Strands and sheets of neoplastic squamous cells are seen invading the submucosa and the muscle layers of the vaginal wall. (H&E. ×120)

276 Squamous cell carcinoma of the vagina
Two small islands of neoplastic cells appear to lie within the lymphatic channels. (H&E. ×50)

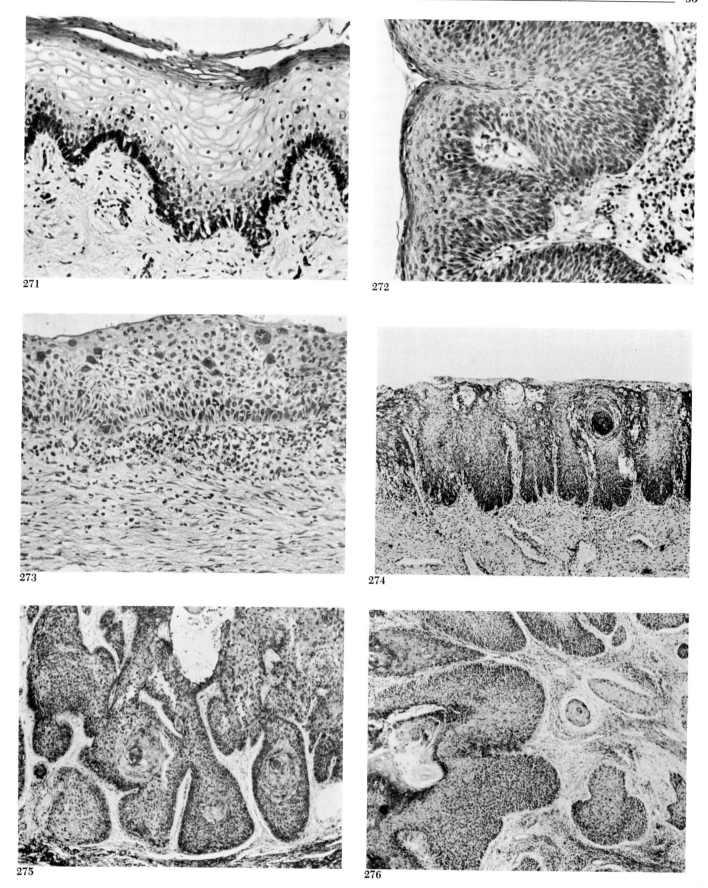

271

272

273

274

275

276

277   Squamous cell carcinoma of the vagina
The invading tumor is characterized by numerous small and large nests of neoplastic squamous cells with a tendency for horn-pearl formation. (H&E. ×80)

278   Mesonephric adenocarcinoma of the vagina
The tumor is developing from mesonephric rests (Wolffian or Gartner's) of the vaginal wall. Aggregates of glandlike structures are seen. The submucosa and the muscle coats are invaded. The overlying squamous epithelium is normal. (H&E. ×50)

279   Adenocarcinoma of the vestibular glands of the vagina
The tumor is composed of irregular glandular structures and scanty stroma infiltrated with inflammatory cells. (H&E. ×50)

280   Adenocarcinoma of the vestibular glands of the vagina
The glands show greater irregularity than in the preceding picture. They are lined by cuboidal cells with scanty cytoplasm and prominent hyperchromatic nuclei. Mitoses are frequent. In same lumens of the glandular acini, a mucinous material is detected. (H&E. ×125)

281   Adenoid cystic type adenocarcinoma of the vagina
Glandular tumor structures are seen in concentric arrangement. The lumen of a ductlike structure is filled by an island of tumor cells with microcystic areas. The neoplastic cells are cuboidal with round hyperchromatic nuclei. Vestibular glands, Müllerian-paramesonephric rests, and ectopic vulvar glands are possible origins of the tumor. (H&E. ×125)

282   Cribriform type adenocarcinoma of the vagina
The tumor shows numerous cystic dilated glandular acini. The intervening connective tissue stroma is scanty. (H&E. ×50)

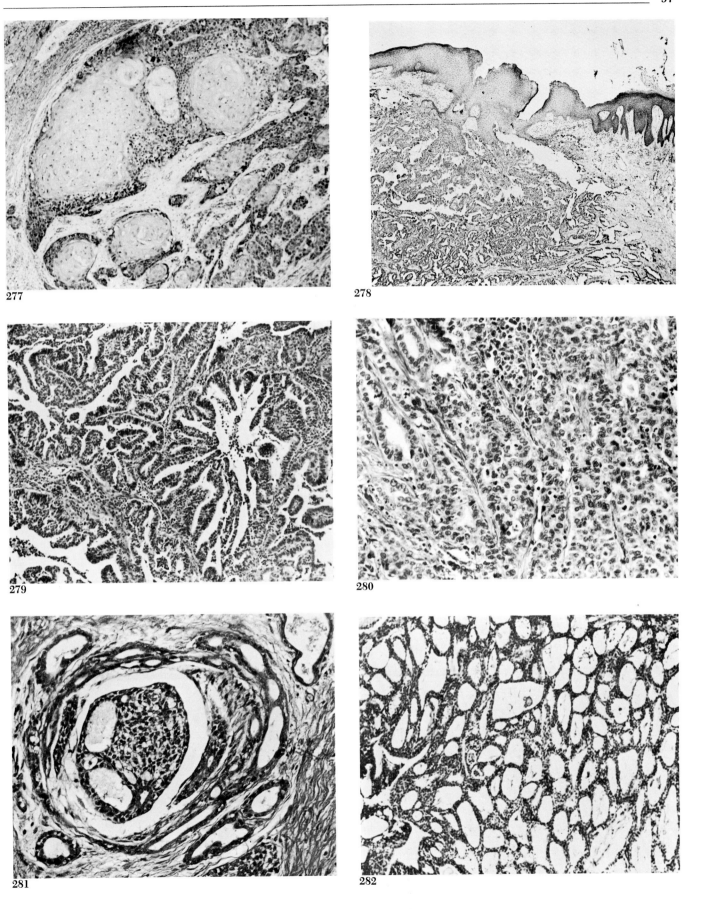

277

278

279

280

281

282

283   Sarcoma botryoides of the vagina
Pedunculated grapelike masses of tumor tissue are seen arising from the upper vaginal wall. (H&E. ×3)

284   Sarcoma botryoides of the vagina
High magnification of Fig. 283. The squamous epithelium of the vagina is invaded by sarcoma. The neoplasm consists of an extensive growth of immature cells with characteristic distinction between the submucosal "cambium" layer and the less cellular central area. (H&E. ×125)

285   Sarcoma botryoides of the vagina
High magnification of Fig. 283. The squamous vaginal epithelium is invaded by sarcoma cells. The submucosa is replaced by densely packed relatively small tumor cells. (H&E. ×225)

286   Sarcoma botryoides of the vagina
High magnification of Fig. 283. Cells with round nuclei and scanty cytoplasm and stellate cells with polyhedral nuclei and delicate cytoplasmic processes form the matrix; an occasional bipolar cell is seen. (H&E. ×250)

287   Sarcoma botryoides of the vagina
Dense cellularity and pronounced pleomorphism are frequently encountered in the tumor (H&E. ×125)

288   Sarcoma botryoides of the vagina
A single elongated neoplastic muscle cell with cross striation is surrounded by several pleomorphic tumor cells. (H&E. ×1000)

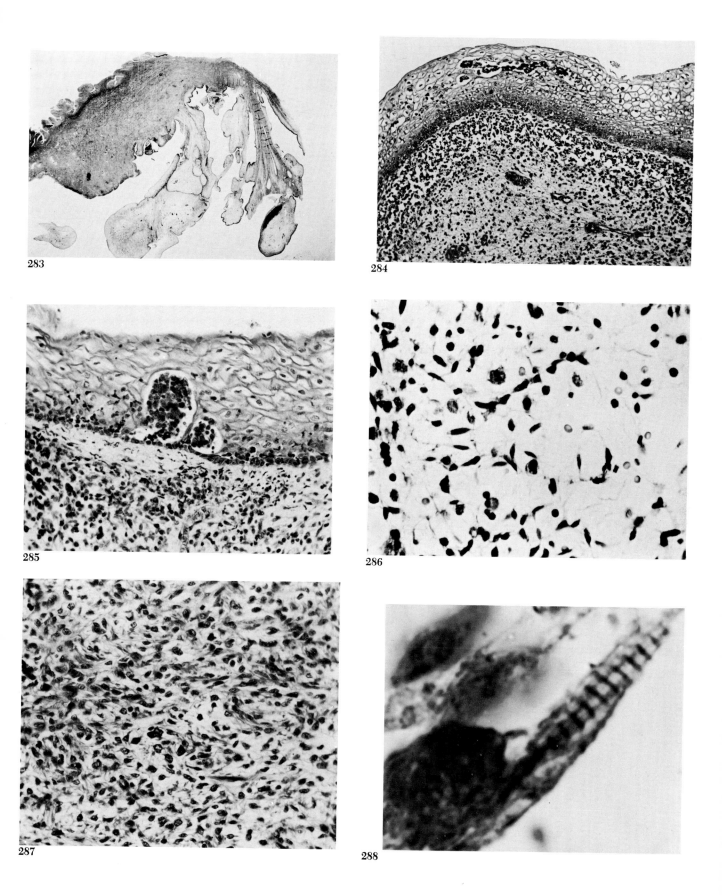

283

284

285

286

287

288

289 Leiomyosarcoma of the vagina
The cellular pleomorphism and the presence of large, irregular, partly hyperchromatic nuclei with prominent nucleoli are striking features. Blunt ends of nuclei are frequent findings in leiomyosarcoma. (H&E. ×325)

290 Malignant melanoma of the vagina
There is diffuse infiltration of the squamous epithelium and the submucosa by irregular pigment-containing neoplastic cells. (H&E. ×80)

291 Malignant melanoma of the vagina
High magnification of Fig. 290. Pigment-containing ovoid to fusiform tumor cells are located at the junction of the squamous epithelium and the lamina propria. The tumor cells migrate into the stratum germinativum and downward into the submucosa. Inflammatory cells are seen in the papillary bodies. (H&E. ×150)

292 Carcinoma of the kidney metastatic to the vagina
A renal carcinoma (hypernephroma) is seen metastasizing by retrograde venous route. There is alveolar arrangement of clear tumor cells. (H&E. ×155)

294 Hemorrhagic chorionic nodule of the vagina
This chorionic nodule is composed of hydropic chorionic villus, proliferated cytotrophoblasts and syncytiotrophoblasts, and a large area of hemorrhagic necrosis of the vaginal wall. Such nodules are observed in normal pregnancy, following abortion, in association with hydatidiform mole and chorioadenoma destruens. (H&E. ×14)

293 Squamous cell carcinoma of the cervix metastatic to the vagina
The squamous cell carcinoma of the cervix may metastasize to the vagina by direct extension or via lymphatic channels. Two metastatic islands are located in the submucosa. (H&E. ×80)

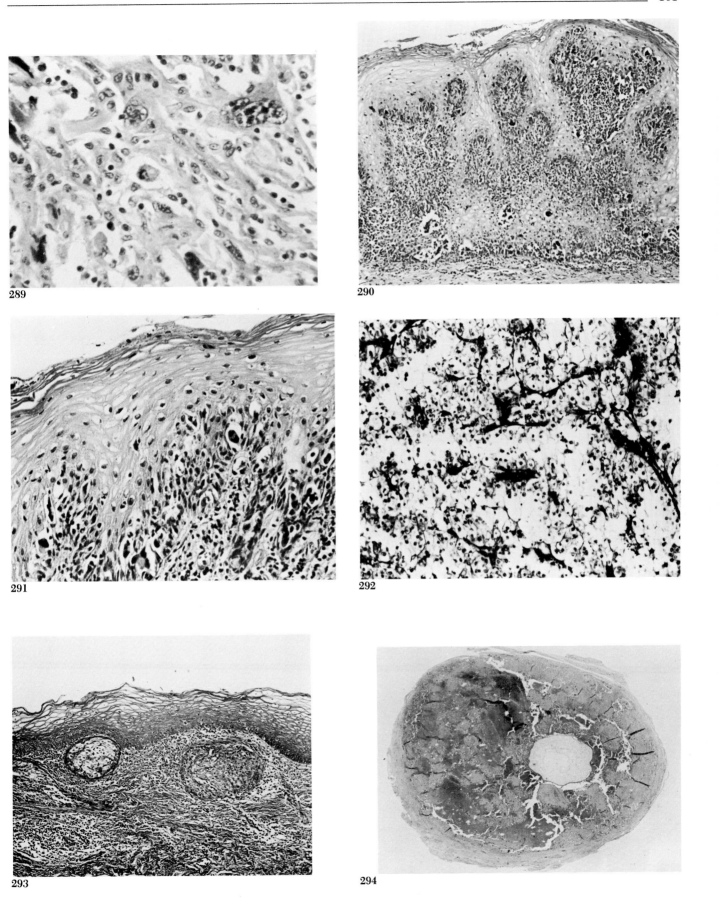

289

290

291

292

293

294

295 Hemorrhagic chorionic nodule of the vagina

High magnification of Fig. 294. Proliferating trophoblastic cells surround hydropic, avascular villus. The presence of a chorionic villus distinguishes this nodule from metastatic choriocarcinoma. In a chorionic nodule, the syncytial cells dominate the histologic picture. (H&E. ×100)

296 Choriocarcinoma uteri metastatic to the vagina

The hemorrhagic nodule is covered by intact stratified squamous epithelium. The muscle layers of the vaginal wall show extensive hemorrhagic necrosis and islands of invading trophoblastic cells. As a rule, there is absence of chorionic villi. The metastasis to the vagina is by a retrograde venous route. (H&E. ×8)

297 Choriocarcinoma uteri metastatic to the vagina

High magnification of Fig. 296. Metastatic tumor islands are seen plugging the vascular channels. The trophoblastic tissue consists of Langhans' cells and syncytiotrophoblasts. Differentiation into these two cell types is characteristic of metastatic choriocarcinoma, although the cytotrophoblasts may dominate the histologic picture. (H&E. ×75)

298 Acute radiation vaginitis

The necrosis of the lining squamous epithelium and the upper portion of the submucosa followed intravaginal radium application (3,400 mg per hr). The acute inflammatory exudate extends deep into the muscular coats. (H&E. ×50)

299 Chronic radiation vaginitis

Complete regeneration of the squamous epithelium is evident. The submucosa and muscular layers show extensive fibrosis with vascular telangiectasis and in places vascular obliteration. Mild chronic inflammation is present. The biopsy was taken 1 year following radium therapy for carcinoma of the cervix. (H&E. ×50)

300 Vascular changes in chronic radiation vaginitis

The wall of a large vessel, located in the vaginal wall, shows fibrosis of the tunica media with the subendothelial appearance of large foam cells. (H&E. ×100)

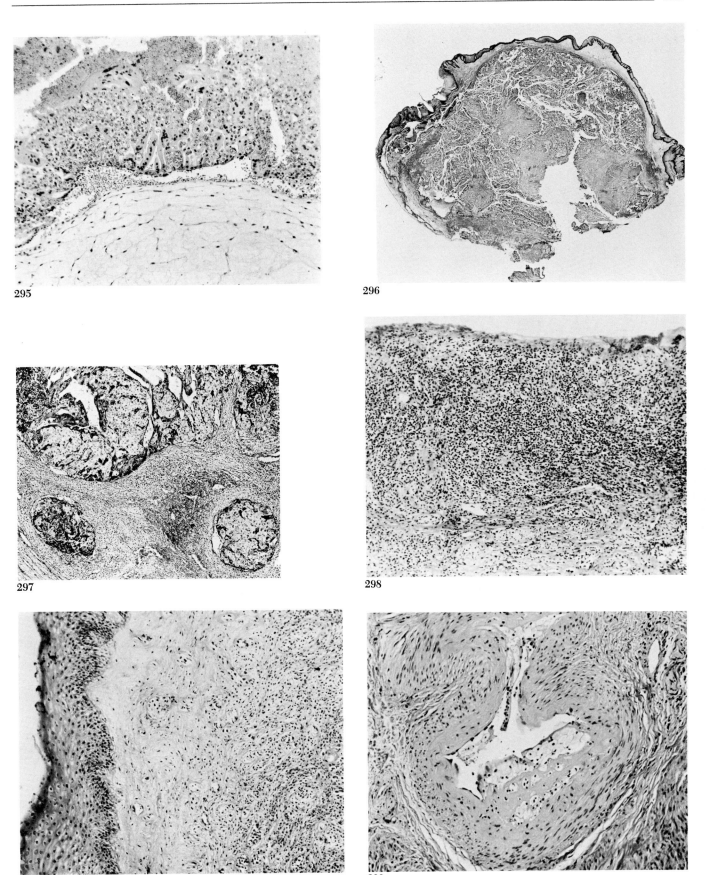

295

296

297

298

299

300

COLOR PLATES
Chapter 2
Diseases of the Vagina
Plate 4

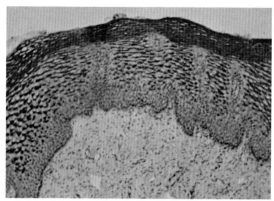

19 Normal vaginal epithelium in a woman of reproductive age The epithelial cells contain a large amount of glycogen. (PAS reaction. ×100)

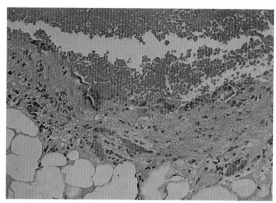

20 Vaginitis emphysematosa The emphysematous cyst of the vaginal wall is filled with blood. The cystic cavity is lined by foreign-body giant cells. (H&E. ×160)

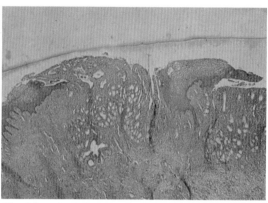

21 Adenosis of the vagina The surface epithelium of the vagina shows a defect through which protrudes tissue composed of glandular elements. Glandular elements of Müllerian type epithelium are scattered through the vaginal wall. (H&E. ×50)

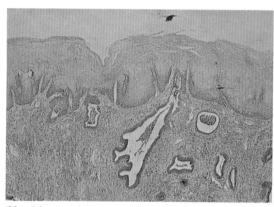

22 Adenosis of the vagina Mucin-secreting glands similar if not identical with endocervical glands are seen irregularly scattered throughout the vaginal wall. The glands are of various sizes and may be accompanied by a mild inflammatory reaction. In places these glands may assume an adenomatous character. (PAS reaction. ×70)

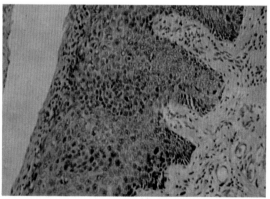

23 Marked dysplasia of the vaginal mucosa There is hyperkeratosis and parakeratosis of superficial cell layers of the squamous epithelium. Rete ridges show irregular downward growth. Cells with atypical hyperchromatic nuclei are present in the stratum germinativum. The authors prefer the term dysplasia for these morphologic changes rather than leukoplakia. (H&E. ×70)

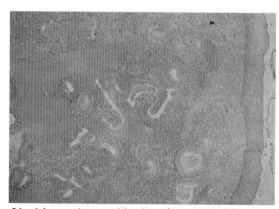

24 Adenocarcinoma arising in endometriosis of the vagina Beneath the normal vaginal mucosal epithelium lies a tumor composed of neoplastic glandular structures resembling an endometrial carcinoma. (H&E. ×80)

Plate 4

3

Diseases of the Cervix Uteri
(Exocervix and Endocervix)

301 Cervix uteri in a 2-month-old infant
Note the squamocolumnar junction located in the exocervix. Multiple rugae are seen in the fornices and vaginal walls. (H&E. ×11)

302 Normal exocervix and endocervix in a woman of reproductive age
Note the squamocolumnar junction now in the endocervical canal. (H&E. ×8)

303 Normal squamous epithelium of the exocervix
Three groups of cells are recognized: (1) basal cells, (2) intermediate cells, and (3) "cornified" cells. True cornification is usually not present. The term "cornified" is rather inaccurate. (H&E. ×120)

304 Leukoparakeratosis of the exocervix
Marked parakeratosis of the exocervical squamous epithelium is seen. Colposcopic findings in such cases are those of "leukoplakia." (H&E. ×125)

306 Papillary leukoparakeratosis of the exocervix
There is marked parakeratosis and acanthosis of exocervical squamous epithelium. Elongation of the rete ridges is seen. Chronic inflammatory cells are present in connective tissue stroma and in transepidermal migration. (H&E. ×125)

305 Hyperkeratosis of the exocervix
There is marked cornification of the exocervical epithelium with formation of a keratin layer. (H&E. ×125)

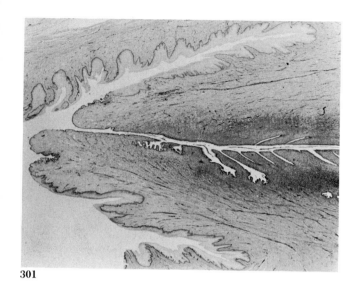

301

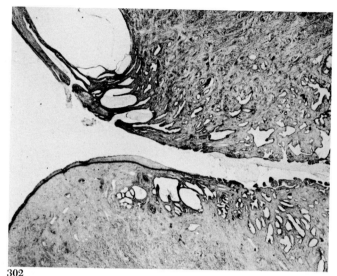

302

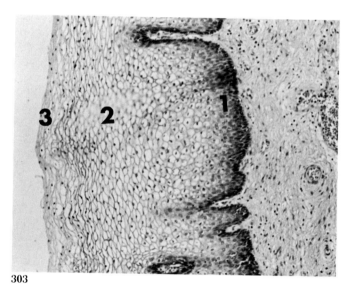

303

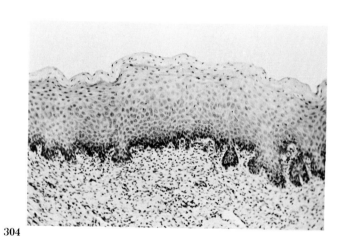

304

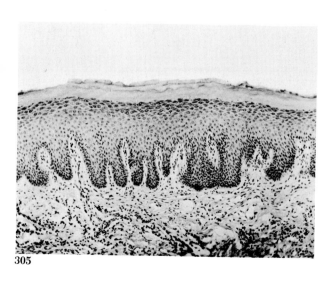

305

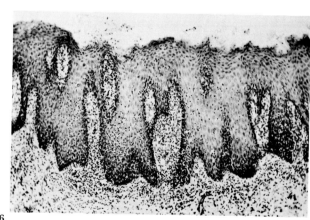

306

307 Papillary leukoparakeratosis simulating carcinoma of the exocervix, tangential section
Note the absence of cellular and nuclear atypism. (H&E. ×80)

308 Decubital ulcer of the exocervix
The margin of the decubital ulcer of the portio vaginalis can be observed in cervical prolapse and following the use of a pessary. (H&E. ×20)

309 Glandular erosion of the exocervix
The squamous epithelium of the exocervix is replaced by columnar endocervical epithelium with gland-like formations. This glandular erosion is frequently acquired and occasionally seen as a congenital lesion. (H&E. ×50)

310 Healed erosion of the exocervix
A healed erosion is covered by somewhat irregular squamous epithelium. This is brought about by epidermidization of the eroded area. (H&E. ×120)

311 Healed erosion of the exocervix with formation of endocervical retention cysts (so-called Nabothian cysts)
(H&E. ×20)

312 Squamocolumnar junction of the cervix
(H&E. ×50)

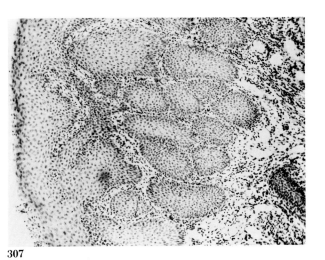

307

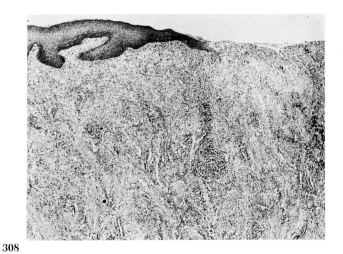

308

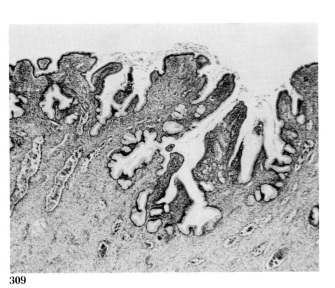

309

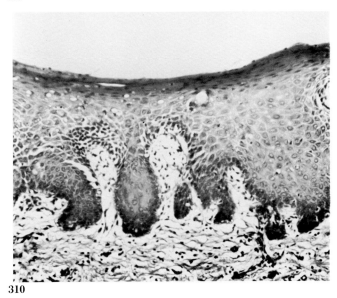

310

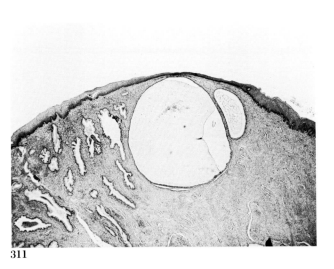

311

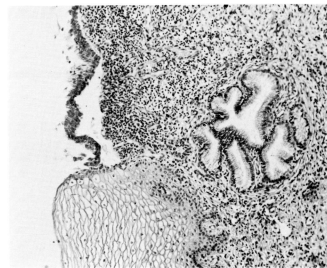

312

313 Normal infantile endocervix
(H&E. ×20)

314 Normal endocervix in a woman of reproductive age
(H&E. ×50)

315 Endocervical gland
High magnification of Fig. 314. Note the single row of tall columnar mucin-producing epithelium with clear cytoplasm and the nuclei placed at the base. (H&E. ×250)

316 Metaplasia of endocervical glandular epithelium, stage I
The nuclei are in midcell position. Note the appearance of the individual reserve cells at the basement membrane. These cells are cuboidal with scant cytoplasm and dense round nuclei. They do not stain for mucopolysaccharides. (H&E. ×120)

317 Metaplasia of endocervical glandular epithelium, stage II
The surface columnar epithelium shows disturbance of normal arrangement. Underlying is a well-developed row of cuboidal reserve cells. (H&E. ×180)

318 Metaplasia of endocervical glandular epithelium, stage III
Replacement of cuboidal epithelium by proliferated reserve cells is seen. At this stage, the cuboidal reserve cells show stratification and early differentiation into squamous epithelial cells. (H&E. ×180)

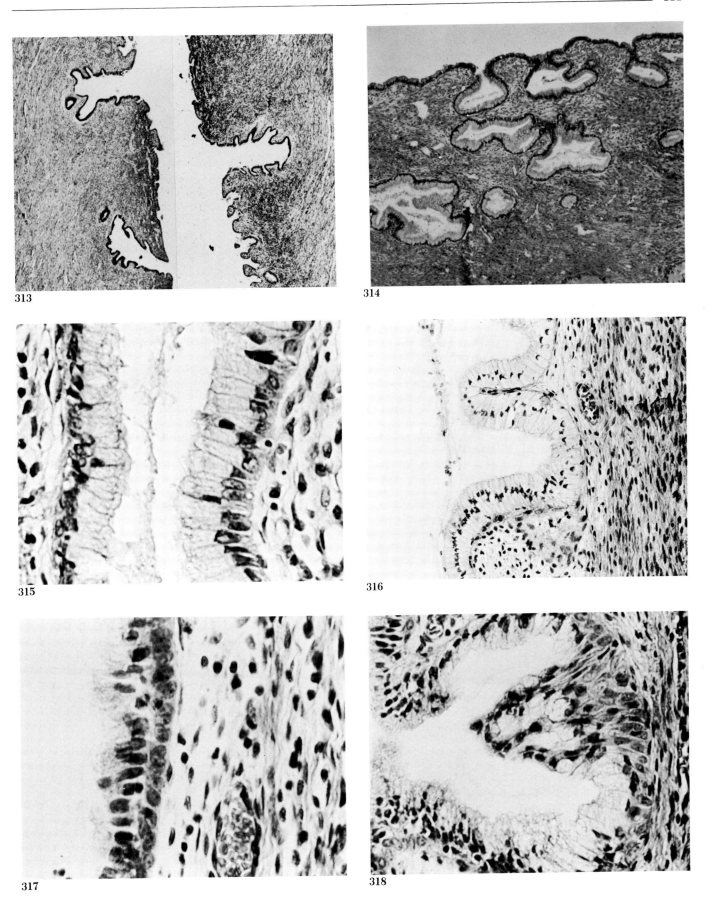

313

314

315

316

317

318

319 Metaplasia of endocervical glandular epithelium, stage IV
The fragmentary mucin-secreting endocervical epithelial cells are surrounded by squamous epithelium with early keratinization. (H&E. ×150)

320 Extensive squamous metaplasia of the endocervix, showing variations of stages (H&E. ×130)

321 Squamous epithelial nodule of the cervix of disontogenetic origin
This nodule may develop from paramesonephric or mesonephric cervical rests. It is also referred to as Walthard cell rest of the cervix. (H&E. ×125)

322 Polyp of the endocervix
The polyp consists of numerous endocervical glands and supporting fibrous connective tissue stroma. It is covered by a layer of columnar epithelium. The stroma is highly vascular. (H&E. ×80)

324 Squamous metaplasia in a fibrous polyp of the endocervix
The polyp consists mainly of edematous and vascular connective tissue stroma. The overlying endocervical epithelium shows squamous metaplasia. (H&E. ×15)

323 Squamous metaplasia occurring in a polyp of the endocervix
(H&E. ×120)

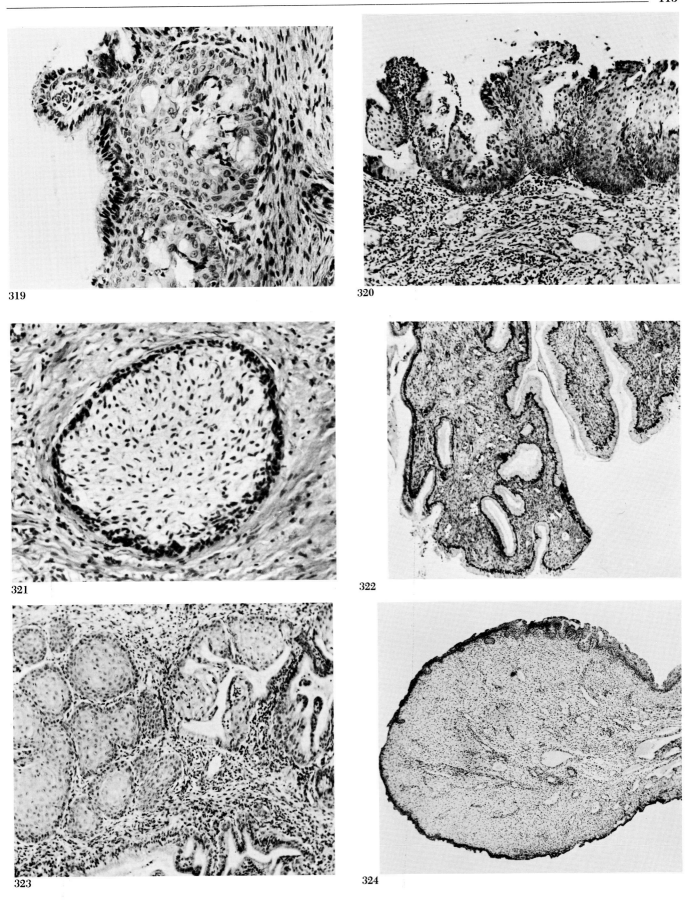

319

320

321

322

323

324

325   Acute nonspecific exocervicitis
The connective tissue stroma and the squamous epithelium are infiltrated with acute and chronic inflammatory cells. (H&E. ×150)

326   Subacute endocervicitis with early squamous metaplasia
(H&E. ×100)

328   Russell bodies in an endocervical polyp with inflammatory changes
The Russell bodies are polygonal to ovoid in shape and markedly eosinophilic. They can be identified in routine H&E sections of nearly 50 per cent of endocervical polyps. They are occasionally mistaken for foreign bodies. Russell bodies are composed of neutral mucopolysaccharides. (H&E. ×220)

327   Inflammatory polyp of the cervix
The polyp is formed by inflammatory granulation tissue. (H&E. ×70)

329   Russell bodies in an endocervical polyp with inflammatory changes
Intracellular Russell bodies reacted with Gram's iodine. The prevalence of Russell bodies in endocervical polyps probably indicates the presence of an active immunologic process. (Brown and Brenn's stain. ×380)

330   Chronic follicular endocervicitis
Periglandular formation of lymphoid follicle is visible in the connective tissue stroma of the cervix. (H&E. ×50)

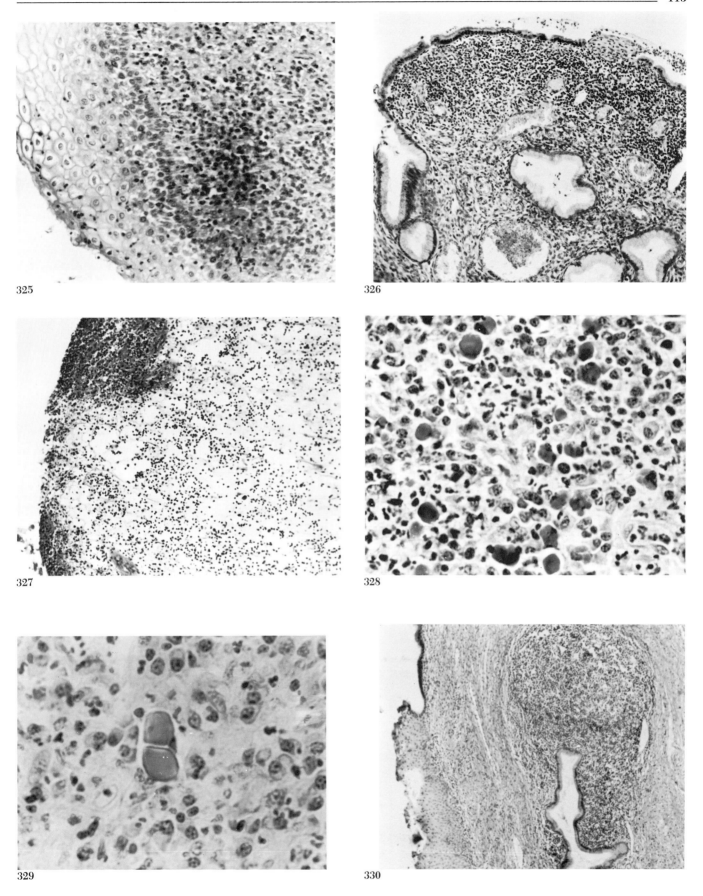

325

326

327

328

329

330

331 Schistosomiasis (bilharziasis) of the cervix
The pseudotubercle formation shows ova of *Schistosoma mansoni* and foreign-body giant cells. (H&E. ×120)

332 Schistosomiasis (bilharziasis) of the cervix
High magnification of Fig. 331. (H&E. ×310)

333 Sarcoidosis (Boeck's sarcoid) of the cervix
This Negress, 32 years of age, has advanced systemic sarcoidosis. Discrete, noncaseating epithelioid tubercles are present in the connective tissue stroma of the cervix. (H&E. ×60)

334 Sarcoidosis (Boeck's sarcoid) of the cervix
High magnification of Fig. 333. The tubercle is formed by epithelioid cells and a single giant cell. The peripheral accumulation of lymphocytes is inconspicuous. (H&E. ×180)

335 Tuberculous endocervicitis
The tubercle is formed by epithelioid cells, Langhans' giant cells, and a central area of caseation necrosis. The tubercle is located in the connective tissue stroma. Endocervical glands are preserved. (H&E. ×125)

336 Tuberculous endocervicitis
High magnification of Fig. 335. There is typical tuberculous granulation tissue with epithelioid cells, Langhans' giant cells, central caseation necrosis, and diffuse lymphocytic infiltration. Acid-fast organisms were found. (H&E. ×200)

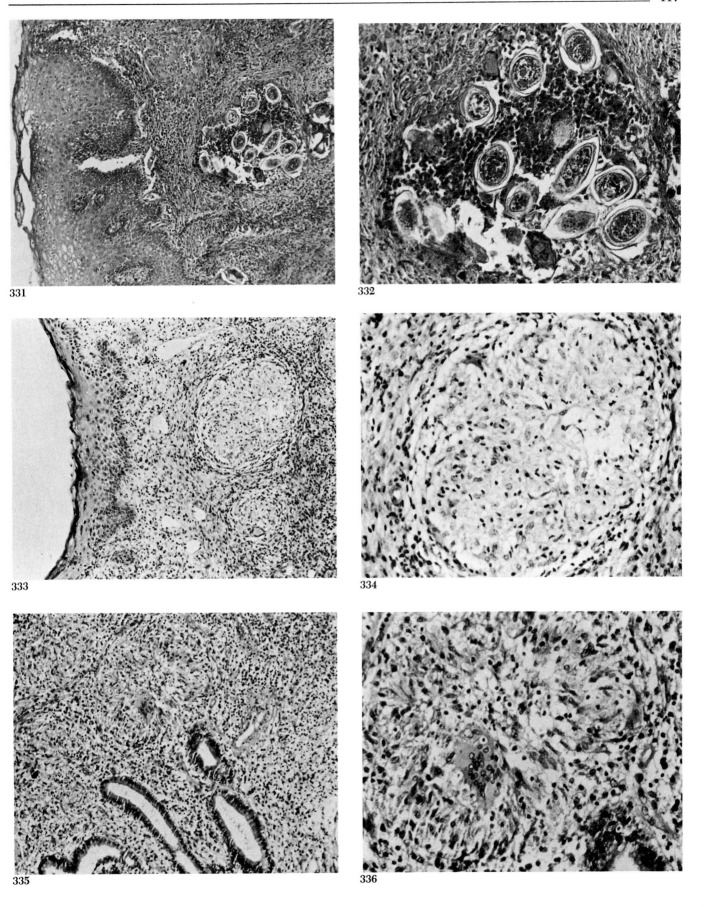

331

332

333

334

335

336

337   Late secondary syphilis of the cervix
Multiple perivascular granulomas are seen localized in the cervix. The granulomas are composed of endothelial proliferation and plasma cells. They show a tendency for conglomeration. A special stain shows spirochetes. (H&E. ×80)

338   Late secondary syphilis of the cervix
The granuloma is formed by epithelioid cells and giant cells with no evidence of necrosis. There is marked mononuclear cell infiltration. The patient, 22 years of age, had a positive serologic reaction. (H&E. ×150)

339   Cytomegalic inclusion disease of the endocervix
Within the cytoplasm of the columnar endocervical epithelium are numerous eosinophilic homogeneous inclusion bodies. (H&E. ×60)

340   Cytomegalic inclusion disease of the endocervix
High magnification of Fig. 339. Numerous large, round, doubly contoured inclusion bodies are seen within the cytoplasm of endocervical epithelial cells. (H&E. ×320)

341   Condyloma acuminatum of the exocervix
There is papillomatosis with pronounced acanthosis. The connective tissue core shows branching and is covered with a thick layer of squamous epithelium. (H&E. ×24)

342   Adenomatous hyperplasia of the endocervix
There is marked adenomatous hyperplasia of endocervical glands. Different degrees of cystic dilatations are seen. There is an increase of mucin production. (H&E. ×15)

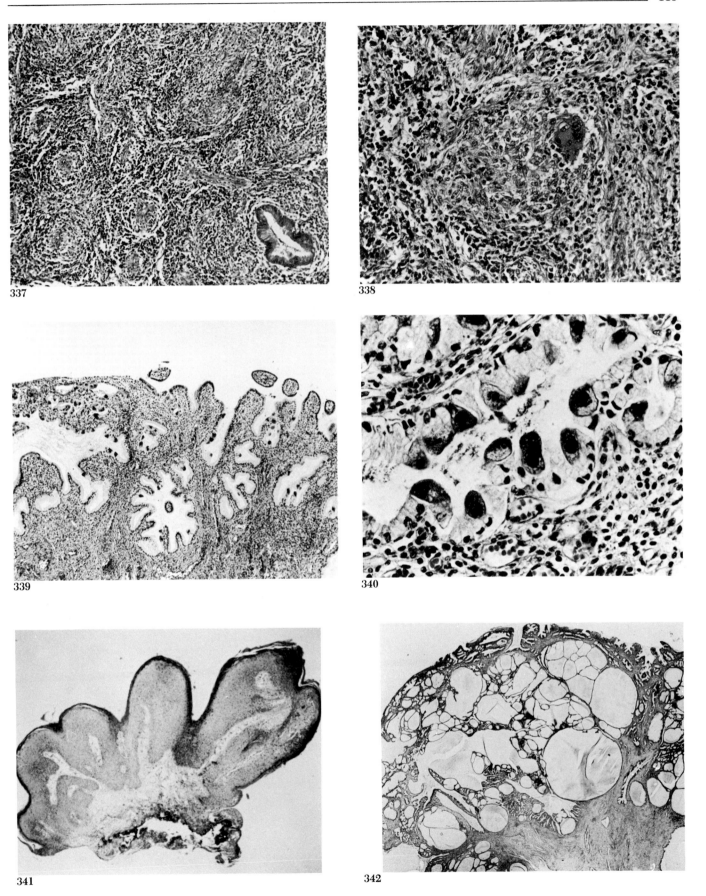

337

338

339

340

341

342

343   Focal adenomatous hyperplasia (tunnel clusters) of the endocervix
The normal endocervical gland to the left is surrounded by numerous glandular structures with flattened lining epithelium. The name "tunnel clusters" has been applied to such changes occurring in the endocervix. Such tunnel clusters may be associated with a relatively large retention cyst and suggest obstruction of the drainage pathways. (H&E. ×50)

344   Circumscribed adenosis of the cervix
Circumscribed accumulation of newly formed glandular structures is seen. There are duct formations and communications with exocervical surface epithelium. This lesion should be differentiated from mesonephric rests. (H&E. ×30)

345   Circumscribed adenosis of the cervix
High magnification of Fig. 344. The glands vary in size and shape. Some form cystlike spaces which contain discrete amounts of mucin. The lining epithelium of the glands is cuboidal, with round prominent nuclei. The glands are probably modified paramesonephric (Müllerian) epithelium. (H&E. ×100)

346   Diffuse adenosis of the cervix
There is marked increase of cervical connective tissue in association with numerous glandular structures scattered throughout. (H&E. ×15)

347   Diffuse adenosis of the cervix
High magnification of Fig. 346. Numerous glands are lined by cuboidal epithelium with prominent round nuclei. They contain inspissated material. (H&E. ×50)

348   Diffuse adenosis of the cervix
High magnification of Fig. 346. In places, clusters of glands are seen surrounded by fibrous connective tissue. These diffusely, newly formed glands probably represent a modified paramesonephric (Müllerian) epithelium. (H&E. ×150)

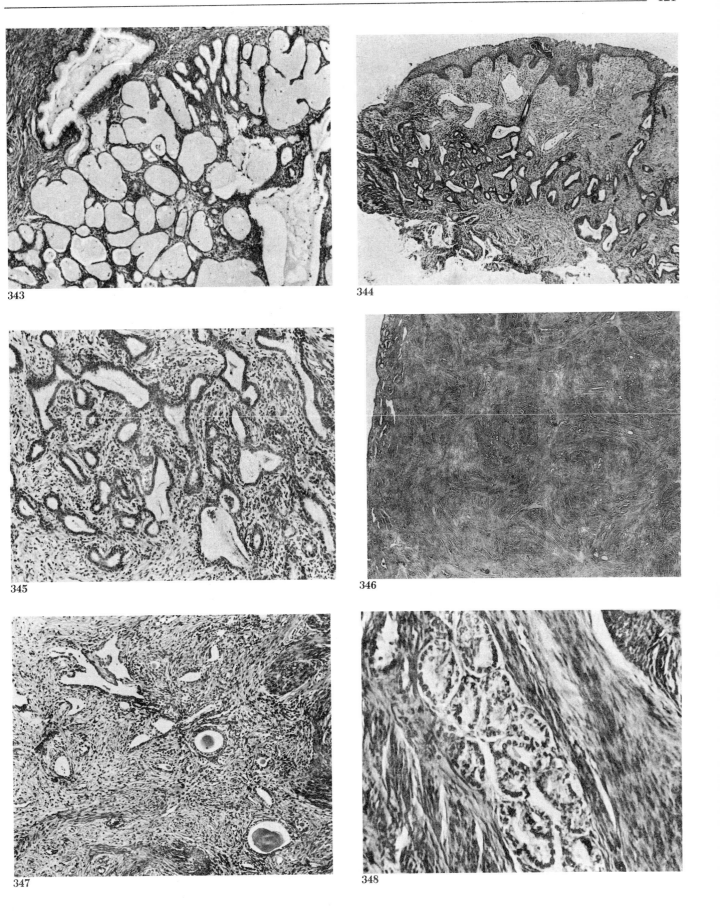

343

344

345

346

347

348

349 Epidermal inclusion cyst of the cervix
The cyst is lined by squamous epithelium and contains keratinized cells. (H&E. ×35)

350 Epidermal inclusion cyst of the cervix
This cervical cyst is lined by squamous epithelium. "Cornified" cells form the cyst content. (H&E. ×30)

351 Paramesonephric dysontogenetic cyst of the cervix
This cyst of the cervix is lined by oviductlike epithelium. (H&E. ×125)

352 Mesonephric dysontogenetic cyst of the cervix
This cyst of the cervix is lined by mesonephric type of epithelium. Low columnar epithelial cells with dark nuclei rest upon a prominent basement membrane. (H&E. ×50)

353 Squamous papilloma of the cervix
This tumor is composed of numerous villous protrusions formed by squamous epithelial cells. (H&E. ×25)

354 Metabolic calcification of endocervical glands
Deposition of calcium aggregates in and around the endocervical glands is seen. (H&E. ×100)

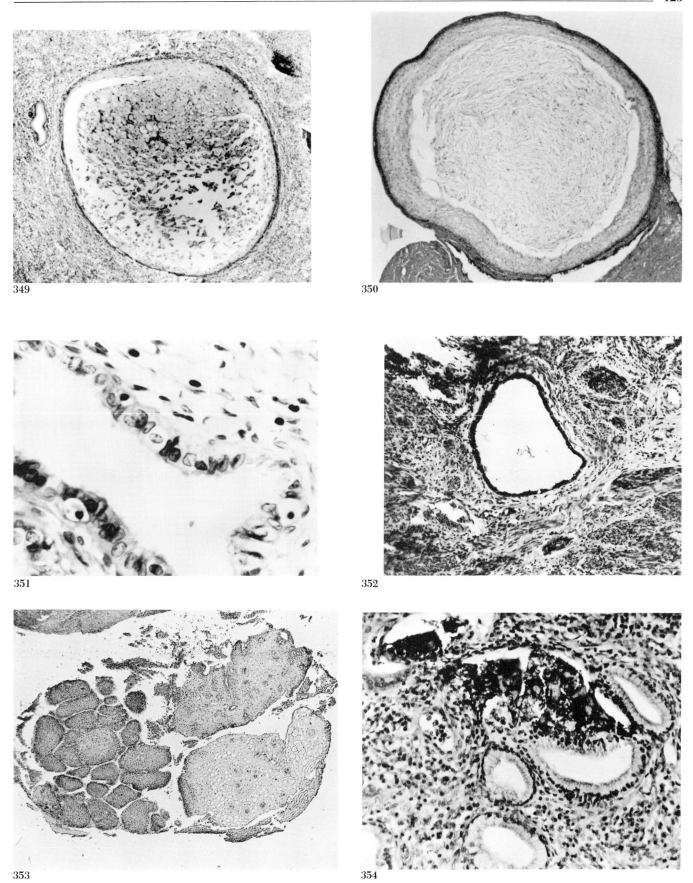

349

350

351

352

353

354

355 Lipoma of the cervix
The circumscribed intramural tumor is formed by mature fat cells. Below the tumor are located two endocervical glands. (H&E. ×40)

356 Heterotopic sebaceous glands in the cervix
(H&E. ×90)

357 Hamartoma of the cervix
This probably represents an anomaly of development rather than a true neoplasm. The non-encapsulated tumor is composed of fibrous connective tissue, hyaline cartilage, and lipid containing histiocytes. (H&E. ×50)

358 Hamartoma of the cervix
High magnification of Fig. 357. (H&E. ×120)

359 Hamartoma of the cervix
High magnification of Fig. 357. The central area of this cervical hamartoma contains lipid histiocytes. (H&E. ×120)

360 Cavernous hemangioma of the cervix
This tumor is formed by widely dilated vascular channels and intervening connective tissue stroma. The endothelium-lined channels contain blood. (H&E. ×50)

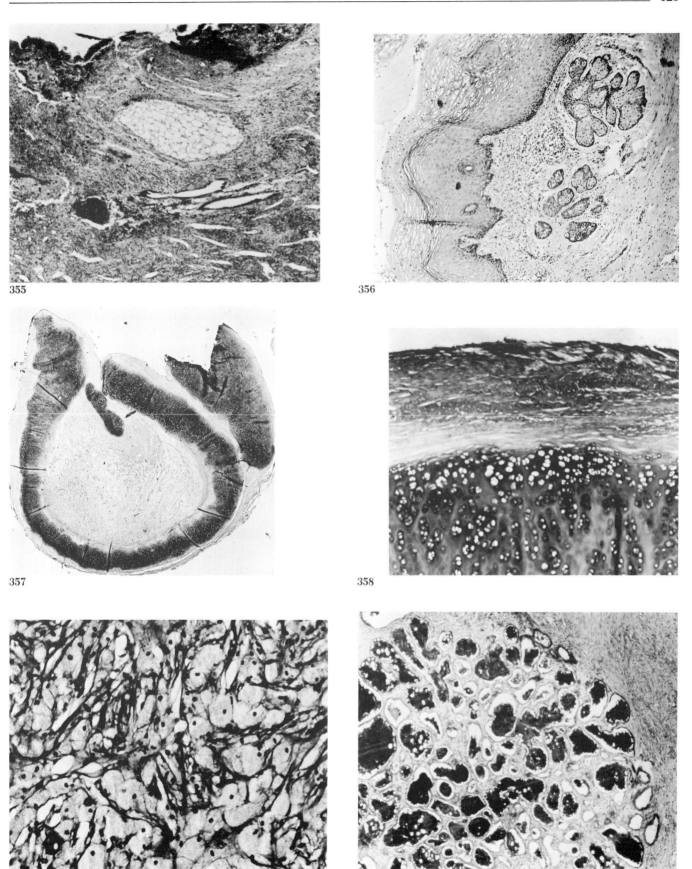

355

356

357

358

359

360

361 Glomus tumor of the cervix
The tumor is formed by compact masses of glomus cells surrounding small vascular channels. (H&E. ×80)

362 Glomus tumor of the cervix
Vascular channels, some with endothelial cells are compressed by proliferating relatively uniform glomus cells. The glomus cells show a characteristic peritheliomatous arrangement. (H&E. ×180)

363 Hemangiopericytoma of the cervix
This tumor is formed by pericytes, the contractile cells of the capillaries. (H&E. ×40)

364 Hemangiopericytoma of the cervix
High magnification of Fig. 363. The vascular channels show perivascular proliferation of tumor cells. (H&E. ×80)

365 Hemangiopericytoma of the cervix
High magnification of Fig. 363. Perivascular proliferation of tumor cells is evident. (H&E. ×280)

366 Leiomyoma of the cervix
There is neoplastic proliferation of smooth muscle fibers. They form interlacing bundles or fascicular structures. The nuclei are long and slender. They appear round on cross section. (H&E. ×120)

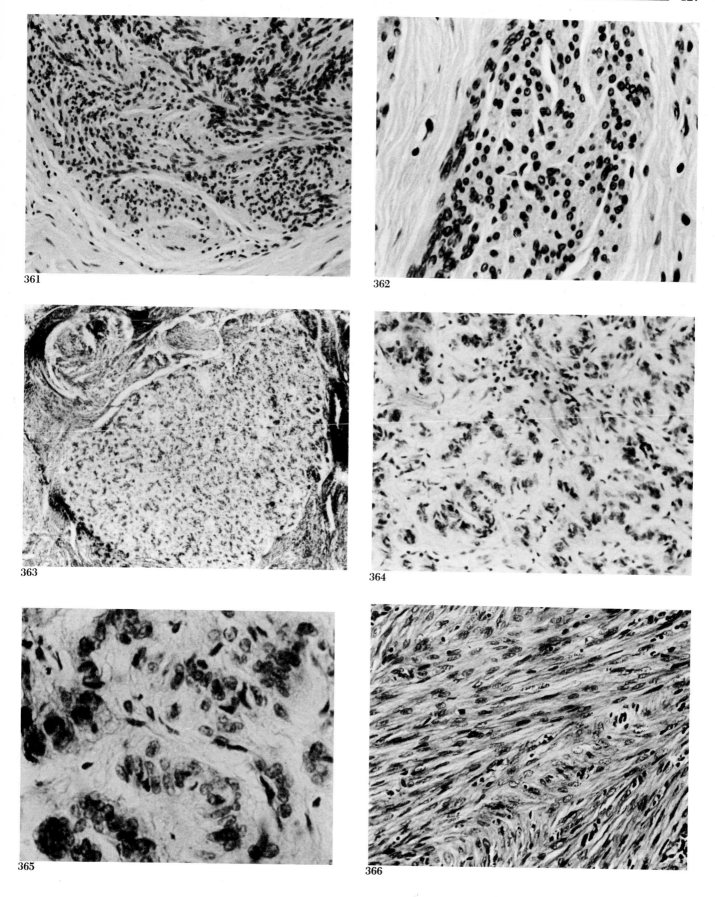

361

362

363

364

365

366

367   **Silver pigment deposition in cervical connective tissue following treatment of exocervical erosion with silver nitrate**
(H&E. ×50)

368   **Hyperplasia of mesonephric rests of the cervix**
There is numerical increase of the glandular elements of the ampullary portion of Gartner's ducts of the cervix. (H&E. ×25)

369   **Hyperplasia of mesonephric rests of the cervix**
The glandular structures are lined by cuboidal epithelial cells with prominent hyperchromatic nuclei. (H&E. ×50)

370   **Hyperplasia of mesonephric rests of the cervix**
High magnification of Fig. 369. A small amount of diastase-resistant, weakly PAS positive, material is present in all mesonephric structures; most probably it is a glucoprotein. Alcian blue and Mayer's mucicarmine stains are uniformly negative in all benign and malignant mesonephric derivatives. (H&E. ×150)

371   **Mesonephric adenoma of the cervix**
The tumor is formed by mesonephric glandular structures lined by a single layer of cuboidal epithelial cells. The nuclei are hyperchromatic and prominent. (H&E. ×120)

372   **Mesonephric papilloma of the cervix and fornix**
The lesion is polypoid in appearance with variation in the size and shape of the papillary structures. (H&E. ×50)

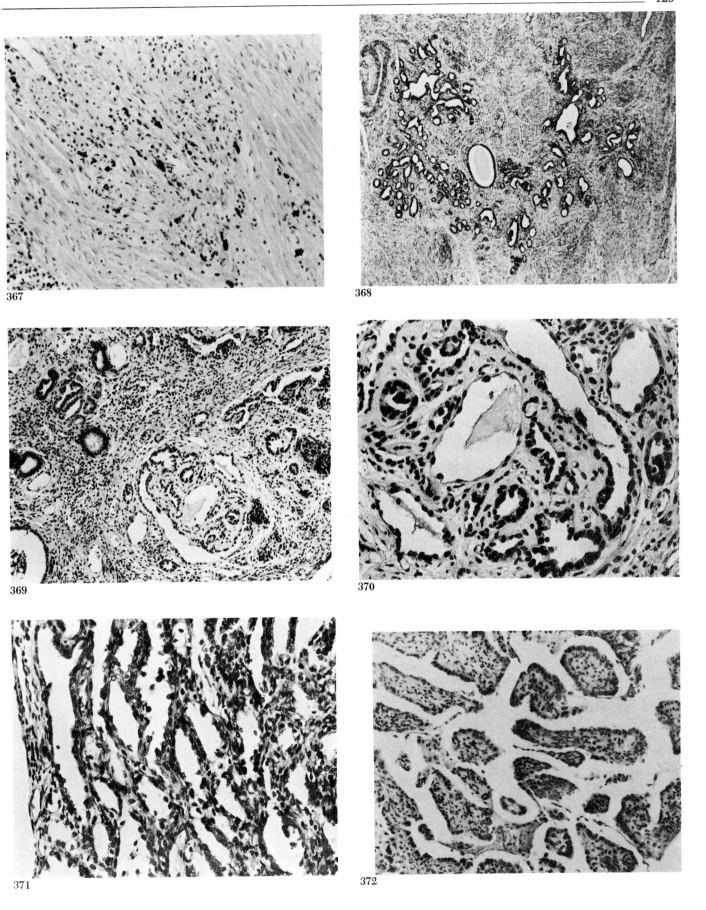

367

368

369

370

371

372

373 Mesonephric papilloma of the cervix and fornix
High magnification of Fig. 372. Calcific deposition is indicated by arrows within the connective tissue stroma of the papillary projections. Note the similarity with the psammoma bodies. (H&E. ×120)

374 Mesonephric papilloma of the cervix and fornix
High magnification of Fig. 372. The papillary structures are lined by uniform cuboidal epithelial cells with prominent round nuclei and indistinct nucleoli. The connective tissue stroma is infiltrated with lymphocytes and polymorphonuclear leukocytes. A moderate degree of stromal edema is present. (H&E. ×150)

375 Proliferating mesonephric papilloma of the cervix without stromal invasion
Benign mesonephric papillary and polypoid tumors of the cervix are, as a rule, encountered in infancy and childhood. They produce clinical symptoms of intermittent and irregular mucosanguineous vaginal discharge. Such tumors represent diagnostic difficulties. (H&E. ×120)

376 Proliferating mesonephric papilloma of the cervix without stromal invasion
High magnification of Fig. 375. Frequently mesonephric papillomas of the cervix and/or fornix are multicentric in origin. If inadequately excised, they invariably recur. (H&E. ×150)

377 Mesonephric carcinoma of the cervix
The tumor is composed of tubular structures which form in places oval and cystic cavities lined by cuboidal epithelium with irregular hyperchromatic nuclei. Some of the epithelial cells show cytoplasmic vacuolization. The other epithelial cells appear as clear cells. There is a striking similarity to an ovarian mesonephroma. (H&E. ×70)

378 Mesonephric carcinoma of the cervix
The tumor is formed by large pleomorphic vacuolated epithelial cells. Cyst formations are present between solid masses of the tumor. (H&E. ×50)

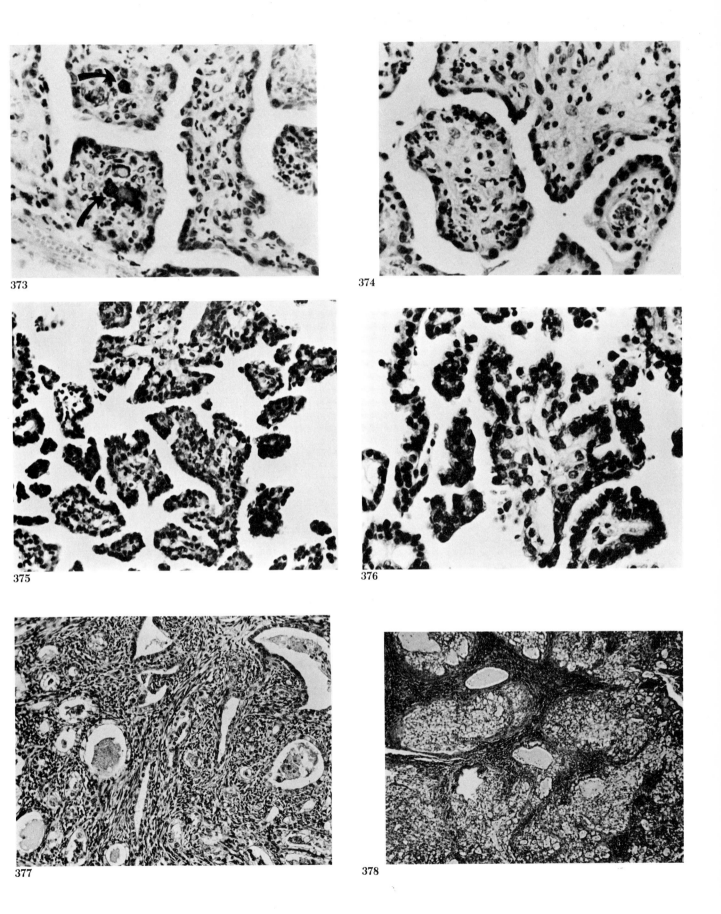

373

374

375

376

377

378

379 Mesonephric carcinoma of the cervix
High magnification of Fig. 378. The tumor cells have irregular hyperchromatic nuclei and cytoplasmic vacuolization. There is a tendency toward coalescence of vacuoles and the formation of cystic spaces. (H&E. ×180)

380 Mesonephric carcinoma of the cervix
High magnification of Fig. 378. In other areas of the tumor presented in Fig. 378, clear cells dominate the morphologic picture. They are large vacuolated cells with irregular hyperchromatic nuclei. (H&E. ×180)

381 Mesonephric papillary carcinoma of the cervix
The tumor is formed by papillary and cystic areas. The tumor develops from the tubular mesonephric rests of the cervix. (H&E. ×60)

382 Mesonephric papillary carcinoma of the cervix
High magnification of Fig. 381. The tumor is composed of papillary conglomerations. The papillary processes are formed by cuboidal and columnar cells with scant eosinophilic cytoplasm and large, prominent, irregular nuclei. (H&E. ×120)

383 Mesonephric papillary carcinoma of the cervix
High magnification of Fig. 381. Some of the tumor cells forming papillary projections show cytoplasmic vacuolization. The connective tissue stroma is sparse. (H&E. ×180)

384 Mesonephric alveolar carcinoma of the cervix
This mesonephric tumor is composed of alveolar structures which vary in size. Single cells and clusters of cells lie free in the glandular spaces. The lining epithelium does not stain with alcian blue nor with Mayer's mucicarmine stain. (H&E. ×180)

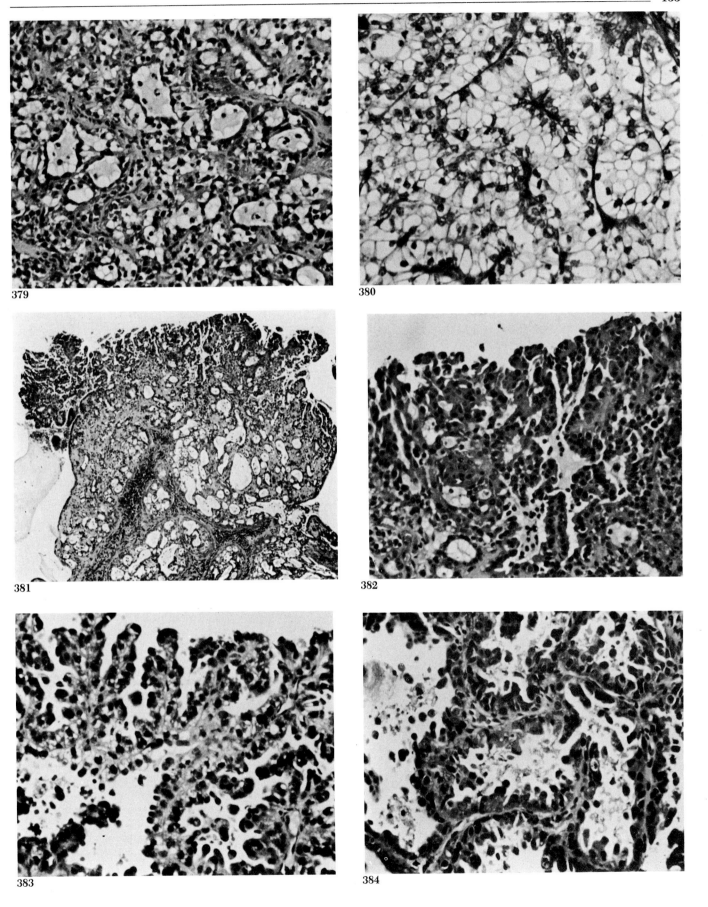

379

380

381

382

383

384

385 Simple basal cell hyperplasia (dysplasia) of the cervix

The mucosal epithelium shows hyperplasia of basal cells along with midzonal appearance of irregular shaped cells with hyperchromatic nuclei. The maturation of the cells as they approach the surface is preserved. (H&E. ×100)

386 Simple basal cell hyperplasia (dysplasia) of the cervix

Note the marked hyperplasia and thickening of the basal cell layer of the cervical mucosal epithelium. The superficial epithelial layer shows parakeratosis. (H&E. ×100)

387 Atypical basal cell hyperplasia (dysplasia) of the cervix

The hyperplasia of the basal cells involves almost the entire thickness of the exocervical epithelium. The surface epithelium shows maturation. (H&E. ×120)

388 Atypical basal cell hyperplasia (dysplasia) of the cervix

Marked basal cell hyperplasia and the appearance of small immature cells with frequent mitotic figures can be seen. Maturation of the cells is preserved at the surface. (H&E. ×120)

389 Basal cell hyperplasia (dysplasia) occurring in the endocervical gland

(H&E. ×120)

390 Basal cell hyperplasia (dysplasia) occurring in the endocervical gland

Actually there is hyperplasia of reserve cells with basilar dysplasia and a tendency to luminal squamous cell differentiation. (H&E. ×150)

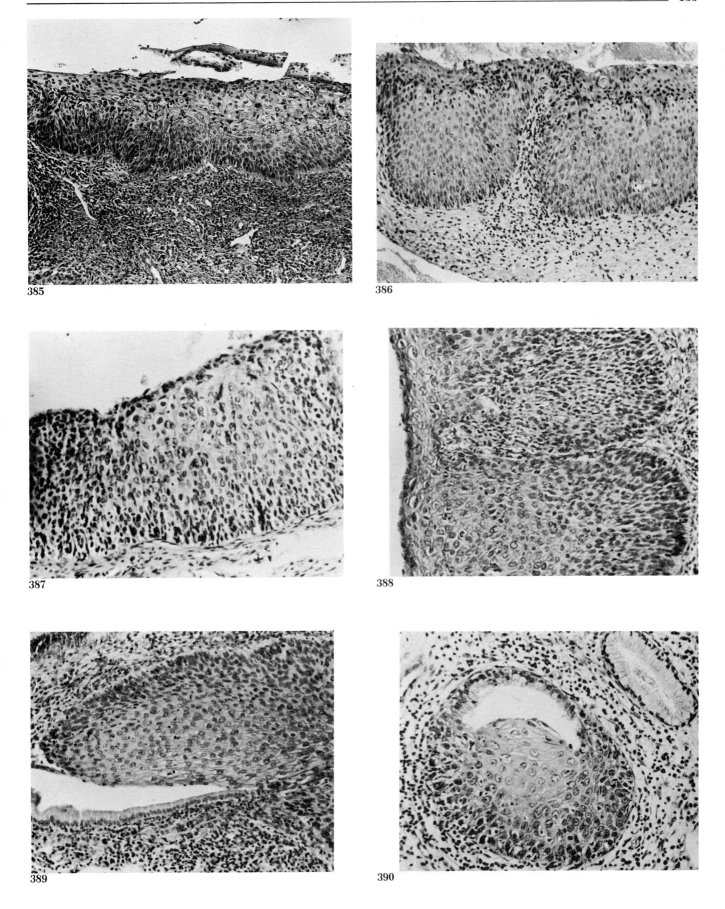

385

386

387

388

389

390

391 Intraepithelial carcinoma (carcinoma in situ) of the cervix

There is loss of stratification, cellular differentiation, and polarity. Nuclear hyperchromasia and mitotic figures are prominent. The lack of any cellular maturation is striking. The basement membrane is stretched but intact. This condition is known as *simple replacement*. (H&E. ×250)

392 Intraepithelial carcinoma (carcinoma in situ) of the cervix

The progressive numerical increase of malignant neoplastic cells results in an undulating basement membrane. This condition is known as *bulky outgrowth*. (H&E. ×100)

393 Intraepithelial carcinoma (carcinoma in situ) of the cervix

The neoplastic changes extend through the full thickness of the epithelium with a loss of cellular polarity and irreversible alterations of cellular characteristics. The cells are pleomorphic, and the nuclei are irregular, large, and hyperchromatic with frequent mitotic activity. The basement membrane is intact. The subepithelial inflammatory reactions vary. (H&E. ×150)

394 Intraepithelial carcinoma (carcinoma in situ) of the cervix

The characteristic changes of a malignant neoplasm are evident: loss of cellular polarity, abnormal mitoses, change in the cytoplasmic-nuclear ratio, and lack of any maturation. The basement membrane is intact. (H&E. ×150)

395 Intraepithelial carcinoma (carcinoma in situ) of the cervix

There is prominent variation in the size and shape of the cells and severe distortion of the architectural pattern. The basement membrane is intact. Exfoliation of neoplastic cells is evident. (H&E. ×150)

396 Intraepithelial carcinoma (carcinoma in situ) of the cervix

Marked intercellular edema and cellular pleomorphism is seen. There is infiltration of the underlying connective tissue and neoplastic epithelium by inflammatory cells. The basement membrane is intact. (H&E. ×280)

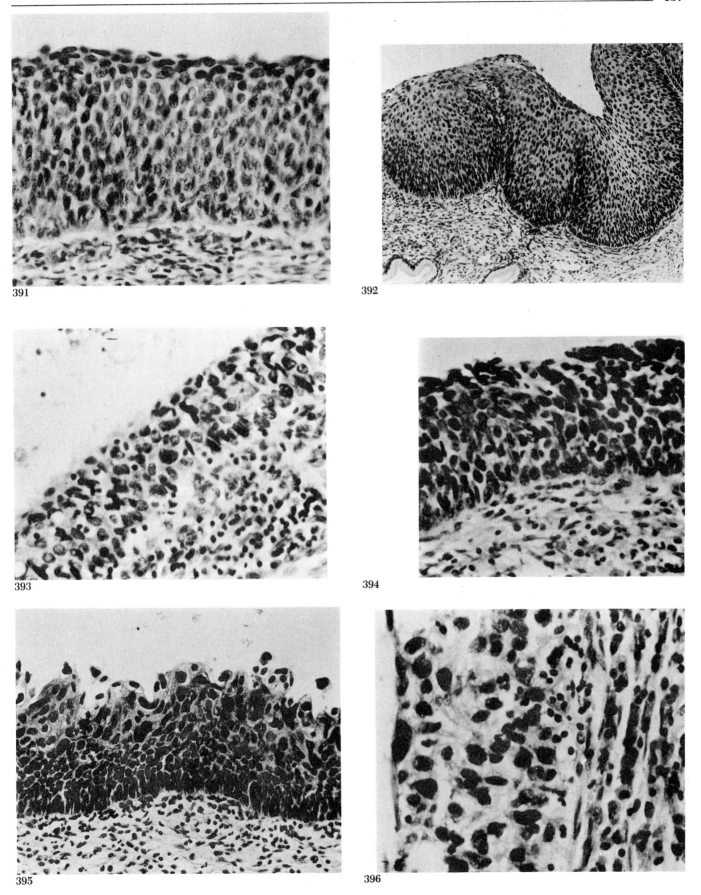

391

392

393

394

395

396

397 Intraepithelial carcinoma (carcinoma in situ) of the cervix

The tumor is formed by well differentiated cells with a tendency toward keratinization. The cellular atypism, pleomorphism, and nuclear hyperchromatism are striking. There is severe subepithelial inflammation. (H&E. ×100)

398 Intraepithelial carcinoma (carcinoma in situ) of the endocervix, with glandular involvement

The neoplastic cells are seen pushing their way into endocervical glands or crypts. (H&E. ×100)

399 Intraepithelial carcinoma (carcinoma in situ) of the endocervix, with massive glandular involvement

Although there may be extensive, if not complete, replacement of the glandular epithelium by neoplastic cells, there is still neither a break in the basement membrane nor frank invasion. (H&E. ×50)

400 Microcarcinoma or carcinoma of the cervix, with early stromal invasion, (Ia_1) stage of minimal invasion

The basement membrane has been disrupted, and the neoplastic cells appear to have invaded the underlying connective tissue. (H&E. ×130)

401 Microcarcinoma or carcinoma of the cervix with early stromal invasion, (Ia_1) stage of minimal invasion

The apparent invasion of the connective tissue stroma has not progressed beyond a depth of 3 mm from the basement membrane. (H&E. ×130)

402 Microcarcinoma or carcinoma of the cervix, with early stromal invasion, (Ia_1) stage of minimal invasion

Sectioning and examining of the entire specimen is mandatory if microcarcinomas are to be detected. (H&E. ×130)

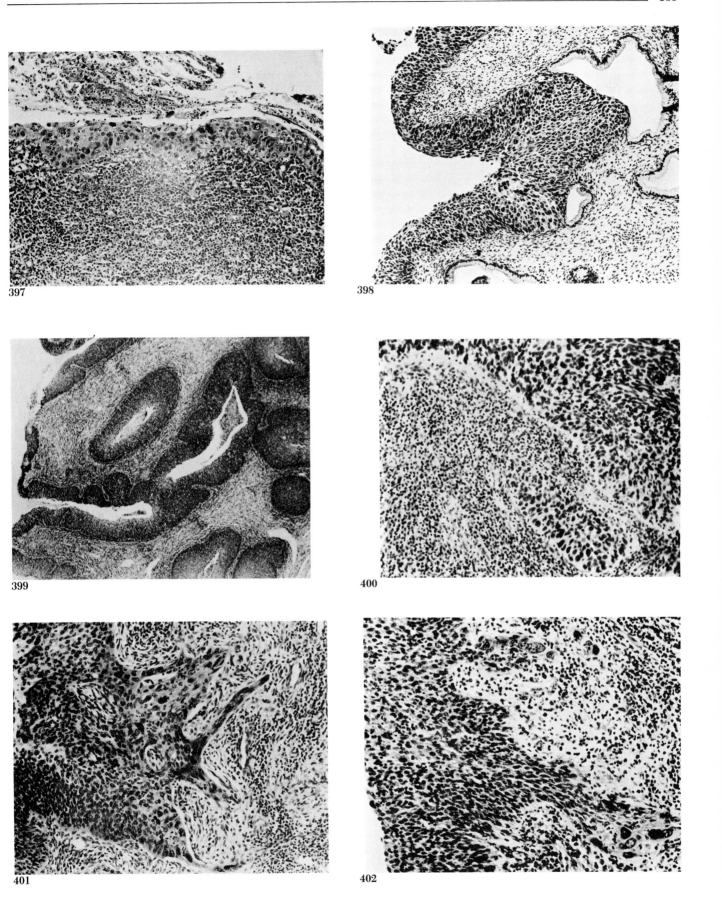

397

398

399

400

401

402

403   **Microcarcinoma or carcinoma of the cervix, with early stromal invasion, (Ia₁) stage of minimal invasion**
(H&E. ×180)

404   **Microcarcinoma or carcinoma of the cervix, with early stromal invasion, (Ia₂) stage of superficial invasion**
The basement membrane is disrupted, and the invasion of neoplastic cells extends at least 3 mm but not more than 5 mm from the basement membrane. (H&E. ×120)

405   **Microcarcinoma or carcinoma of the cervix, with early stromal invasion, (Ia₂) stage of superficial invasion**
Careful examination of lymphatic channels and venous sinusoids is mandatory in superficial microcarcinoma. If there is doubt of lymphatic involvement for clinical purposes, the tumor should be treated as unequivocally invasive. (H&E. ×100)

406   **Microcarcinoma or carcinoma of the cervix, with early stromal invasion, (Ia₂) stage of superficial invasion**
(H&E. ×60)

407   **Microcarcinoma or carcinoma of the cervix, with early stromal invasion, (Ia₂) stage of superficial invasion**
There is superficial infiltration of cervical connective tissue stroma by neoplastic islands. The infiltration extends 5 mm below the basement membrane. (H&E. ×50)

408   **Invasive squamous cell carcinoma of the cervix**
There is infiltration of the entire field (measuring 6 mm in diameter) by islands of neoplastic epithelial cells. This tumor is clinically classified as Ia. (H&E. ×50)

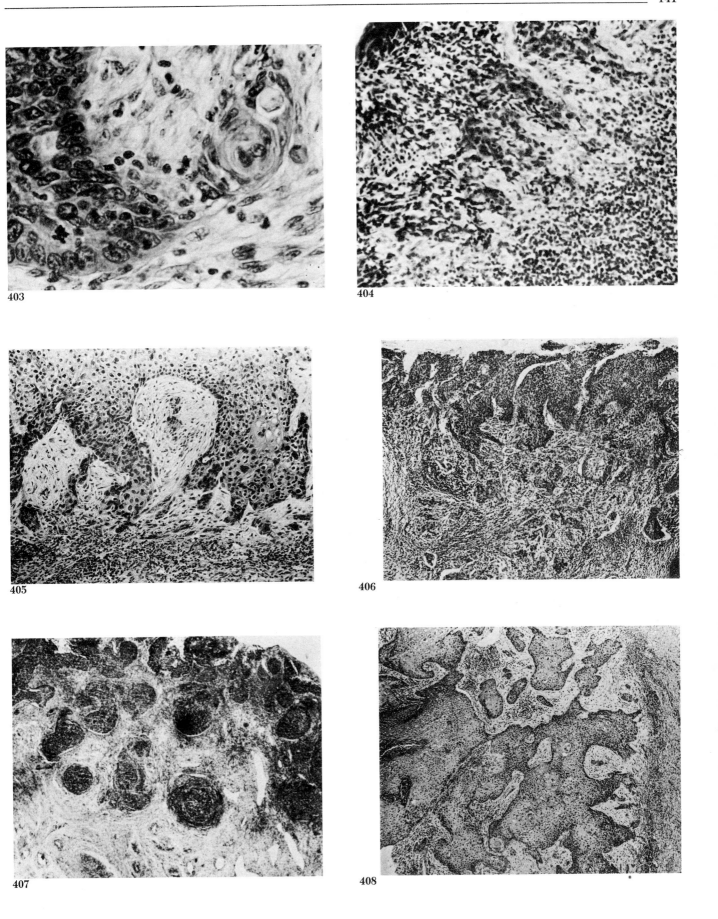

403

404

405

406

407

408

409 Invasive squamous cell carcinoma of the cervix
A typical invasive carcinoma of the cervix with plexiform masses is seen. (H&E. ×50)

410 Poorly differentiated squamous cell carcinoma of the cervix
(H&E. ×120)

411 Anaplastic carcinoma of the cervix
This tumor is of the undifferentiated or unripe cell variety. (H&E. ×180)

412 Anaplastic carcinoma of the cervix
This highly undifferentiated cervical carcinoma has a sarcoma-like appearance. (H&E. ×280)

413 Anaplastic carcinoma of the cervix
This undifferentiated cervical carcinoma shows bizarre cells and mitoses. (H&E. ×340)

414 Poorly differentiated scirrhous carcinoma of the cervix
These poorly differentiated squamous carcinoma cells show a marked desmoplastic reaction of connective tissue stroma. (H&E. ×120)

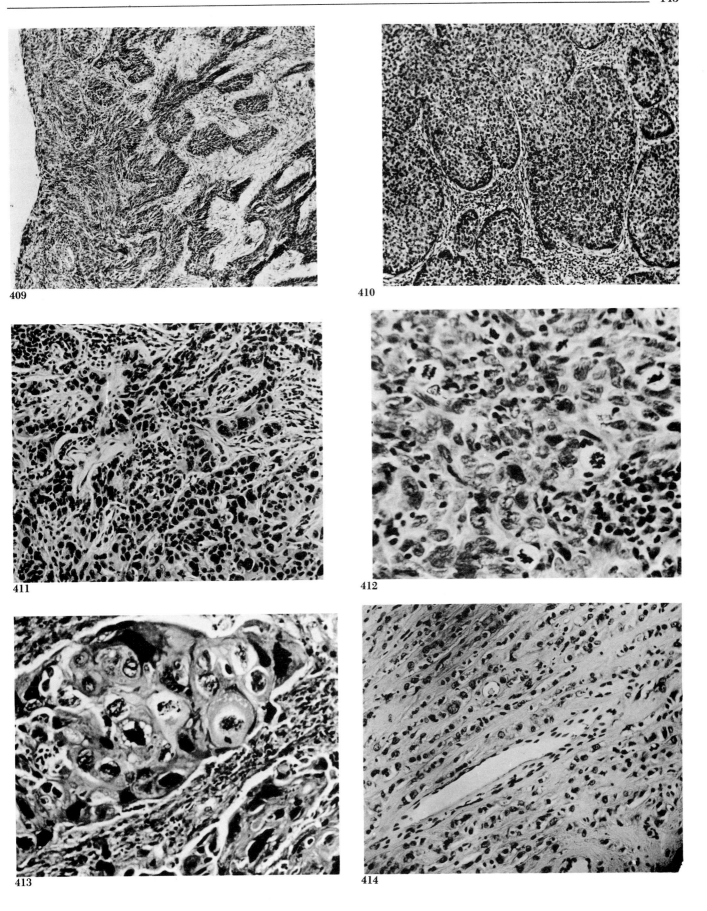

409

410

411

412

413

414

415 Occult, invasive, carcinoma of the cervix
Note intact overlying squamous epithelium and islands of squamous cell carcinoma invading cervical stroma. (H&E. ×20)

416 Squamous carcinoma developing in the endocervical canal
This tumor is sometimes difficult to detect and occasionally is an incidental finding in a hysterectomy specimen. (H&E. ×5)

417 Papillary adenocarcinoma of the endocervix
This is a general view of a papillary endocervical carcinoma. (H&E. ×5)

418 Well-differentiated adenocarcinoma of the endocervix
Note the neoplastic proliferation and stromal invasion by well formed glandular structures. There is slight to moderate cellular atypism. The neoplastic epithelial cells are mucin-producing. (H&E. ×180)

419 Well-differentiated adenocarcinoma of the endocervix
There is moderate irregularity of the endocervical glands. The epithelial cells lining the glands show atypism and are mucin-producing. Sometimes in well-differentiated tumors, the diagnosis of carcinoma is difficult. (H&E. ×140)

420 Moderately well differentiated adenocarcinoma of the endocervix
The glandular character of the tumor is partly preserved. Mucinous material is secreted by the neoplastic cells. (H&E. ×250)

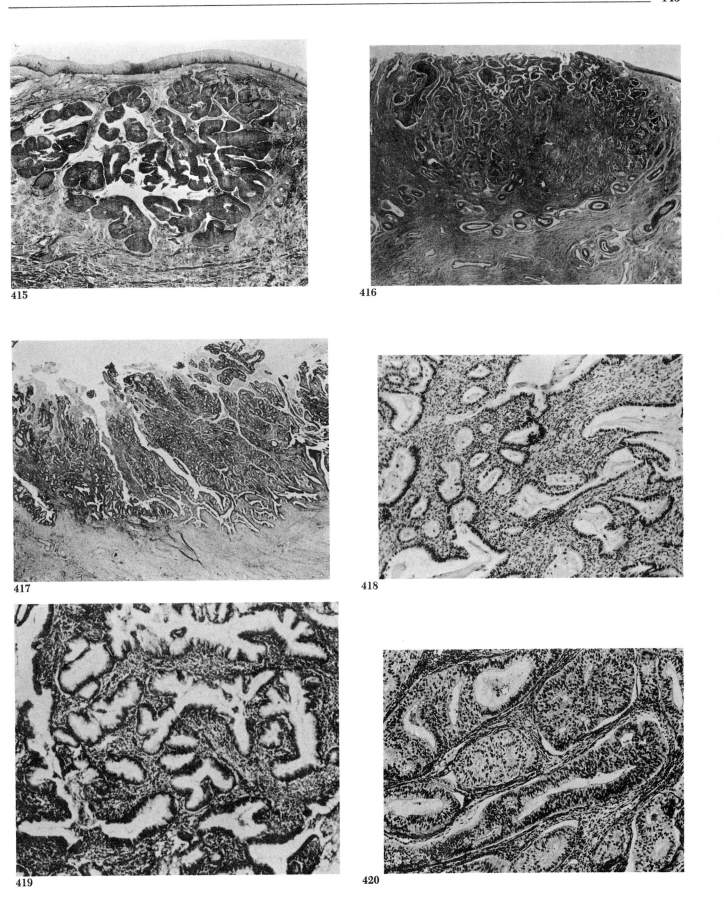

415

416

417

418

419

420

421 Papillary adenocarcinoma of the endo-cervix
This tumor is formed by papillary structures with piling of highly anaplastic epithelial cells. (H&E. ×250)

422 Papillary adenocarcinoma of the endo-cervix
High magnification of Fig. 421. Note the papillary fold with the thin stromal core and stratified round to elongated neoplastic cells. (H&E. ×320)

423 Papillary adenocarcinoma of the endo-cervix
Some of the cells lining papillary projections maintain their mucus-secreting property. (H&E. ×320)

424 Poorly differentiated adenocarcinoma of the endocervix
The pleomorphic cells with irregular shaped nuclei form abortive glandular structures. (H&E. ×280)

425 Adenoacanthoma of the endocervix
This tumor is formed by glandular structures which are interspersed with and partly lined by strands of neoplastic squamous epithelium. Not to be misconstrued as collision tumor. (H&E. ×80)

426 Adenocystic carcinoma of the endocervix
This tumor is formed by sheets of cuboidal cells and cystlike structures. (H&E. ×80)

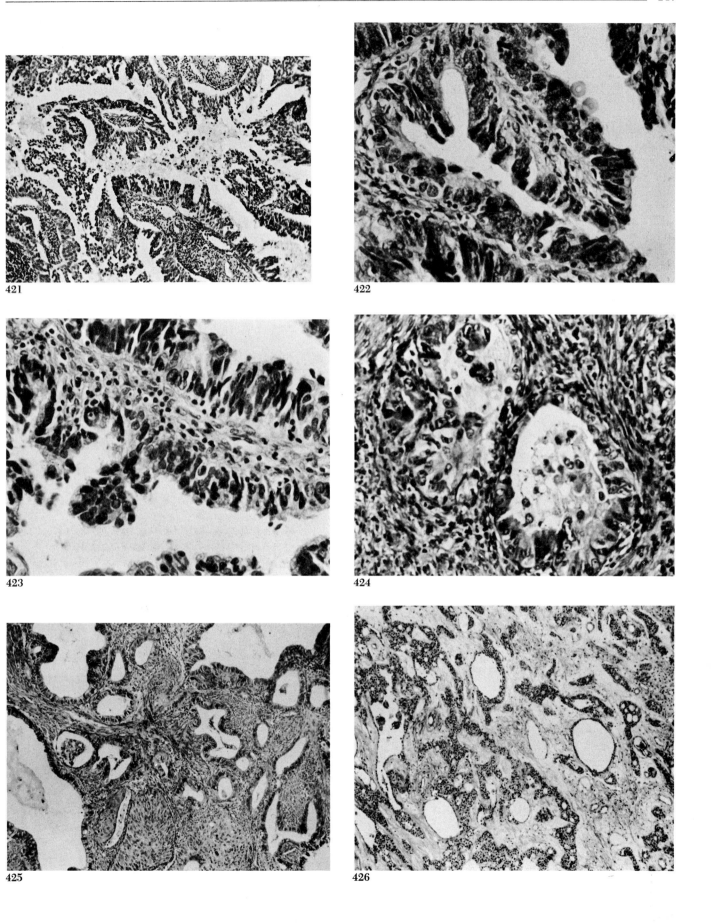

421

422

423

424

425

426

427 Adenocystic carcinoma of the endocervix
High magnification of Fig. 426. There are islands of cuboidal cells with formation of microcysts. Mucin is detected in some of the cells. (H&E. ×180)

428 Adenocystic carcinoma of the endocervix
High magnification of Fig. 427. Microcyst formation is seen. Cuboidal epithelial cells show ovoid hyperchromatic nuclei and cytoplasmic vacuolization. Mucinous material is present in the cuboidal cells. (H&E. ×340)

429 Cylindromatous adenocarcinoma of the endocervix
This tumor is composed of small nests and strands of neoplastic, highly basophilic cells. Microcysts are noted in some of the epithelial islands. (H&E. ×40)

430 Cylindromatous adenocarcinoma of the endocervix
High magnification of Fig. 429. Within the microcysts, mucin is detected. Although mitotic figures are rare and the tumor appears rather benign, metastases are frequent. (H&E. ×80)

431 Cylindromatous adenocarcinoma of the endocervix
High magnification of Fig. 430. Compact islands of basophilic cells with multiple mucin-containing microcyst formations are seen. (H&E. ×150)

432 Gelatinous carcinoma of the endocervix
This is a highly undifferentiated carcinoma of endocervical glands. There is diffuse arrangement of mucin-producing neoplastic epithelial cells. (H&E. ×200)

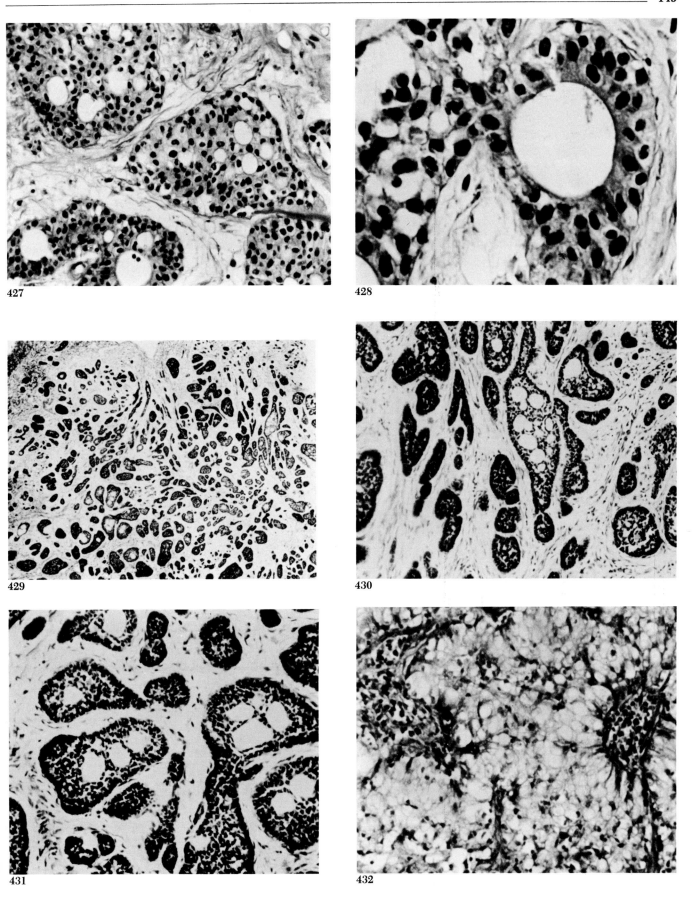

427

428

429

430

431

432

433   Gelatinous carcinoma of the endocervix
This highly anaplastic endocervical carcinoma is composed of large, mucin-containing cells. Because of degeneration of the neoplastic cells, the mucin may be liberated and can be detected free in connective tissue stroma. (H&E. ×180)

434   Lymphatic spread of squamous cell carcinoma of the cervix
Distant metastases occur late in the disease process. In adenocarcinoma of the endocervix, metastases occur early. (H&E. ×200)

435   Carcinosarcoma of the cervix
This tumor is formed by islands of squamous cell carcinoma and sarcomatous connective tissue stroma. There is intimate admixture of the two tumors. (H&E. ×80)

436   Sarcoma botryoides of the cervix
Intact squamous epithelium overlies the edematous cellular tumor of the exocervix. (H&E. ×10)

437   Sarcoma botryoides of the cervix
High magnification of Fig. 436. Densely cellular and highly pleomorphic tumor areas are contrasted with areas that are sparse in cells. (H&E. ×80)

438   Sarcoma botryoides of the cervix
The tumor is formed by clusters of elongated, partly irregular cells of embryonic mesodermal type. The surrounding stroma is myxomatous. (H&E. ×280)

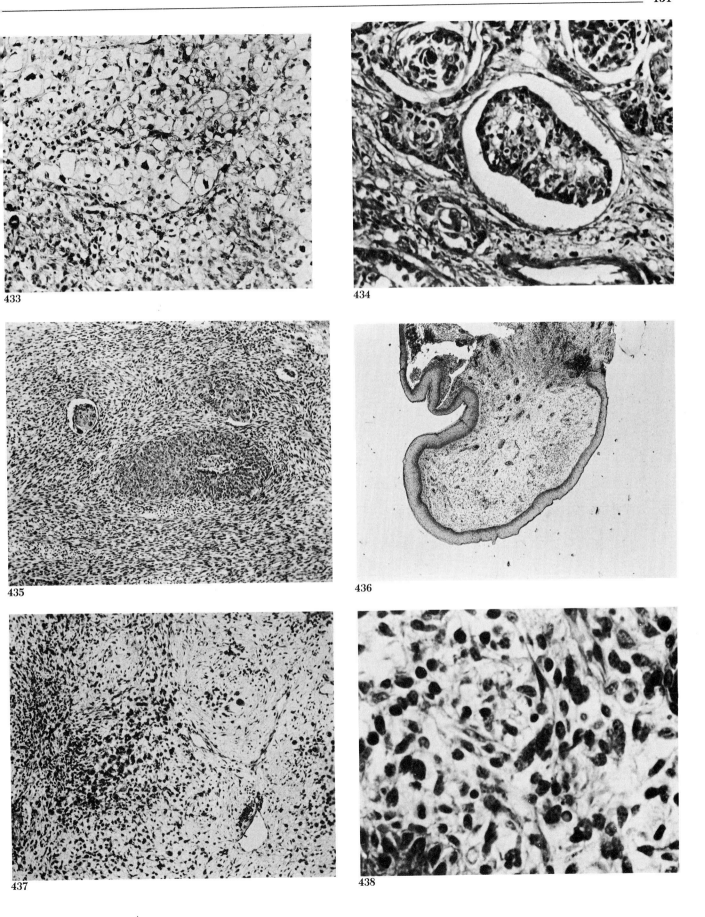

433

434

435

436

437

438

439   Sarcoma botryoides of the cervix
Neoplastic muscle cells with cross striations are seen in myxomatous stroma. (H&E. ×350) AFIP Acc #233038

440   Sarcoma botryoides of the cervix
The tumor is formed by elongated cells with spindle nuclei. The eosinophilic cytoplasm is fairly prominent in these cells. They are identified as myoblasts. Cross striation is not seen in these cells. (H&E. ×350)

441   Choriocarcinoma of the uterus, metastatic to the cervix
There is cervical stromal invasion by choriocarcinoma. This is either by direct extension or by metastatic deposit. (H&E. ×100)

442   Malignant   lymphoma   (lymphoblastic lymphosarcoma) of the cervix
The tumor is composed of round cells of uniform size which are seen diffusely infiltrating the connective tissue stroma of the cervix. Differentiation from lymphatic leukemia may be difficult. (H&E. ×180)

443   Hodgkin's disease of the cervix
The tumor is composed of many cell types including lymphocytes, neutrophils, eosinophils, plasma cells, reticulum cells, fibroblasts, and Reed-Sternberg giant cells. There is massive infiltration of the cervix by tumor cells. (H&E. ×100)

444   Chronic   lymphocytic   leukemia   of   the cervix
Marked infiltration of the cervical connective tissue stroma by lymphocytic aggregates is present. (H&E. ×200)

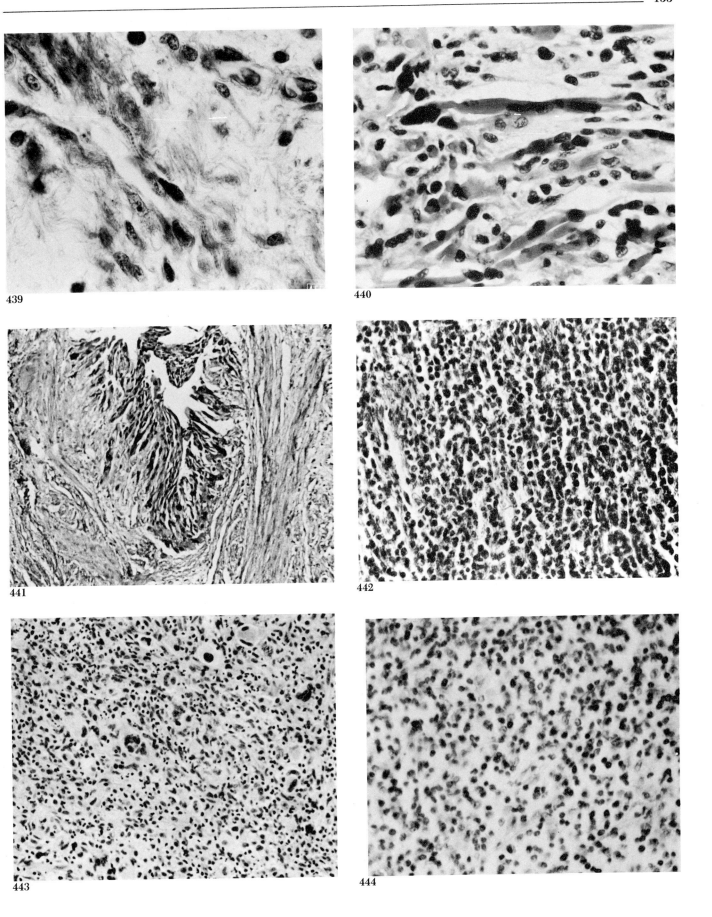

439

440

441

442

443

444

445   Granulocytic leukemia of the cervix
The cervical connective tissue stroma is diffusely infiltrated with relatively large granulocytes and neutrophilic myelocytes. (H&E. ×200)

446   Preradiation invasive squamous cell carcinoma of the cervix
This biopsy specimen shows invasive squamous cell carcinoma before radiation. (H&E. ×120)

447   Invasive squamous cell carcinoma 2 weeks after radiation of the cervix
This patient received 1,000 r by external radiation prior to biopsy. There is arrest of mitotic activity. The nuclei are large and show marked hyperchromatism. Some of the nuclei show pyknosis. There is an overall increase in the size of the tumor cells. (H&E. ×120)

448   Invasive squamous cell carcinoma 4 weeks after radiation of the cervix
This patient received 3,000 r by external radiation prior to biopsy. Note the severe cellular degeneration and disintegration. There is marked vacuolar degeneration of individual neoplastic cells and progressive cytolysis. (H&E. ×120)

449   Pseudosarcomatous changes in the cervix following irradiation
A biopsy was taken 9 months after completion of internal and external radiotherapy for a stage I squamous cell carcinoma of the cervix. The estimated total dose to point A was 9,300 r. Note the marked proliferation of cervical connective tissue cells with cellular elongation, nuclear hyperchromatism, and increased deposition of collagen. (H&E. ×100)

450   Pseudosarcomatous changes in the cervix following irradiation
The alarmingly irregular cellular pattern and disorientation of the cells is characteristic of post-irradiation pseudosarcoma of the cervix. Mitotic figures are infrequent or absent. (H&E. ×250)

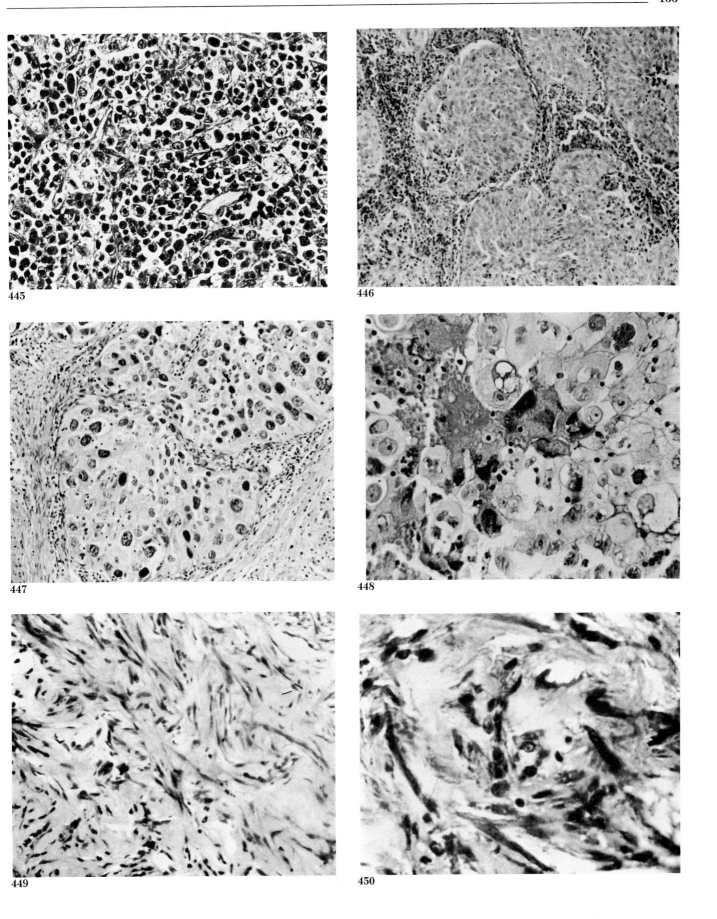

445

446

447

448

449

450

COLOR PLATES
Chapter 3
Diseases of the Cervix Uteri
Plates 5, 6

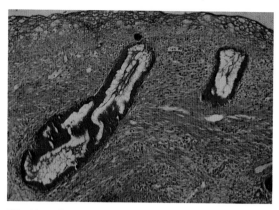

25 Normal exocervix and endocervix in a woman of reproductive age Neutral mucopolysaccharides are distributed in endocervical epithelial cells. (PAS stain. ×90)

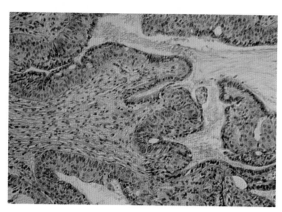

26 Squamous metaplasia of the endocervix in an infant Squamous metaplasia is seen in the endocervix of an infant. (H&E. ×100)

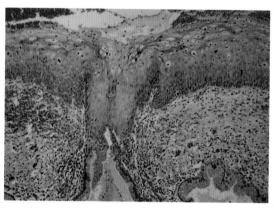

27 Epidermization of the endocervix An erosion is healing by a process of covering or of becoming covered with exocervical squamous epithelium. Epidermization should be differentiated from squamous metaplasia or epidermidalization. (H&E. ×75)

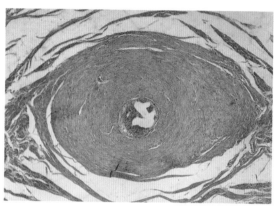

28 Gartner's duct of the cervix (H&E. ×55)

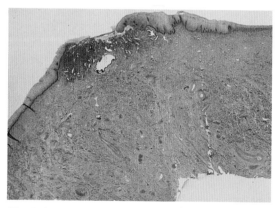

29 Endometriosis of the exocervix Note the eroded exocervix. The underlying connective tissue contains endometrial glands and dense endometrial stromal cells. Some of the endometrial glands are cystic. (H&E. ×24)

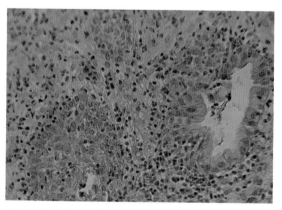

30 Eosinophilia of the endocervix There is marked infiltration of the cervical connective tissue stroma by eosinophilic leukocytes. The possibility that the presence of eosinophilia in tissue represents a local allergic response, although highly selective, to breakdown of tissue due to neoplasia, bacterial inflammation, or previous surgical procedure should be taken into consideration. (H&E. ×100)

Plate 5

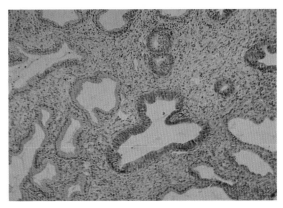

31 Adenomatous hyperplasia of the endocervix The isolated endocervical glands show hyperplasia of the lining epithelium. (H&E. ×75)

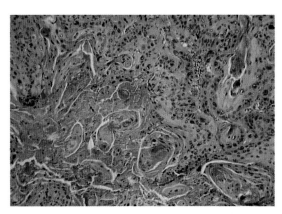

32 Keratinizing squamous cell carcinoma of the cervix This well-differentiated invasive squamous cell carcinoma of the cervix shows massive keratinization and formation of horn pearls. (H&E. ×75)

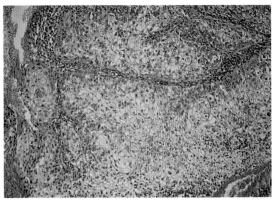

33 Clear cell carcinoma of the cervix This so-called clear cell carcinoma of the cervix represents a form of relatively poorly differentiated squamous cell carcinoma with irregular cells, pale-staining cytoplasm, and large hyperchromatic nuclei. (H&E. ×133)

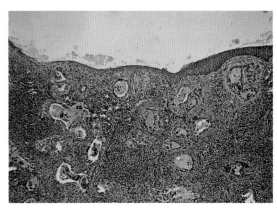

34 Poorly differentiated adenocarcinoma of the endocervix Invasion of endocervical stroma by numerous abortive glandular structures is seen. Heaps of atypical, sometimes mucin-producing, neoplastic cells line the glands. (H&E. ×62)

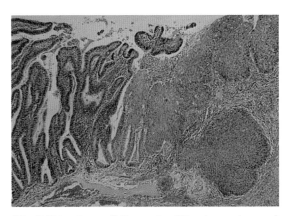

35 Collision tumor of the cervix This adenocarcinoma of the endocervix is colliding with a squamous cell carcinoma of the exocervix. Two independent cancers are arising in adjacent tissue of the same organ and invading each other. Not to be confused with adenoacanthoma of the endocervix. (H&E. ×70)

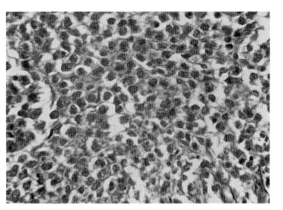

36 Reticulum cell sarcoma of the cervix The connective tissue stroma is diffusely infiltrated with large reticulum cells. They show pleomorphic nuclei and accentuated nucleoli. (H&E. ×450)

Plate 6

4

Diseases of the Endometrium

451   Endometrial cavity of a 2-month-old infant
This longitudinal section through the uterus of a 2-month-old infant shows a relatively thin, undeveloped mucosa with endometrial glands developing from clefts extending downward from the surface. (H&E. ×11)

452   Endometrium of a 2-month-old infant
High magnification of Fig. 451. The endometrium of a 2-month-old infant shows a relatively poorly developed endometrial gland with subnuclear vacuolation. (H&E. ×155)

453   Cross section of the uterus of a 7-year-old child
The cross section through the uterus of a 7-year-old child shows a well-developed cavum uteri lined by a thin mucosa. The myometrium is relatively thick. (H&E. ×6)

454   Endometrium of a 7-year-old child
High magnification of Fig. 453. The endometrium of a 7-year-old child shows somewhat complex endometrial glands. However, there is no evidence of secretory activity. (H&E. ×50)

455   Prepubertal endometrium at 14 years of age
The endometrial glands show active proliferation, and the stroma is quite cellular. (H&E. ×125)

456   Early proliferative endometrium (5th to 7th day of the cycle)
The surface epithelium is thin and delicate. The glands are sparse and straight. (H&E. ×30)

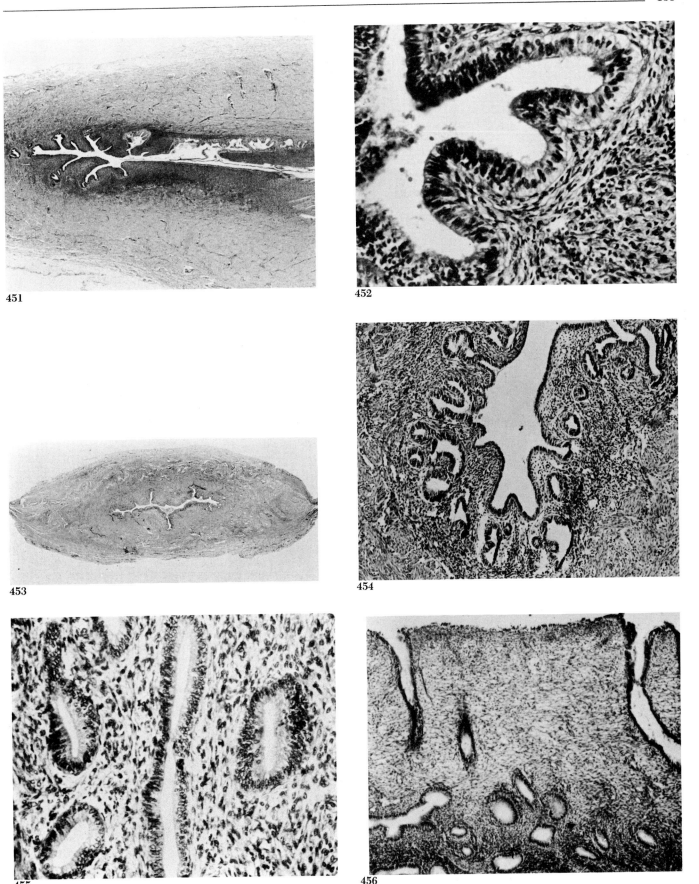

451

452

453

454

455

456

457 Early proliferative endometrium (5th to 7th day of the cycle)
High magnification of Fig. 456.

458 Midproliferative endometrium (8th to 12th day of the cycle)
The endometrium in the proliferative (estrogenic) phase of the menstrual cycle shows tubular glands with abundant mitoses embedded in a compact, cellular stroma. (H&E. ×125)

459 Midproliferative endometrium (8th to 12th day of the cycle)
High magnification of Fig. 458. Dense stroma and many glandular mitoses are seen. (H&E. ×200)

460 Late proliferative endometrium (13th to 14th day of the cycle)
The dense stroma shows tortuous glands lined by pseudostratified epithelial cells. (H&E. ×130)

461 Late proliferative endometrium (13th to 15th day of the cycle)
The endometrial glands are lined by columnar epithelium. The term proliferative endometrium is used from cessation of menstruation to the time of ovulation. Details of the endometrial glands are shown. (H&E. ×150)

462 Secretory endometrium, 16th day (2d postovulatory day)
Note the glandular coiling and relatively dense stroma. (H&E. ×30)

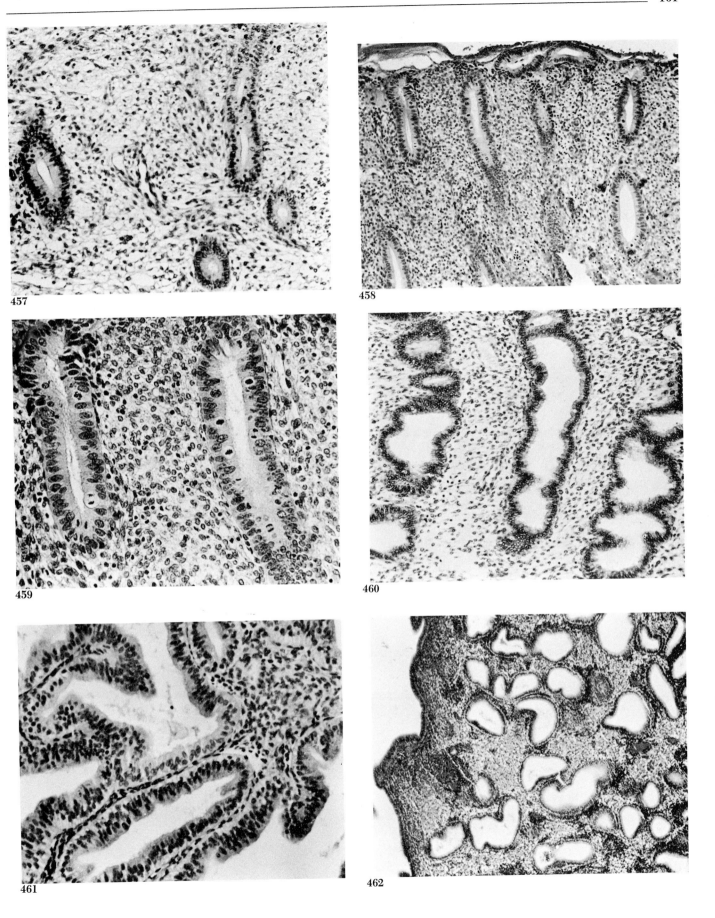

457

458

459

460

461

462

463   Secretory endometrium, 16th day (2d post-ovulatory day)

High magnification of Fig. 462. The earliest secretory phase change is subnuclear vacuolation in glandular epithelium. There are no more glandular mitoses. (H&E. ×150)

464   Secretory endometrium, 18th day (4th postovulatory day)

The subnuclear vacuoles are larger, and the nuclei of the glandular epithelium are pushed up to midcell position. The stroma shows early edema. (H&E. ×30)

465   Secretory endometrium, 18th day (4th post-ovulatory day)

High magnification of Fig. 464. There is palisading of subnuclear vacuoles and nuclei as well as increased tortuosity of the glandular contour. (H&E. ×135)

466   Secretory endometrium, 20th day (6th post-ovulatory day)

The products of secretion have been partly extruded into the glandular lumens, and there is a pronounced degree of stromal edema. (H&E. ×80)

467   Secretory endometrium, 20th day (6th post-ovulatory day)

High magnification of Fig. 466. Secretion having been discharged, the gland nuclei have returned to the basal position. There is no increase in the cytoplasm of stromal cells. (H&E. ×150)

468   Secretory endometrium, 22d day (8th postovulatory day)

The glandular lumens contain products of secretion. Stromal edema has receded. (H&E. ×62)

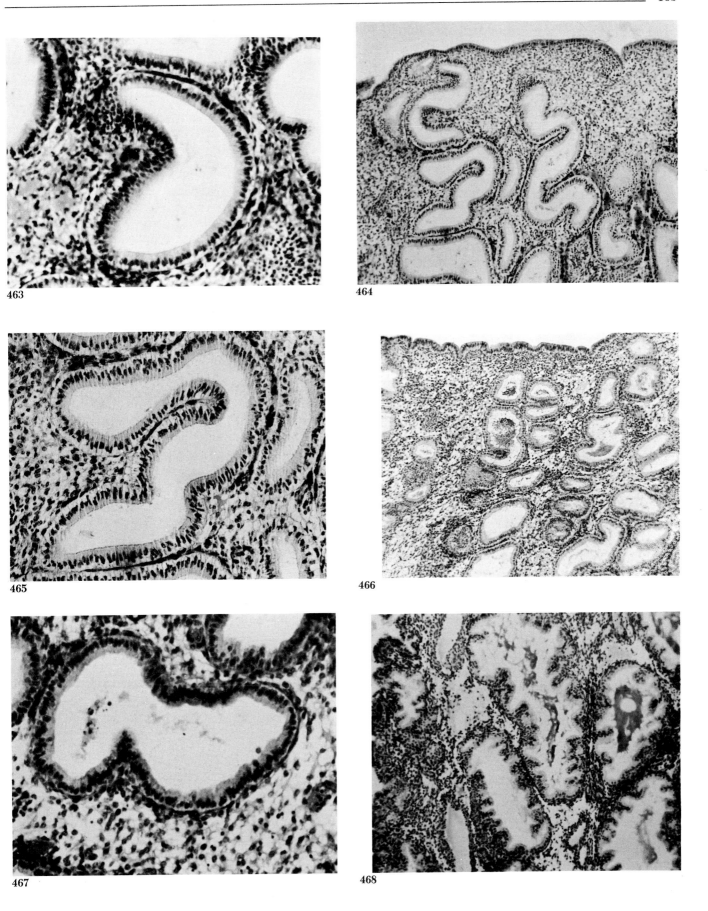

463

464

465

466

467

468

469   Secretory endometrium, 22d day (8th post-ovulatory day)
High magnification of Fig. 468. There are margins of glands with regression of secretory activity. Spiral arterioles are just beginning to develop. (H&E. ×180)

470   Secretory endometrium, 24th day (10th postovulatory day)
The appearance of the glands is not essentially different from that seen on the twentieth to twenty-second day, but spiral arterioles have developed and are surrounded by condensation of predecidually transformed stromal cells. (H&E. ×30)

471   Secretory endometrium, 24th day (10th postovulatory day)
High magnification of Fig. 470. There is regression of glandular secretion and increase of cytoplasm in the cells surrounding the spiral arterioles. (H&E. ×125)

472   Secretory endometrium, 26th day (12th postovulatory day)
Regression of secretion in the dentate glands is accompanied by a diffuse predecidual stromal reaction extending outward from spiral arterioles and becoming confluent. (H&E. ×90)

473   Secretory endometrium, 26th day (12th postovulatory day)
High magnification of Fig. 472. There is almost complete exhaustion of glandular activity. Note the relative size of the predecidual stromal cells. (H&E. ×200)

474   Secretory endometrium, 27th day (13th postovulatory day)
The predecidual reaction fills the interglandular spaces in the superficial layer of the mucosa, and leukocytic infiltration presages the onset of menstrual dissolution. (H&E. ×35)

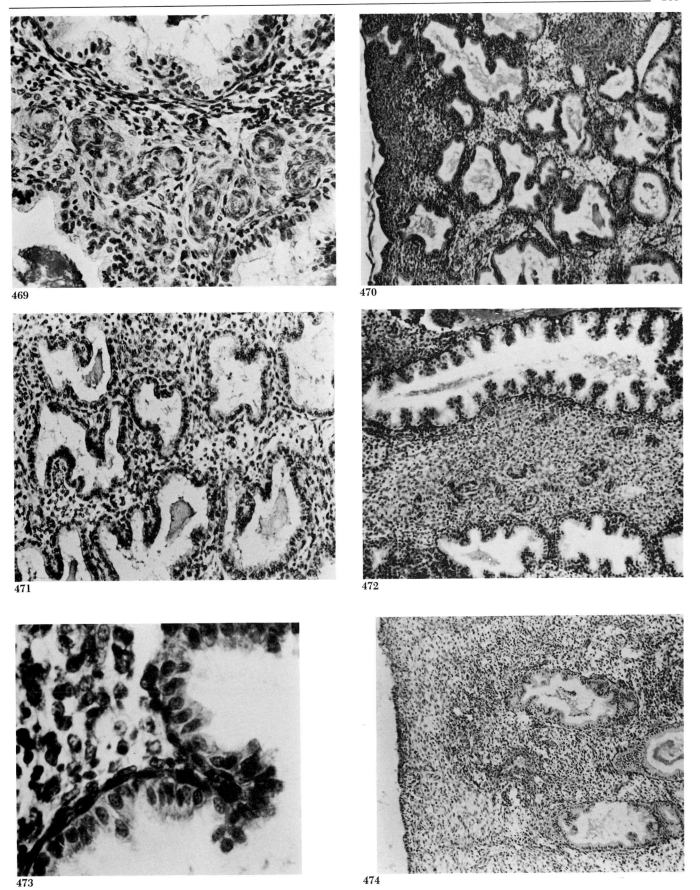

469

470

471

472

473

474

475 Menstrual endometrium, established
The stroma has undergone dissolution and is largely replaced by polymorphonuclear leukocytes. The persistence of glandular vacuolation is a minor abnormality. (H&E. ×125)

476 Menstrual endometrium with fibrin thrombi
(H&E. ×50)

477 Early menstrual endometrium (1st day of the cycle)
Deposition of fibrin in a focus of stromal lysis is shown. (H&E. ×125)

478 Menstrual endometrium (2d day of the cycle)
Note the advanced stromal and glandular dissolution. Curettings. (H&E. ×60)

479 Menstrual endometrium (3d to 4th day of the cycle)
There is advanced endometrial dissolution with marked cellular debris. Curettings. (H&E. ×50)

480 Differential behavioral pattern of superficial and glandular secretory endometrium
Secretory endometrium, on the twenty-second day of cycle, shows products of secretion in the glandular lumens and recession of gland nuclei to a basal level. The surface epithelium, especially on the left, shows a subnuclear clear zone and nuclei at the midcell position. (H&E. ×125)

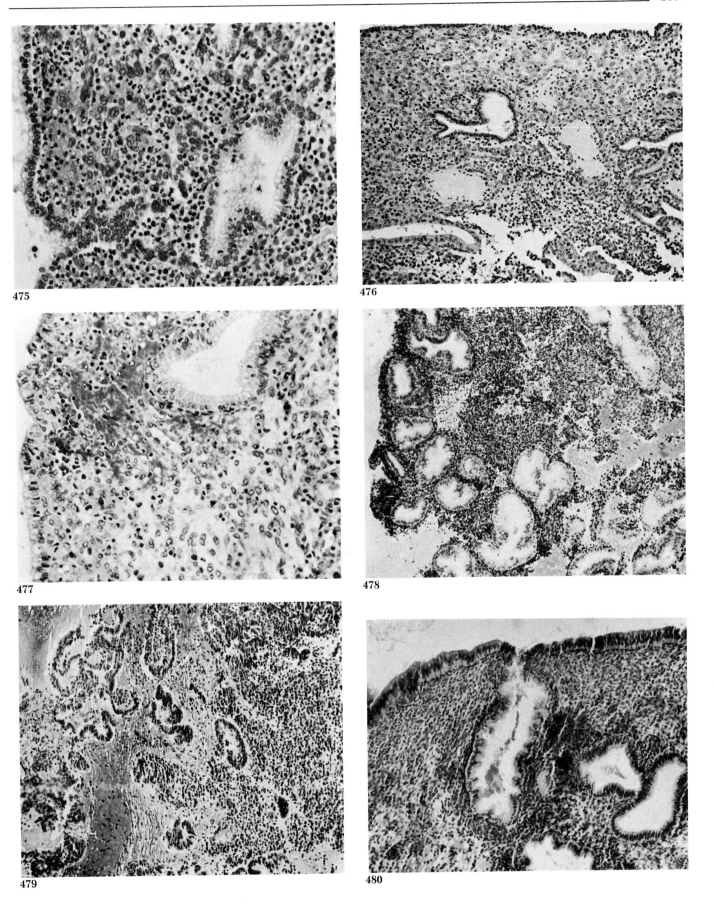

475

476

477

478

479

480

481 Differential behavioral pattern of super-ficial and glandular secretory endometrium
High magnification of Fig. 480. The surface epithelial cells are almost twice as tall as the glandular epithelial cells. Detail of the clear subnuclear zone and the intact brush border is also shown. In general, the surface epithelium lags behind the glandular epithelium as a target for steroid hormones. (H&E. ×600)

482 Isolated clear cells in the endometrial gland ("helle Zellen," Feyrter)
Isolated clear cells are seen in endometrial glands. They are ovoid, with clear cytoplasm and round prominent nuclei. They may appear in normal, hyperplastic, or neoplastic epithelium. The origin of these cells is undetermined, although the possibility of tubal epithelial metaplasia has been considered. (H&E. ×250)

483 Senile atrophy of the endometrium
The endometrium shows a thin mucosa with small tubular glands in compact, cellular stroma. (H&E. ×60)

484 Senile atrophy of the endometrium
High magnification of Fig. 483. Note the inert glands and inert stroma. (H&E. ×125)

485 Senile atrophy of the endometrium with cystic glandular dilatation
The mucosa contains small tubular glands as well as cystically dilated glands lined by a flat epithelium and containing inspissated secretion. (H&E. ×60)

486 Regenerating endometrium 4 days after curettage
Young, poorly developed endometrial glands are seen in loose fibroblastic stroma. (H&E. ×40)

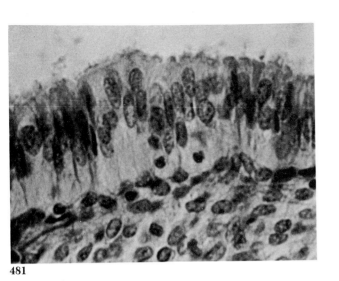

481

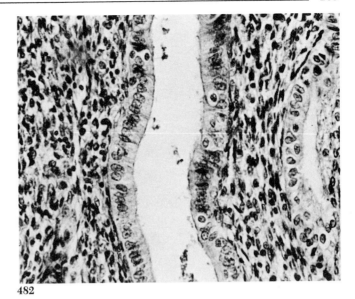

482

483

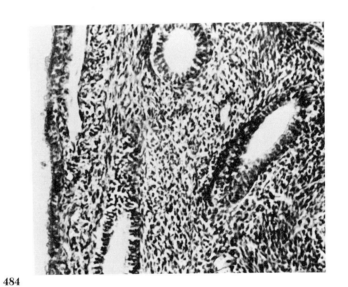

484

485

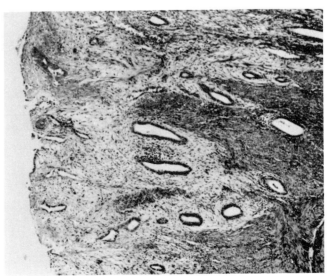

486

487 Regenerating endometrium 4 days after curettage

High magnification of Fig. 486. Irregular, immature glandular nuclei, fibroblastic stroma, and a thrombosed arteriole are visible. (H&E. ×125)

488 Cervical squamous cell epithelium in endometrial curettings

Uterine curettings show an admixture of endometrium and detached fragments of exocervix. This represents an artefact of the mechanics of curettage and is not to be misconstrued as squamous metaplasia or carcinoma. (H&E. ×50)

489 Endometrial curettings simulating adenocarcinoma

Endometrial curettings show degenerative, autolytic, and shrinkage changes due to delay in fixation and poor fixation. Such changes can be misinterpreted as endometrial adenocarcinoma. (H&E. ×200)

490 Menstrual endometrium simulating carcinoma of the endometrium

Menstrual endometrium is frequently misdiagnosed as endometrial carcinoma by beginners. (H&E. ×125)

491 Curettings of edematous and compressed menstrual endometrium

These findings are sometimes mistaken for neoplasm. (H&E. ×180)

492 Invagination and pseudopapillary formation, an artefact of curettings

So-called invagination of endometrial glands is seen as an artefact of endometrial tissue produced by dehydration, poor and inadequate fixation. (H&E. ×50)

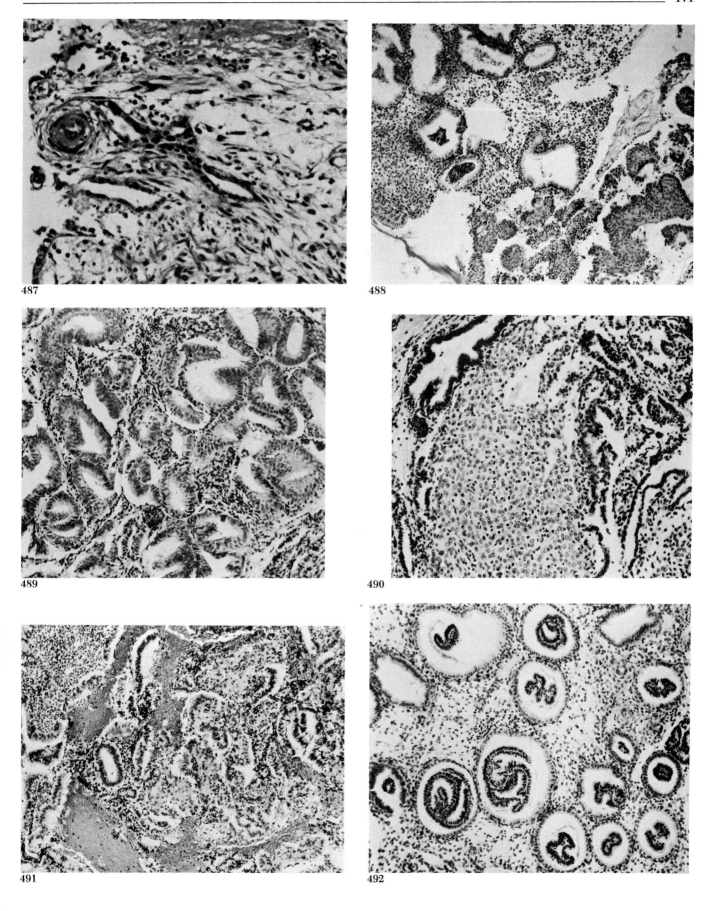

487

488

489

490

491

492

493 Invagination and pseudopapillary formation, an artefact of endometrial curettings
High magnification of Fig. 492. Pseudointraglandular papillomatosis is seen as an artefact of an improper handling of endometrial curetting material. (H&E. ×155)

494 Membranous dysmenorrhea
Tissue resembling an endometrial cast is passed showing focal necrosis, degenerated secretory endometrial glands, areas of hemorrhage, and mild inflammatory infiltration. (H&E. ×40)

495 Edema of endometrial stroma in fibro-congestive syndrome – Taylor (metropathia uteri)
The mucosa is twice the normal thickness because of excessive edema, but the glands, stroma, and vasculature seem normal. (H&E. ×29)

496 Secretory endometrium in an inadequate biphasic cycle (inadequate secretory endometrium)
Patient with eighteen- to twenty-day cycle. Curettage was done on the first day of menstrual flow. The endometrial glands and stroma correspond to the sixteen- to seventeen-day normal endometrium. The progestational phase is poorly developed. (H&E. ×120)

497 Delayed desquamation of secretory endometrium
This patient had excessive and prolonged menstrual type of bleeding. (A) Biopsy taken on the first day of menstrual flow. Note the secretory endometrium with early dissolution. (B) Biopsy taken on the fifth day. Note the persistence of secretory endometrium with progressive dissolution. *There is no evidence of endometrial regeneration.* A possible cause for delayed desquamation is persistence of the corpus luteum. (H&E. ×150)

498 Premenopausal endometrium (inadequately stimulated endometrium)
The cystic gland is lined by cuboidal nonsecreting epithelium. The surrounding endometrial glands show secretory changes corresponding to the twenty-second to twenty-fourth day of the cycle. (H&E. ×150)

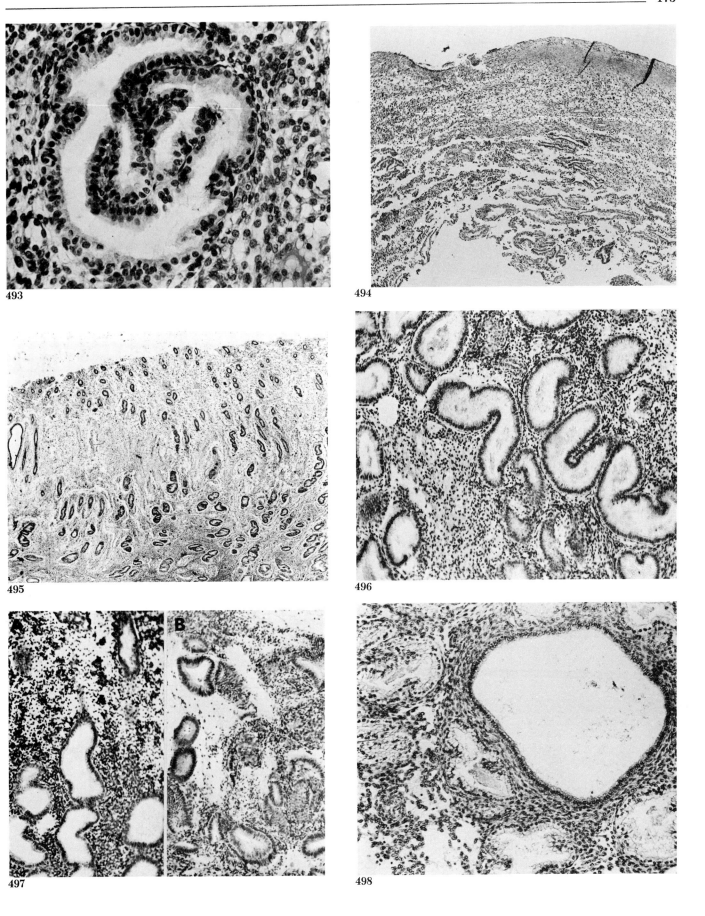

493

494

495

496

497

498

499 Anovulatory endometrium
The endometrial glands are small and in the proliferative phase. The endometrial stroma is edematous and shows early dissolution. These curettings were taken on the first day of menstrual flow in a patient with a monophasic temperature curve. (H&E. ×62)

500 Anovulatory endometrium
This endometrial biopsy was taken on the third day of the menstrual flow in a patient with a twenty-eight-day cycle. The fragments of proliferative endometrium show areas of dissolution. (H&E. ×180)

501 Hypoplasia of the endometrium
This endometrial biopsy specimen was taken from a patient with secondary amenorrhea. Such moderately well-developed proliferative endometrium is also observed in a subthreshold cycle. (H&E. ×150)

502 Atrophy of the endometrium
This endometrial biopsy specimen was taken from a patient with secondary amenorrhea. A poorly developed proliferative endometrium is seen. (H&E. ×150)

503 Atrophy of the endometrium in Sheehan's syndrome
These curettings of endometrium were taken 1 year post partum. The glands are sparsely distributed and inert. The stroma is thin and fibroblastic in character. (H&E. ×125)

504 Cystic glandular hyperplasia of the endometrium from a patient with granulosa—theca cell tumor of the ovary
(H&E. ×90)

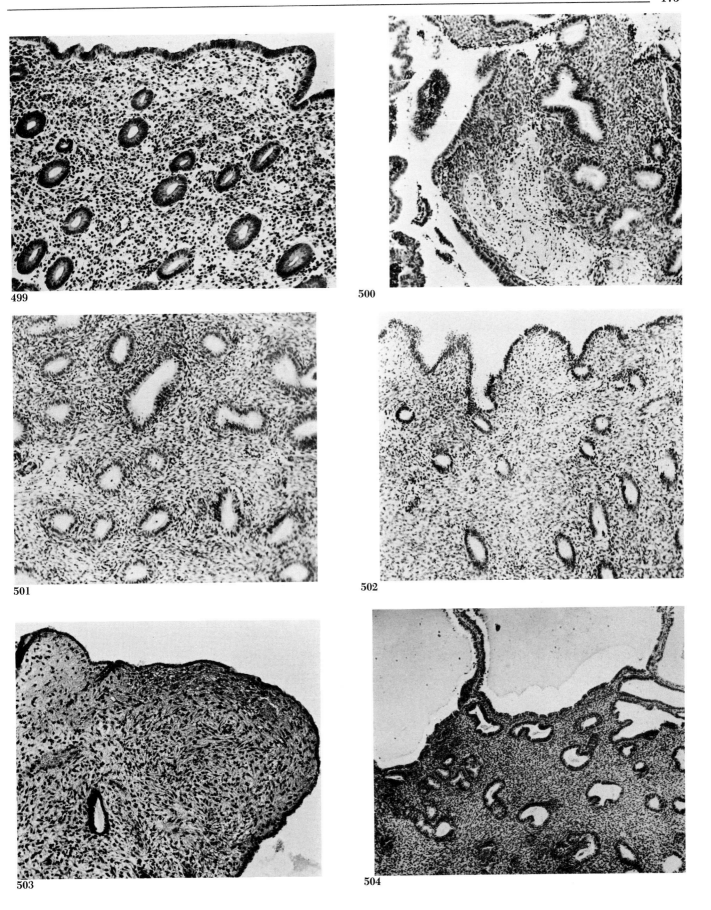

499

500

501

502

503

504

505 Pseudodecidual reaction of the endometrium associated with Krukenberg's tumor of the ovary

Decidual transformation of the endometrium is seen in a patient with Krukenberg's tumor of the ovary and clinical evidence of androgenization. (H&E. ×30)

506 Pseudodecidual reaction of endometrium associated with Krukenberg's tumor of the ovary

High magnification of Fig. 505. Details of the decidual reaction are shown. (H&E. ×150)

507 Pseudosarcomatous changes of the endometrial stroma following norethindrone therapy

This patient, 25 years of age, was treated for 3 months with 10 mg daily of norethindrone (17 alpha-ethinyl-19 nortestosterone), a semisynthetic progestational agent. (H&E. ×150)

508 Pseudosarcomatous changes of the endometrial stroma following norethindrone therapy

A moderate degree of nuclear variability should not be construed as sarcoma. This is a florid decidual reaction to a synthetic progestagen. (H&E. ×150)

509 Endometrial changes following administration of Enovid for 1 year

Endometrial changes are shown following administration of Enovid for 1 year in a patient with endometriosis. The glands are small and tubular; there is a diffuse decidual transformation of the stroma; dilated venules are prominent. (H&E. ×30)

510 Endometrial changes following Enovid administration for 1 year

High magnification of Fig. 509. There is suppression of glandular activity. The plump, sharply outlined decidual cells are arranged in a pavement fashion. Enovid is a brand of norethynodrel with mestranol. The patient received 20 mg daily for 1 year. (H&E. ×125)

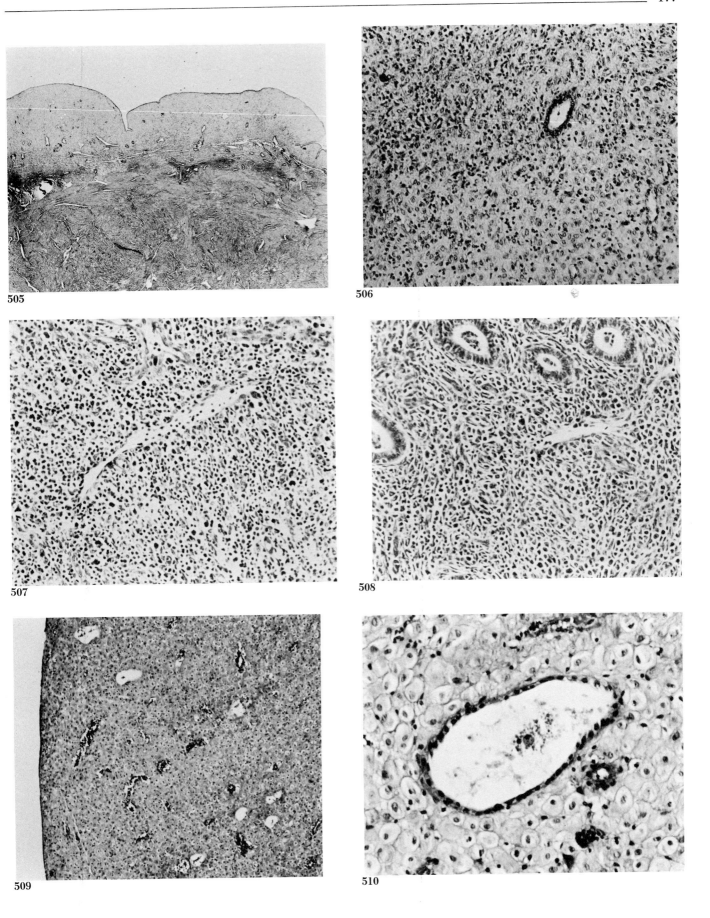

505

506

507

508

509

510

511 Squamous metaplasia of the endometrium
The glands are increased in number and complexity. Scattered nests of squamous cells are in continuity with glands deep in the substance of the mucosa. (H&E. ×100)

512 Squamous metaplasia of the endometrium
An island of squamous epithelium is seen in juxtaposition with a normal endometrial gland. The stroma around it is compressed, but there is no invasion. The squamous cells show moderate nuclear variation. (H&E. ×130)

513 Myelinated nerve in the endometrium
Endometrium from a woman, 35 years of age, showing a myelinated nerve at the endomyometrial junction. (H&E. ×125)

514 Endometrial inspissation with the formation of a concretion
The endometrial gland shows inspissated secretion resembling corpus amylaceum of the prostate. (H&E. ×200)

515 Lipoid macrophages within the lumen of an endometrial gland
(H&E. ×125)

516 Lipoid macrophages within the lumen of an endometrial gland
High magnification of Fig. 515. Multivacuolated cytoplasm of macrophages is shown. (H&E. ×312)

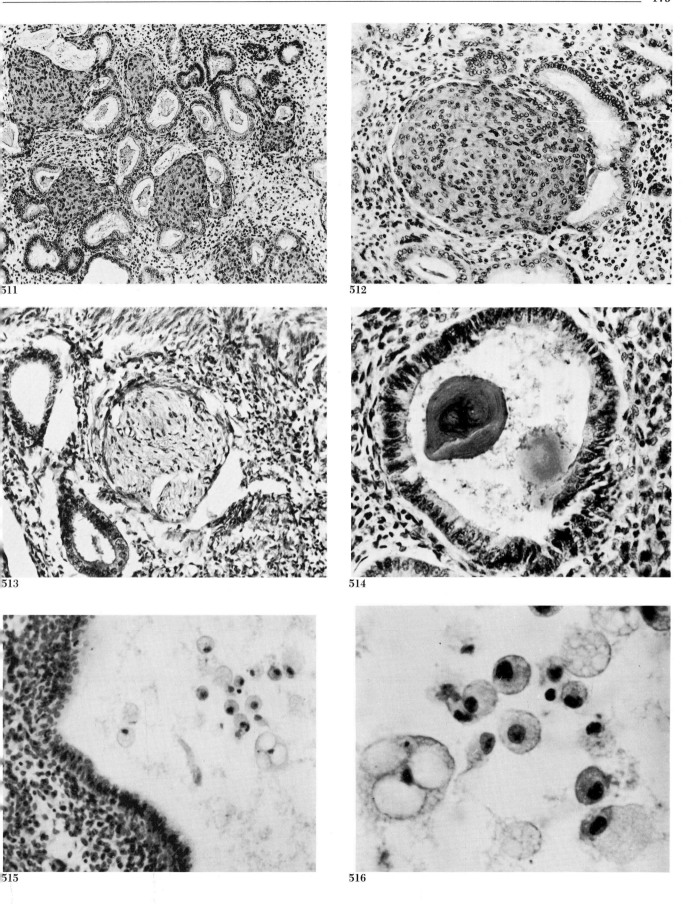

511

512

513

514

515

516

517 Uterus subseptus
The septum is seen partly dividing a uterine cavity. (H&E. ×5) AFIP Acc #218754

518 Cystic glandular hyperplasia of the endometrium
The cystically dilated glands are lined by cuboidal or low columnar epithelial cells. Note that not all the glands are cystic. Some are small and atrophic. (H&E. ×90)

519 Cystic glandular hyperplasia of the endometrium
High magnification of Fig. 518. (H&E. ×180)

520 Cystic glandular hyperplasia of the endometrium
The cystic changes are diffuse. Similar changes are observed in patients indulging in self-medication with estrogens. There is an increase in the number of the endometrial glands which show cystic dilatation. The endometrial stroma is also increased. There is no evidence of secretory activity. See also Fig. 504. (H&E. ×30)

521 Cystic glandular hyperplasia of the endometrium
High magnification of Fig. 520. Portions of the flat lining epithelium of two glands are shown; the intervening stroma is inert, even quasi-fibrotic. (H&E. ×150)

522 Cystic glandular hyperplasia of the endometrium with hemorrhage
(H&E. ×35)

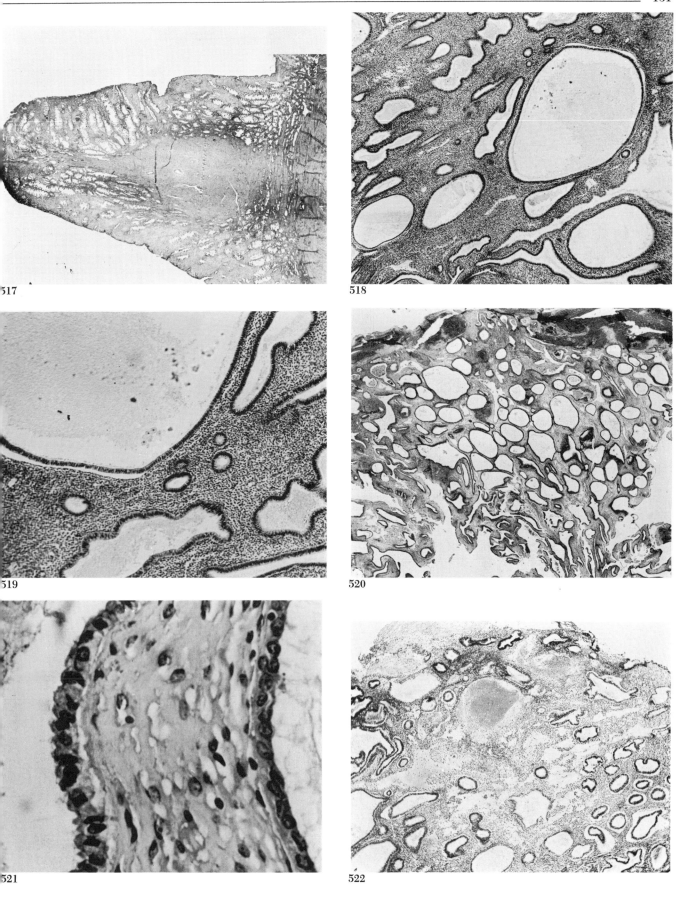

517

518

519

520

521

522

523 Cystic glandular hyperplasia of the endometrium with hemorrhage
High magnification of Fig. 522. There is a dilated sinusoid structure with a loose thrombus. (H&E. ×90)

524 Cystic glandular hyperplasia of the endometrium with oviduct-like epithelium lining cystic glands
(H&E. ×125)

525 Cystic glandular hyperplasia of the endometrium accompanied by secretory changes and predecidual stromal reaction
Though hyperplastic, the endometrium shows response to cyclical ovarian steroid hormones. (H&E. ×200)

526 Adenomatous hyperplasia of the endometrium
The glands are not especially dilated but are lined by a tall columnar epithelium with nuclear crowding and accentuated pseudostratification. (H&E. ×62)

527 Adenomatous hyperplasia of the endometrium
Adenomatous hyperplasia of the endometrium shows the so-called back-to-back pattern of glands, an effect of stromal compression by increased glandular tortuosity. This pattern per se is not evidence of malignant changes. The hyperplastic glands exhibit multilayering but no increase in mitotic activity. (H&E. ×125)

528 Adenomatous hyperplasia of the endometrium
Despite piling up, the glandular epithelial cells are relatively uniform and only an occasional mitosis is observed. (H&E. ×500)

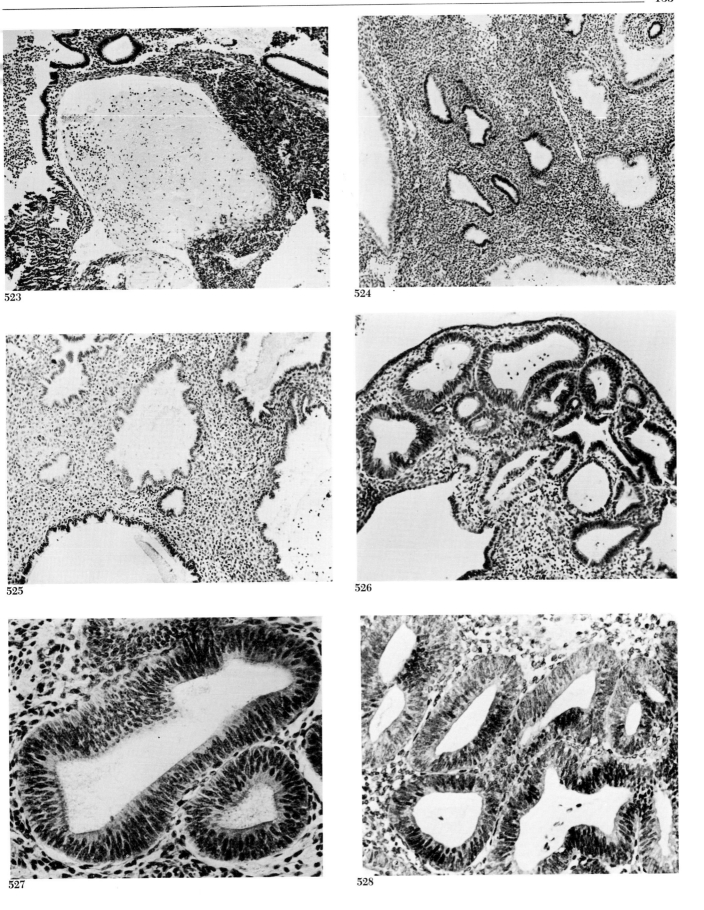

523

524

525

526

527

528

529 Adenomatous hyperplasia of the endometrium with squamous metaplasia
(H&E. ×200)

530 Focal adenomatous hyperplasia of the endometrium
Intraluminal papillation is striking in this particular field, but the remainder of the endometrium was not hyperplastic. (H&E. ×125)

531 Atypical adenomatous hyperplasia of the endometrium
The endometrial glands show cellular atypism and increased mitotic activity. Such a picture may create considerable diagnostic difficulties. (H&E. ×150)

532 Adenomatous endometrial hyperplasia in Stein-Leventhal syndrome (micropolycystic ovary)
Endometrial hyperplasia in a patient with Stein-Leventhal syndrome showing a cystically dilated gland and glands with the back-to-back pattern. Note the presence of lipid macrophages in the lumen of a cystic dilated gland. (H&E. ×62)

533 Adenomatous endometrial hyperplasia in Stein-Leventhal syndrome (micropolycystic ovary)
Note the pronounced degree of glandular crowding and stromal compression. (H&E. ×72)

534 Adenomatous endometrial hyperplasia in Stein-Leventhal syndrome (micropolycystic ovary)
The endometrial hyperplasia in a patient with Stein-Leventhal syndrome shows an extreme degree of piling up by relatively large glandular cells with pallid cytoplasm. Some glands show accessory lumen formation. Some observers feel that this pattern warrants a diagnosis of adenocarcinoma in situ. Following wedge resection of the ovary in the majority of cases, the endometrial changes revert to normal. (H&E. ×125)

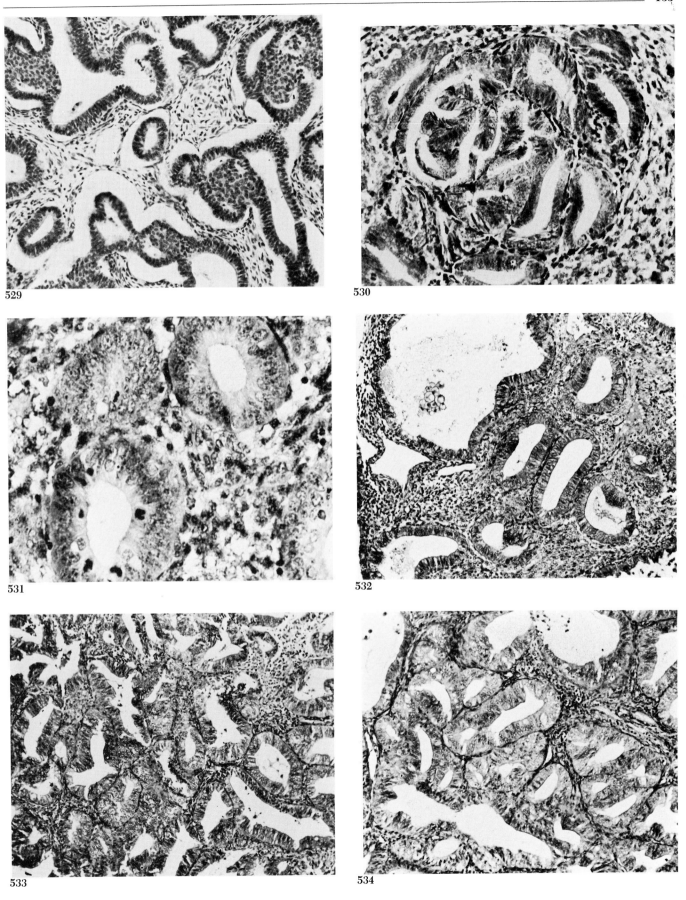

529

530

531

532

533

534

535   Endometrial stromal hyperplasia
There is an increase in the amount of stroma at the expense of glands. The stromal cells lack uniformity. There is absence of mitoses. (H&E. ×125)

536   Endometrial stromal hyperplasia
High magnification of Fig. 535. Note the detail of stromal cell variability and the absence of glands over wide areas. (H&E. ×155)

537   Adenomatous hyperplasia of the endometrium with tubal epithelial metaplasia
The hyperplastic glands lined by hypercellular epithelium are compressing stroma. Intercalated and clear cells are present. (H&E. ×140)

538   Adenomatous hyperplasia of the endometrium with tubal epithelial metaplasia
High magnification of Fig. 537. Note the sharply marginated clear cells in hyperplastic glandular epithelium. (H&E. ×312)

539   Adenomatous hyperplasia of the endometrium with tubal epithelial metaplasia
High magnification of Fig. 537. This detail shows the two forms of glandular epithelium, the crowded elongated cells with normal cytoplasmic density, and the plumper cells with round nuclei and a clear cytoplasm. (H&E. ×450)

540   Acute endometritis
There is stromal edema and diffuse infiltration of glands and stroma by polymorphonuclear leukocytes. (H&E. ×140)

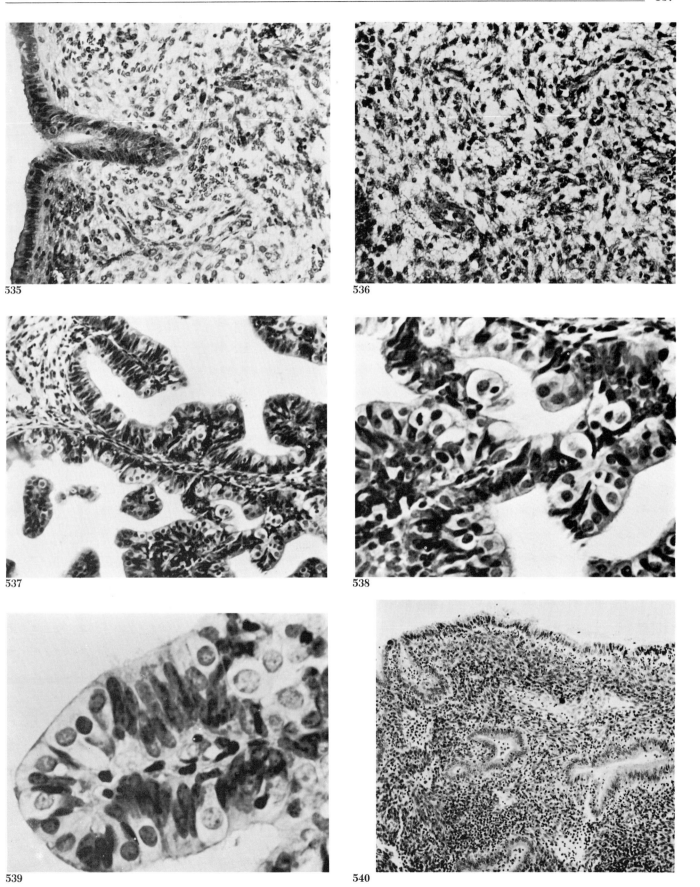

535

536

537

538

539

540

541   Microabscess within a distended endometrial gland
The wall of the distended endometrial gland is necrotic, and the lumen is filled with polymorphonuclear leukocytes. (H&E. ×60)

542   Subacute endometritis
Note the inflammatory debris within the glands and the mixed leukocytic exudate in the stroma (polymorphonuclear leukocytes, lymphocytes, and plasma cells). (H&E. ×62)

543   Chronic endometritis
Diffuse infiltration of the stroma by lymphocytes and plasma cells is seen. (H&E. ×125)

544   Chronic endometritis associated with focal adenomatous hyperplasia
(H&E. ×125)

545   Chronic endometritis in association with submucous leiomyoma
The focal chronic endometritis shows lymphocytic accumulation in the basal layer overlying a submucous leiomyoma. (H&E. ×50)

546   Tuberculous endometritis
Note the discrete and confluent granulomas replacing the mucosa. (H&E. ×50)

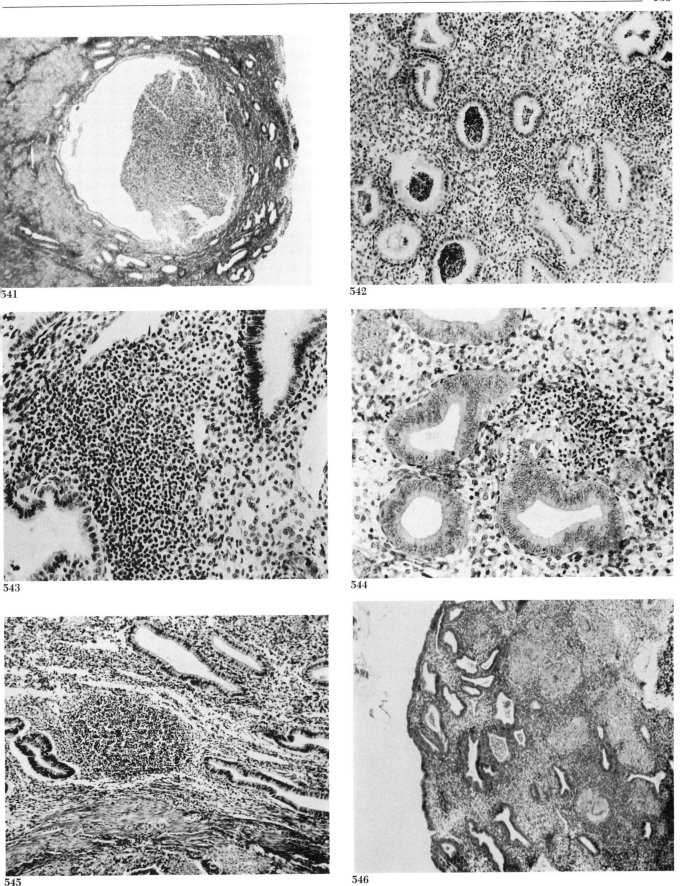

541

542

543

544

545

546

547   Tuberculous endometritis
The granulomas are composed of epithelioid cells and Langhans' giant cells and show lymphocytic infiltration at the periphery. (H&E. ×180)

548   Adenomatous polyp of the endometrium
There is haphazard arrangement of glands within the polyp. Compared with normal endometrium to the right, the stroma of the polyp is relatively dense. The polyp is formed by basalis of the endometrium. (H&E. ×10)

549   Adenomatous polyp of the endometrium
This is a high magnification of the central portion of an adenomatous polyp. (H&E. ×40)

550   Polyp of the endometrium, with diffuse cystic changes of glands
(H&E. ×15)

551   Multiple adenomatous polyps with cystic changes of the glands of the endometrium as seen in curettements
(H&E. ×16)

552   Polyp of the endometrium in Stein-Leventhal syndrome (micropolycystic ovary) with squamous metaplasia
(H&E. ×50)

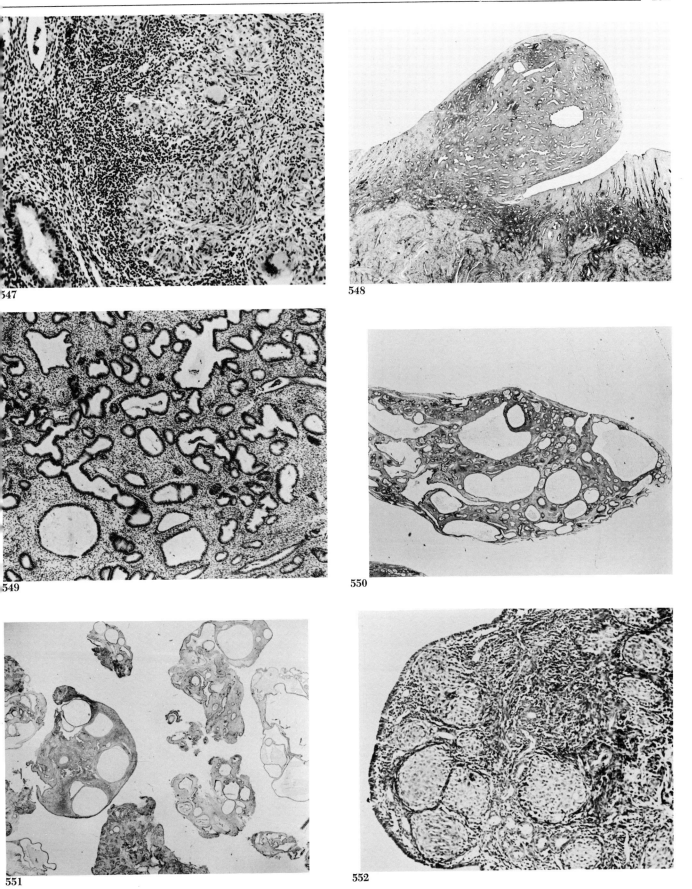

547

548

549

550

551

552

553 Senile endometrial polyp with cystic glandular dilatation
So-called matron's polyp. The remaining endometrial mucosa shows cystic glandular dilatation and atrophy. (H&E. ×8)

554 Stromal polyp of the endometrium
This stromal polyp of the endometrium shows edematous stroma underlying the thin surface epithelium; almost no glands are present in the substance of the lesion. (H&E. ×155)

555 Adenomyomatous polyp of the endometrium
This polypoid structure is formed of endometrial elements and myometrial fibers. (H&E. ×13)

556 Adenomyomatous polyp of the endometrium
High magnification of Fig. 555. Note the smooth muscle fibers interspersed in the endometrial stroma. The endometrial glands are small and show no evidence of secretions. (H&E. ×50)

557 Early adenocarcinoma of the endometrium
The neoplastic process is apparently limited to the endometrium. (H&E. ×50)

558 Early adenocarcinoma of the endometrium
High magnification of Fig. 557. The endometrial glands are lined by neoplastic epithelium showing irregular stratification and formation of intraglandular papillae. The cells are atypical and show hyperchromatic nuclei and mitoses. (H&E. ×150)

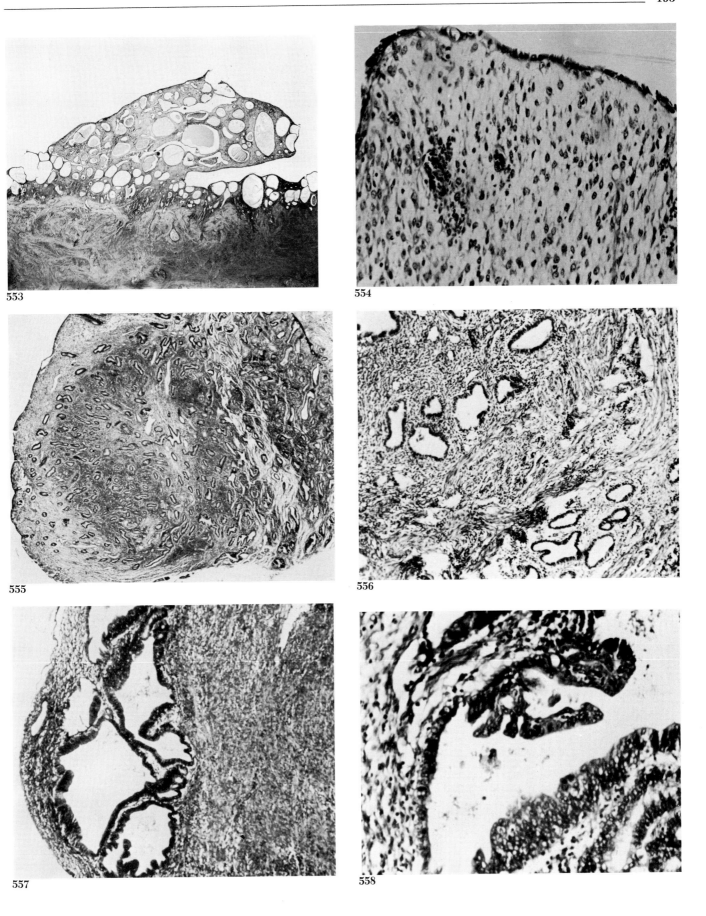

553

554

555

556

557

558

559 Polypoid exophytic adenocarcinoma of the endometrium, general view
(H&E. ×5)

560 Superficial papillary adenocarcinoma of the endometrium
There is papillary neoplastic growth with early superficial myometrial invasion. (H&E. ×10)

561 Adenocarcinoma occurring in a fibroadenomatous isthmic polyp of the endometrium
Note the relatively normal endometrial glands of the polyp to the right. The adenocarcinoma is to the left. (H&E. ×200)

562 Adenocarcinoma developing in mixed cystic glandular and adenomatous hyperplasia of the endometrium
(H&E. ×35)

563 Well-differentiated adenocarcinoma of the endometrium
The tumor is formed of crowded glandular structures lined by one or several layers of well-differentiated epithelial cells. (H&E. ×300)

564 Well-differentiated adenocarcinoma of the endometrium
High magnification of Fig. 563. There is marked stratification of lining epithelium. The epithelial cells show irregular hyperchromatic nuclei with occasional mitotic figures. (H&E. ×600)

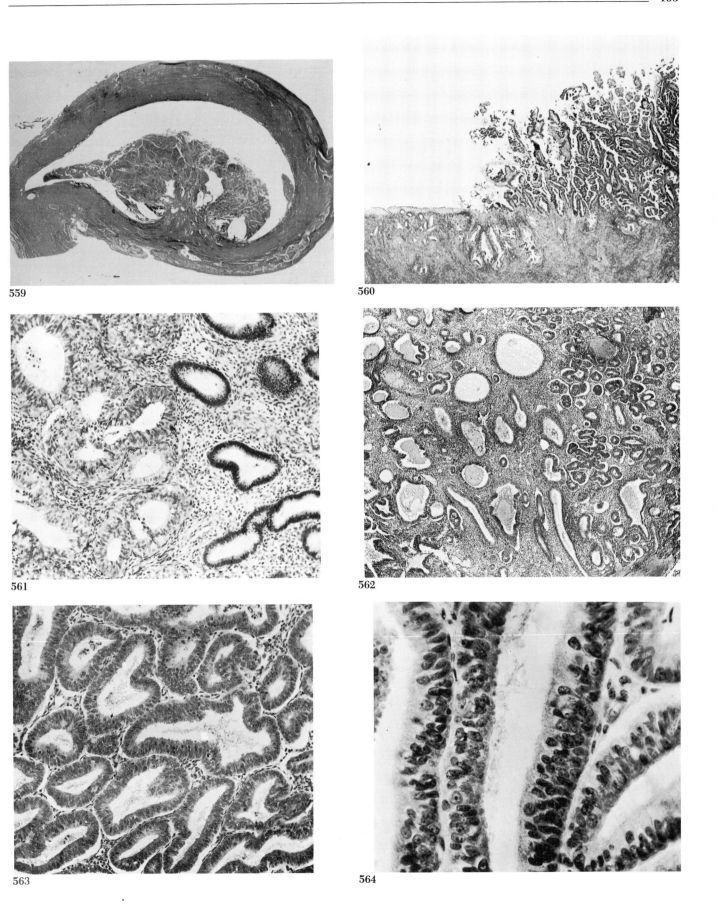

559

560

561

562

563

564

**565 Well-differentiated mucus-secreting ade-
nocarcinoma of the endometrium**
The tumor is formed of well-differentiated,
rather irregular acini lined by mucus-secreting
tall columnar neoplastic cells. (H&E. ×62)

**566 Well-differentiated adenocarcinoma of the
endometrium**
The tumor is formed by closely packed neoplastic glands. They are lined by columnar neoplastic cells with desquamated neoplastic cells
within their lumens. (H&E. ×125)

**567 Secretory adenocarcinoma of the endome-
trium**
This is a highly differentiated adenocarcinoma.
The neoplastic tumor cells show subnuclear
vacuolization, an evidence of partial steroid
stimulation. Such tumors are occasionally observed in young patients and present considerable diagnostic difficulties. (H&E. ×100)

**568 Secretory adenocarcinoma of the endome-
trium**
High magnification of Fig. 567. The neoplastic
endometrial gland shows pronounced subnuclear secretory vacuoles. Areas of epithelial
stratification with mitotic activity are present.
These areas also show connective tissue invasion. (H&E. ×200)

**569 Moderately well-differentiated adeno-
carcinoma of the endometrium**
The tumor is formed of relatively poorly developed neoplastic glands. (H&E. ×180)

**570 Poorly differentiated adenocarcinoma of
the endometrium**
The glandular structure of the tumor is barely
recognizable. The neoplastic epithelial cells are
poorly differentiated. (H&E. ×220)

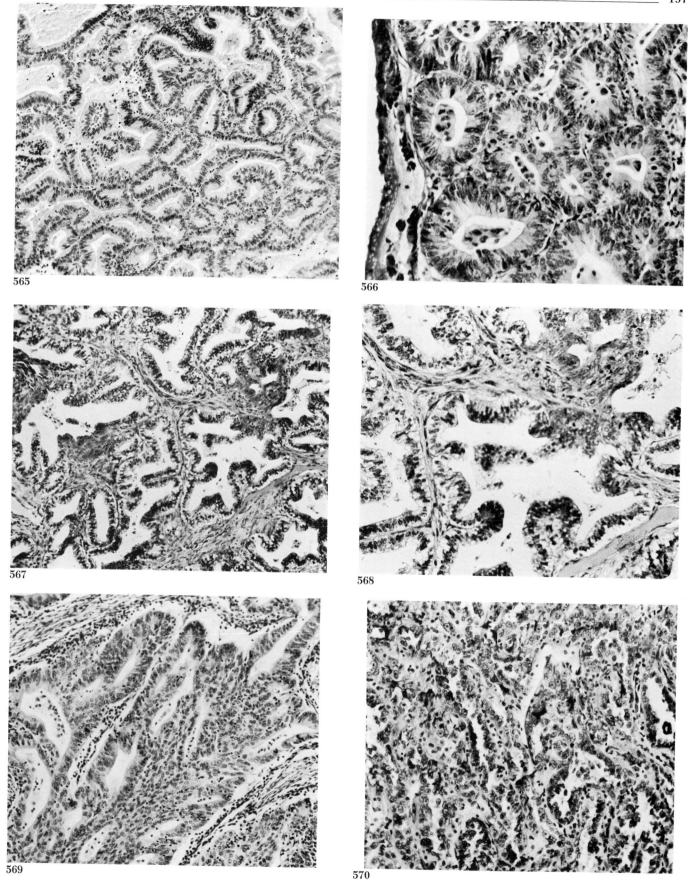

565

566

567

568

569

570

571　Anaplastic carcinoma of the endometrium
This highly undifferentiated tumor shows no evidence of glandular formations. (H&E. ×125)

572　Papillary adenocarcinoma of the endometrium
The tumor is composed of neoplastic glands with dilated lumens and numerous papillary projections. (H&E. ×180)

573　Adenocarcinoma of the endometrium, with solid anaplastic carcinoma
There is transition from a well-differentiated adenocarcinoma into a poorly differentiated, anaplastic solid carcinoma of the endometrium. (H&E. ×180)

574　Adenoacanthoma of the endometrium
Solid nests consisting of neoplastic squamous epithelium have developed within or in juxtaposition to relatively well-developed glands of an endometrial carcinoma. The transition of the epithelial metaplastic changes is sharply delineated. (H&E. ×180)

575　Adenoacanthoma of the endometrium
The glandular structures of an endometrial carcinoma are lined by strands of squamous epithelium. (H&E. ×280)

576　Diffuse adenoacanthoma of the endometrium
The marked diffuse proliferation of squamous epithelium is replacing stroma and compressing well-defined glandular elements. (H&E. ×62)

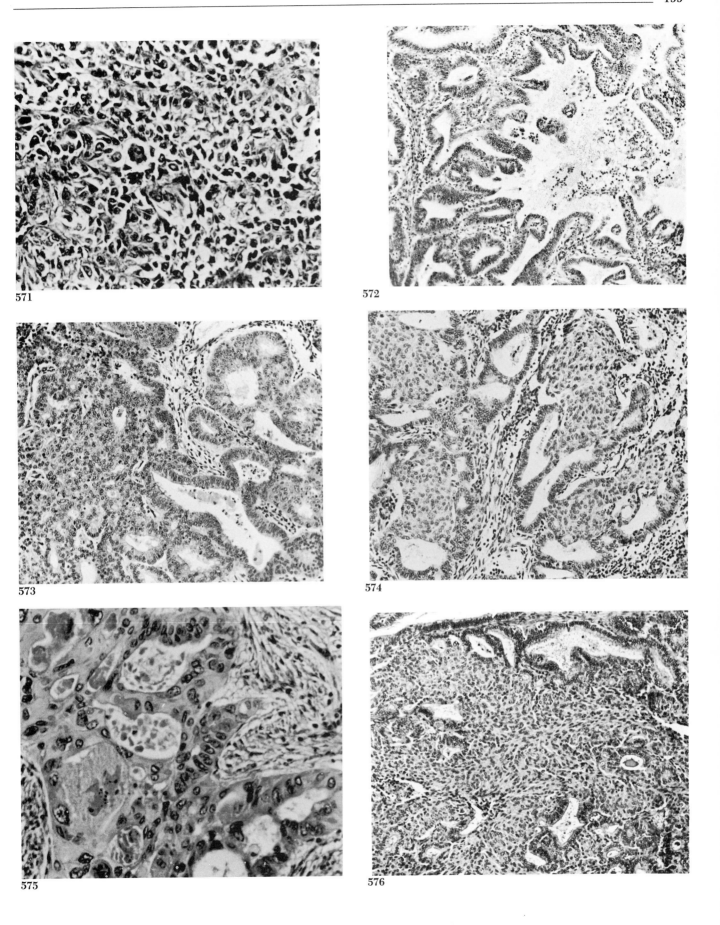

571

572

573

574

575

576

577 Squamous carcinoma of the endometrium
The endometrium is replaced by solid sheets of neoplastic, moderately well-differentiated squamous epithelial cells. (H&E. ×50)

578 Squamous carcinoma of the endometrium
High magnification of Fig. 577. There is complete obliteration of glandular structures by solid growth type of squamous epithelial cells. (H&E. ×150)

579 Carcinosarcoma of the endometrium, general view
(H&E. ×5)

580 Moderately well-differentiated carcinosarcoma of the endometrium
The tumor is formed of neoplastic glands and neoplastic stroma. The carcinomatous elements are of Müllerian origin, and the stromal sarcomatous elements are of mesenchymal origin. (H&E. ×125)

581 Undifferentiated pleomorphic carcinosarcoma of the endometrium
(H&E. ×300)

582 Endometrial stromal sarcoma
There is massive neoplastic proliferation of endometrial stromal cells around normal-appearing endometrial gland. (H&E. ×125)

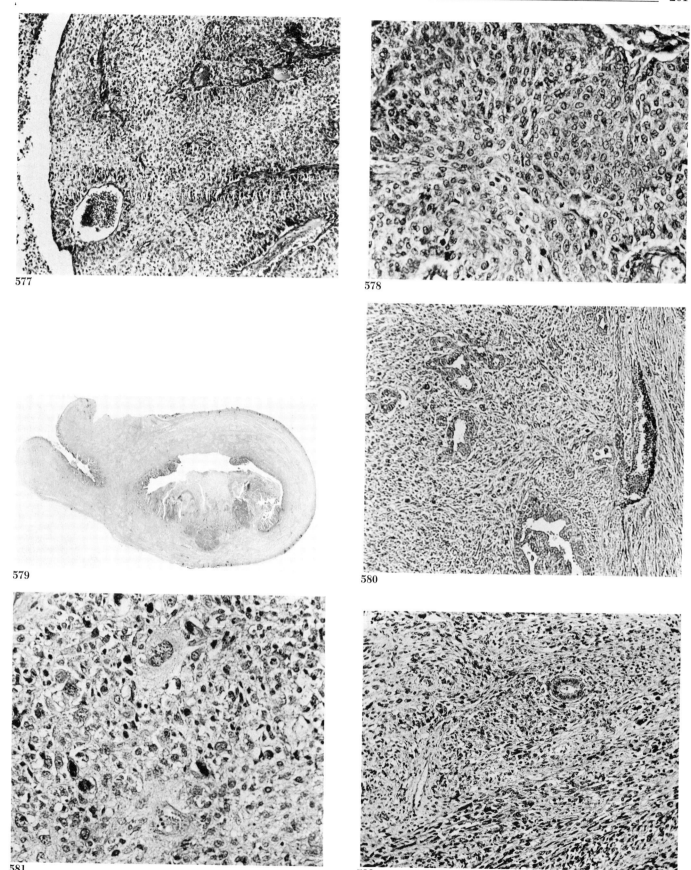

577

578

579

580

581

582

583 Endometrial stromal sarcoma
Proliferated, elongated endometrial stromal cells are shown with hyperchromatic nuclei and frequent atypical mitotic figures. Note the absence of endometrial glands. (H&E. ×140)

584 Endometrial stromal sarcoma
The endometrial stromal cells are assuming a round form with hyperchromatic nuclei and relatively clear cytoplasm. Note the presence of numerous mitoses. (H&E. ×250)

585 Endometrial stromal sarcoma
Predominantly pericellular arrangement of reticulum fibers is seen. (Wilder's reticulum stain. ×250)

586 Mixed mesenchymal sarcoma of the endometrium
There is considerable variation in the structure of the tumor. An island of cartilage is surrounded by sarcomatous stroma. Several glandular structures are formed by highly atypical neoplastic epithelial cells. (H&E. ×125)

587 Mixed mesenchymal sarcoma of the endometrium
The sarcomatous stroma of the tumor shows the presence of numerous rhabdomyoblasts. There are large cells with strongly acidophilic cytoplasm. (H&E. ×150)

588 Mixed mesenchymal sarcoma of the endometrium
Cross-striated muscle fiber (so-called strap cell) is present in a mesodermal mixed tumor. (Heidenhain's iron hematoxylin. ×1,000)

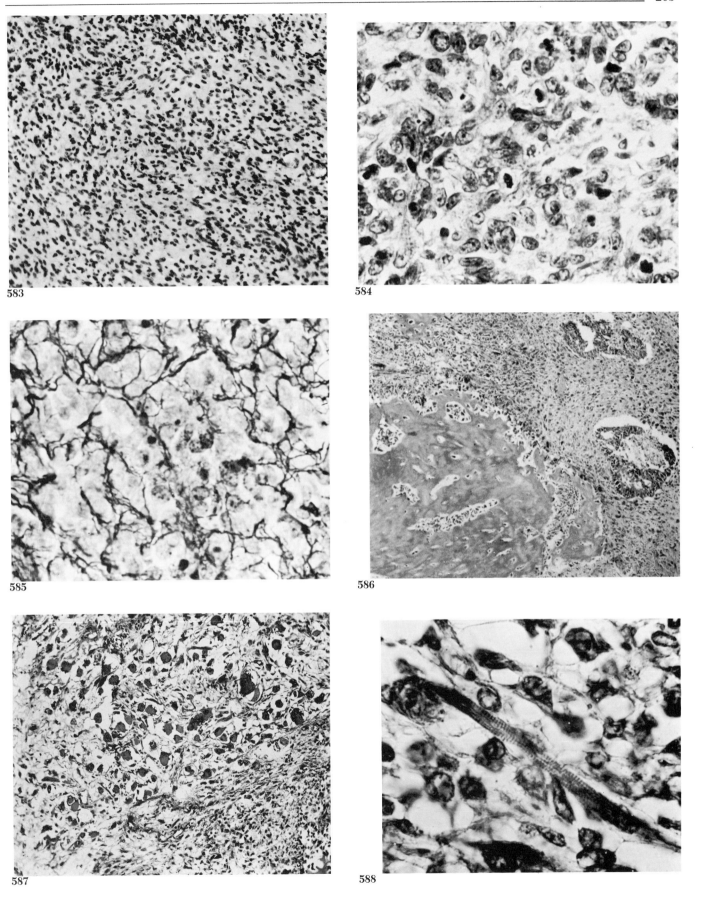

583

584

585

586

587

588

589 Retinal anlage tumor of the endometrium (melanotic progonoma)
The mesenchymal tumor of the endometrium is formed predominantly by fibrocartilaginous elements and intermingled collections of pigmented cells, small round cells, and strands of epithelial cells. (H&E. ×50)

590 Retinal anlage tumor of the endometrium (melanotic progonoma)
High magnification of Fig. 589. Deeply pigmented cells, corresponding to retinal pigment epithelium, are arranged in small clusters and surrounded by fibrocartilaginous tissue. (H&E. ×200)

591 Retinal anlage tumor of the endometrium (melanotic progonoma)
High magnification of Fig. 589. The moderately differentiated retinal cells line the lacunar spaces provided by fibrocartilaginous stroma. There is an abortive attempt of round tumor cells to form Winterstein's rosettes. (H&E. ×200)

592 Chondrosarcoma of the endometrium
The endometrium is replaced by a tumor consisting of large islands of cartilaginous neoplastic tissue. The myometrium is compressed (H&E. ×6)

593 Chondrosarcoma of the endometrium
High magnification of Fig. 592. Cartilaginous tumor tissue is seen at the endomyometrial junction. (H&E. ×50)

594 Chondrosarcoma of the endometrium
High magnification of Fig. 592. The chondrosarcoma of the endometrium represents a form of mesenchymal tumor with predominance of neoplastic cartilaginous tissue. The tumor is formed of pleomorphic cartilage cells and sarcomatous endometrial stroma. (H&E. ×150)

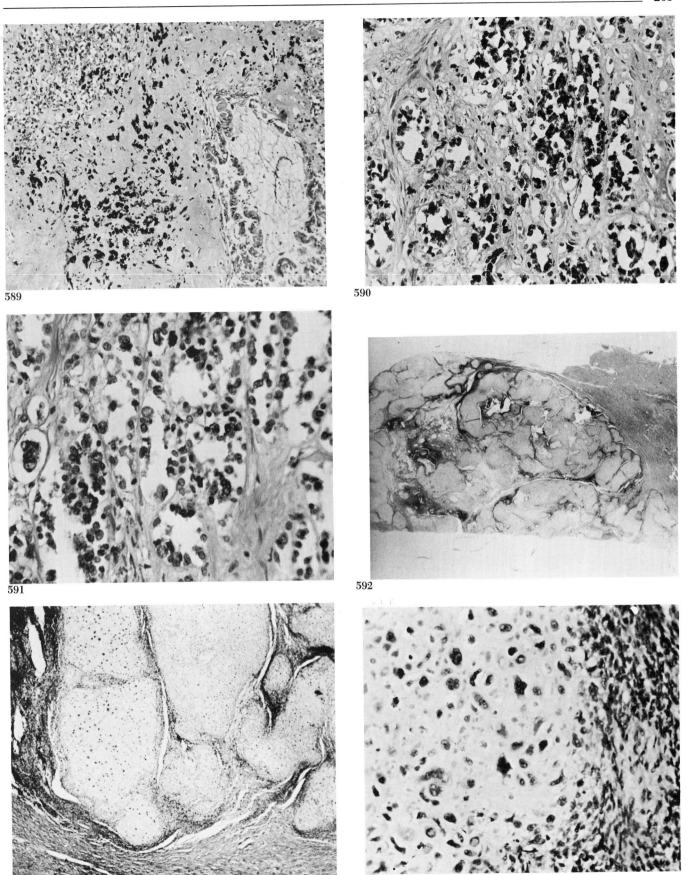

589

590

591

592

593

594

595 Mesonephric carcinoma of the endometrium
The papillary tumor is formed by clear cells with irregular hyperchromatic nuclei. Alcian blue and Mayer's mucicarmine stains were negative, indicating a mesonephric origin of the tumor. The tumor originated in the myometrium, the bulk occupying the endometrial cavity and replacing the endometrium. (H&E. ×150)

596 Malignant lymphoma (lymphoblastic lymphosarcoma) of the endometrium
The endometrium and myometrium are diffusely infiltrated with round cells resembling lymphocytes. Note the isolated, degenerating endometrial glands. (H&E. ×50)

597 Malignant lymphoma (lymphoblastic lymphosarcoma) of the endometrium
High magnification of Fig. 596. The neoplastic cells infiltrating the endometrium are round with prominent dark nuclei. The endometrial stromal cells are sparse. Endometrial glands are absent. (H&E. ×125)

598 Reticulum cell sarcoma of the endometrium
The well-preserved endometrial gland, showing secretory activity, is surrounded by infiltrating pleomorphic neoplastic cells with prominent nucleoli. (H&E. ×180)

599 Reticulum cell sarcoma of the endometrium
There is deposition of reticulum fibers between individual cells and a group of cells. (Wilder's reticulum stain. ×250)

600 Postirradiation endometritis
The patient has been treated with sterilizing dose of intrauterine radium for management of dysfunctional uterine bleeding. The endometrium shows necrosis and infiltration with inflammatory cells. (H&E. ×50)

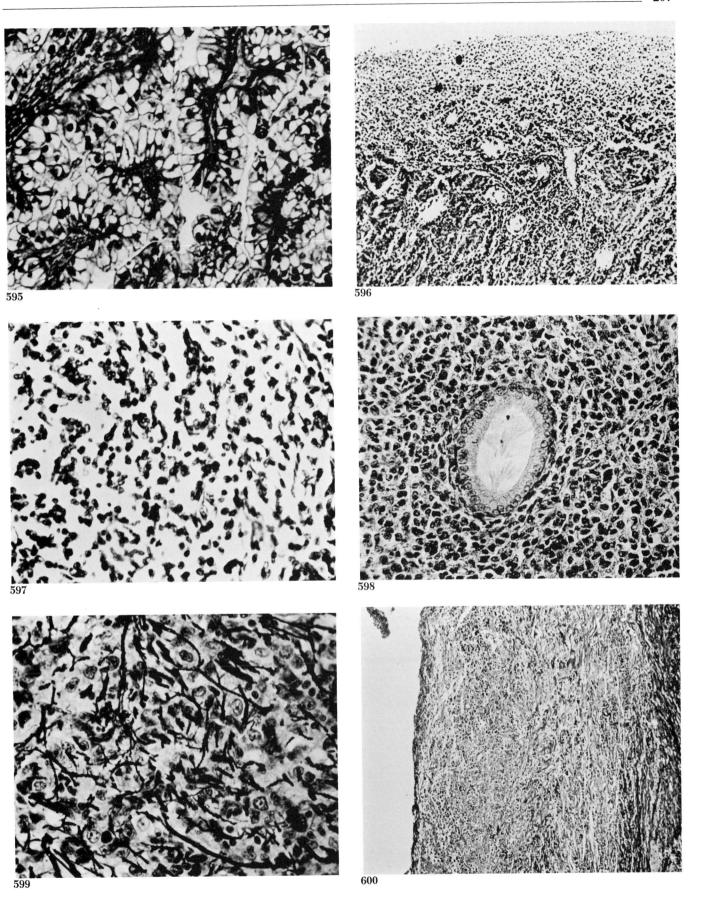

595

596

597

598

599

600

601 Postirradiation endometritis
High magnification of Fig. 600. Note the absence of endometrial glands. The endometrial stroma is mostly replaced by inflammatory cells. Endometrial vessels are dilated and show perivascular hyalinization. (H&E. ×200)

602 Postirradiation atrophy and fibrosis of the endometrium
The atrophy of the endometrium with disappearance of endometrial glands was seen 1 year after x-ray castration. Note the focal stromal hyalinization. (H&E. ×62)

603 Postirradiation atrophy and fibrosis of the endometrium
Massive hyalinization and fibrosis of the endometrium as seen 14 months after x-ray treatment of ovarian tumors. (H&E. ×80)

604 Endometrial adenocarcinoma with irradiation effects
The neoplastic endometrial gland shows dissolution. There is vacuolization of the cytoplasm and necrosis of several neoplastic epithelial cells. This condition was present after intrauterine radium with cancerocidal dose of 6,000 r. (H&E. ×180)

605 Endometrial adenocarcinoma with irradiation effects
There is advanced dissolution of neoplastic tissue with areas of necrosis and inflammatory reaction. The patient had preoperative irradiation with intrauterine radium. (H&E. ×180)

606 Superficial adenomyosis
The superficial myometrial layer is infiltrated by tongues of endometrial tissue extending 3 to 5 mm. (H&E. ×50)

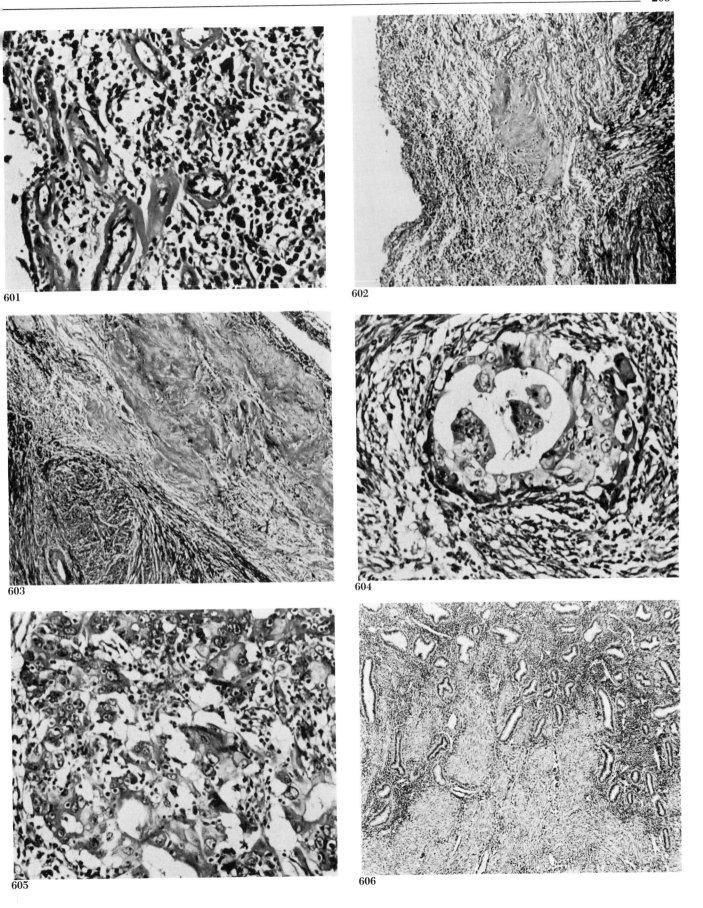

601

602

603

604

605

606

607   Endometriosis of the umbilicus
There are cystically dilated endometrial glands in the connective tissue stroma of the umbilicus. (H&E. ×15)

608   Endometriosis in the vermiform appendix
The lumen of the vermiform appendix is obliterated. Endometrial glands are seen in the connective tissue of subserosa. (H&E. ×12)

609   Endometriosis of the renal pelvis
To the left is renal tissue. To the right, massive endometrial tissue encroaches upon the renal pelvis. The endometrial glands vary in size and show large cystic structures. (H&E. ×8) AFIP Acc #84968

610   Endometriosis of the urinary bladder
Endometrial glands and stroma are scattered throughout the muscle layers of the urinary bladder. Several cystically dilated endometrial glands contain blood. (H&E. ×11)

611   Rectosigmoid endometriosis treated with Enovid
There is a pseudodecidual reaction of endometrial stroma. The endometrial gland is compressed and lined by flattened epithelium. Note the appearance of inflammatory cells around the endometrial gland. (H&E. ×85)

612   Rectosigmoid endometriosis, treated with Enovid
A pseudodecidual reaction of endometrial stromal cells is seen. The endometrial glandular epithelium has undergone degeneration, and it is replaced by inflammatory cells. (H&E. ×125)

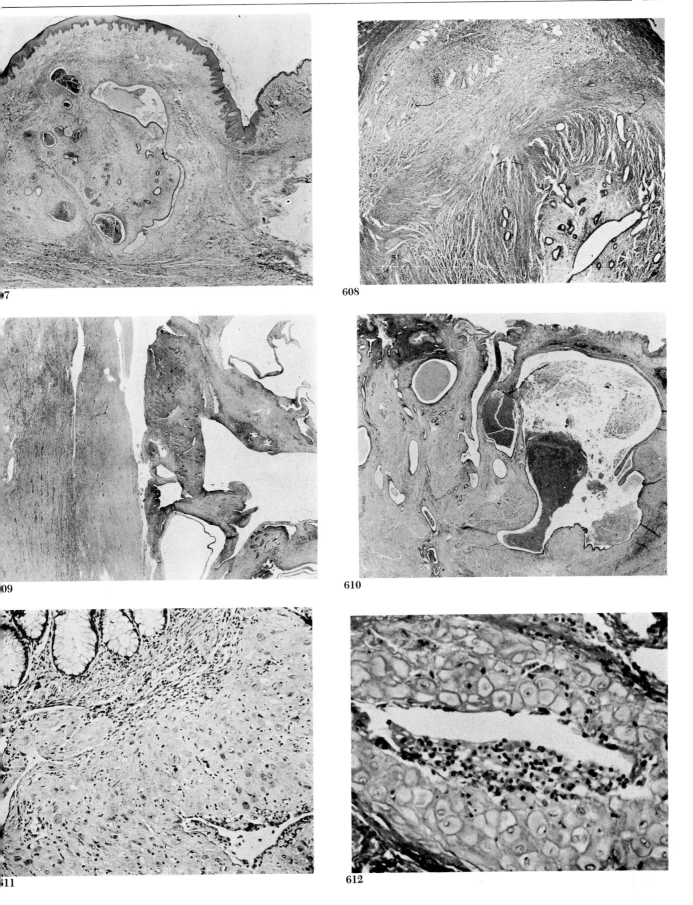

607

608

609

610

611

612

COLOR PLATES
Chapter 4
Diseases of the Endometrium
Plates 7, 8, and 9

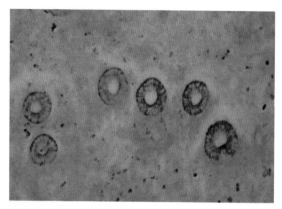

37 Mast cells in proliferative endometrium There are numerous scattered mast cells throughout the stroma of the proliferative endometrium. (Gomori's aldehyde fuchsin. ×120)

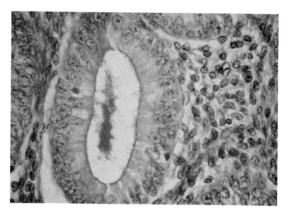

38 Neutral mucopolysaccharides in proliferative endometrium (8th to 10th day of the cycle) Within the lumens of the endometrial glands, in late proliferative endometrium, PAS positive, Alcian blue positive and aldehyde fuchsin positive substances are frequently found. They are identified as neutral, acid, and sulfonated mucopolysaccharides. (PAS with diastase digestion. ×500)

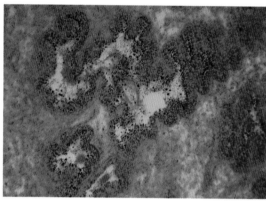

39 Presence of glycogen granules in secretory endometrium (22d day of the cycle) Glycogen granules are seen in the cytoplasm and within the lumens of secretory endometrial glands. (Best's carmine. ×120)

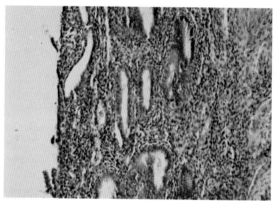

40 Endometrium in ovarian dysgenesis Note the relatively atrophic endometrium with dense endometrial stroma and elongated endometrial glands with a horizontal axis. (H&E. ×62)

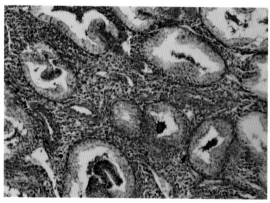

41 Endometrium in induced ovulation with clomiphene citrate Hypersecretory endometrial glands with relatively dense endometrial stroma and early focal predecidual changes are seen after clomiphene citrate therapy, 100 mg daily, for 14 days. (H&E. ×125)

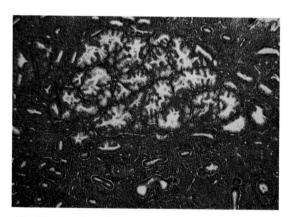

42 Mixed endometrium or irregular ripening of the endometrium Mixed proliferative and secretory endometrium is seen. A complex of actively secreting dentate glands is seen scattered among glands in the proliferative phase. (H&E. ×62)

Plate 7

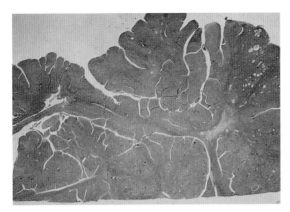

43 Adenofibroma (papillary fibroadenoma) of the endometrium The endometrium is replaced by dense fibromatous connective tissue stroma forming papillary projections. Note the scattered small cystically dilated endometrial glands. The surface epithelium consists of single layer cuboidal epithelium. (H&E. ×20)

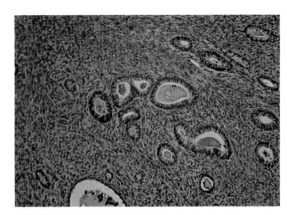

44 Adenofibroma (papillary fibroadenoma) of the endometrium High magnification of Fig. 43. (H&E. ×80)

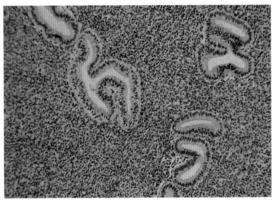

45 Endometrial stromal hyperplasia Relatively normal endometrial glands are surrounded by hyperplastic endometrial stromal cells. The stromal cells are rather uniform and show occasional mitosis. (H&E. ×125)

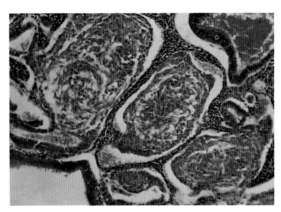

46 Squamous metaplasia in hyperplastic adenomatous endometrium Hyperplastic, adenomatous endometrial glands contain within their lumens islands of metaplastic squamous epithelium. (H&E. ×125)

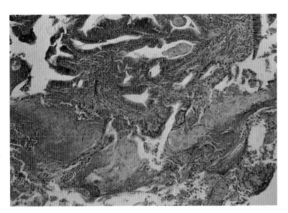

47 Ichthyosis uteri The endometrial glands show well-differentiated adenocarcinoma with focal areas of squamous metaplasia. The surface epithelium of the endometrial cavity is replaced by a thick layer of squamous, keratinizing epithelium. (H&E. ×125)

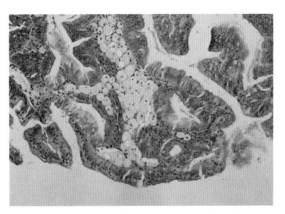

48 Adenocarcinoma of the endometrium with lipid macrophages (foam cells) in connective tissue stroma (H&E. ×150)

Plate 8

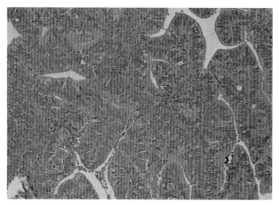

49 Adenocarcinoma of the endometrium with clear cells ("helle Zellen," Feyrter) The tumor is formed by glandular acini lined by stratified columnar epithelium with interspersed chromophobe clear cells. There are round to polygonal cells with clear cytoplasm and round nuclei in the mid-cell position. (H&E. ×180)

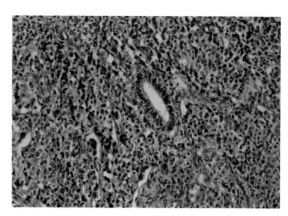

50 Endometrial stromal sarcoma An isolated endometrial gland is seen surrounded by proliferating neoplastic endometrial stromal cells. (H&E. ×125)

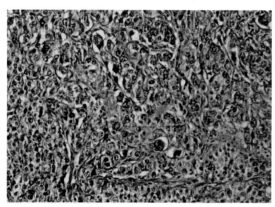

51 Endometrial stromal sarcoma Note the pleomorphic appearance of endometrial stromal sarcoma. (H&E. ×250)

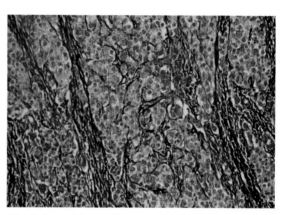

52 Endometrial stromal sarcoma The densely packed round endometrial stromal cells show prominent nuclei and delicate connective tissue fibers. (Wilder's reticulum stain. ×250)

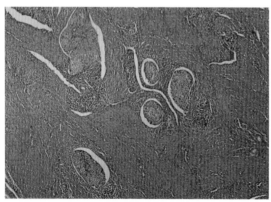

53 Endometrial stromal sarcoma Note the invasion and propagation of sarcomatous endometrial tissue through the lymphatics of the myometrium. (H&E. ×25)

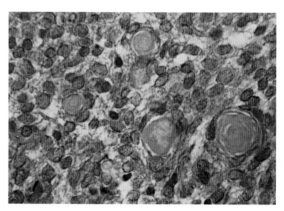

54 Endometrial sarcoma with hyaline bodies (H&E. ×500)

Plate 9

5

Diseases of the Myometrium

613 Idiopathic hypertrophy of the myometrium
The hypertrophy of the myometrium shown here is not associated with pregnancy or with a history of previous pregnancies. The myometrium is thickened 3½ times its normal size. (H&E. ×3)

614 Idiopathic hypertrophy of the myometrium
High magnification of Fig. 613. There is hypertrophy and hyperplasia of the myometrial muscle fibers. (H&E. ×25)

615 Focal hyalinization of the myometrium
The focal area of hyalinization involves smooth muscle fibers and connective tissue and is associated with a mild inflammatory reaction (H&E. ×50)

616 Calcific arteriosclerosis of the myometrium
Calcific sclerosis of the myometrial vessels is observed after the menopause. (H&E. ×50)

617 Paramesonephric dysontogenetic cyst of the myometrium
To the left, a cyst is located in the myometrium. To the right, the cyst lining is formed by oviduct-like epithelium. (H&E. ×20 and ×150)

618 Phlegmonous metritis
There is edema of the myometrium and diffuse infiltration of the uterine wall with acute and chronic inflammatory cells. Note the marked dissociation of the myometrial fibers conditioned by inflammation. (H&E. ×80)

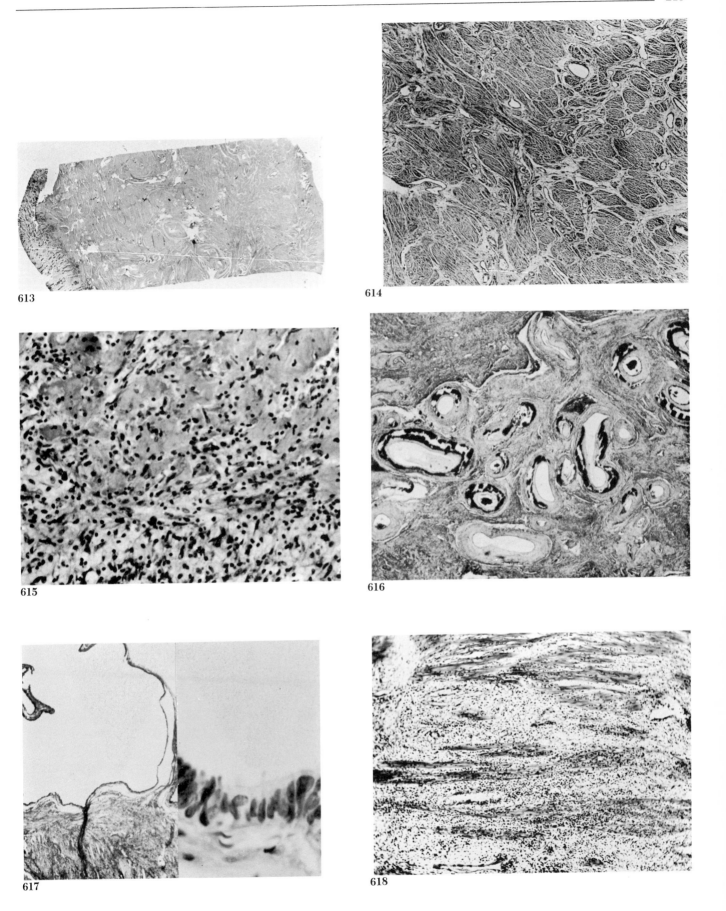

613

614

615

616

617

618

619   Lipomatosis of the myometrium
Diffuse infiltration of the myometrium by single and clusters of fat cells is seen. (H&E. ×50)

620   Lipomatosis of the myometrium
High magnification of Fig. 619. There is fatty replacement of normal myometrial fibers. The cause is undetermined. (H&E. ×175)

621   Xanthogranuloma of the myometrium
Numerous foam cells are seen located within masses of smooth muscle fibers. (H&E. ×85)

622   Xanthogranuloma of the myometrium
High magnification of Fig. 621. The large xanthoma cells or foam cells contain lipid. The nuclei are small, uniform, and dark stained. Occasionally two nuclei are seen in xanthoma cells. (H&E. ×85)

623   Xanthogranuloma of the myometrium
Note the presence of multinucleated giant cells and numerous histiocytes. Abundant lipid material can be demonstrated in a frozen section stained with oil red O or Sudan. (H&E. ×70)

624   Adenomyosis of the myometrium
The myometrial tissue contains several heterotopic endometrial islands formed by endometrial glands and stromal cells. Deep penetration of myometrium by glands of the basal zone of endometrium is well demonstrated in the lower left-hand corner. (H&E. ×6)

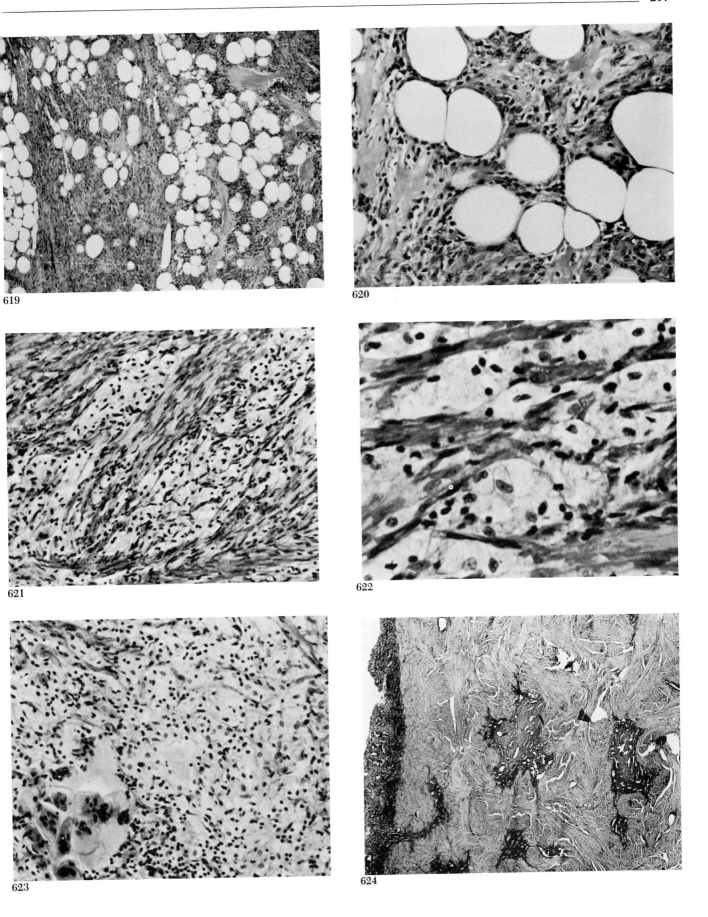

619

620

621

622

623

624

625   Adenomyosis of the myometrium
Scattered isolated endometrial glands are surrounded by endometrial stromal cells (cytogenic stroma or cytogenous mantle) in the myometrium. (H&E. ×50)

626   Adenomyosis of the myometrium
An island of heterotopic endometrial tissue is formed by glandular and stromal components, surrounded by musculature of the uterus. The endometrial glands show no functional activity. (H&E. ×65)

627   Adenomyosis of the myometrium with cyst formations
The cystically dilated endometrial glands are surrounded by sparse stroma. (H&E. ×30)

628   Adenomyosis of the myometrium with endometrial glands in the secretory phase
(H&E. ×50)

629   Adenomyosis of the myometrium with squamous metaplasia
The heterotopic islands of endometrial tissue with squamous metaplasia occur in glands and around glandular structures. (H&E. ×80)

630   Adenomyosis of the myometrium treated with Enovid
The patient received Enovid, 20 mg daily, for 6 months. A pseudodecidual reaction of endometrial stromal cells is seen. The endometrial glands are atrophic. (H&E. ×50)

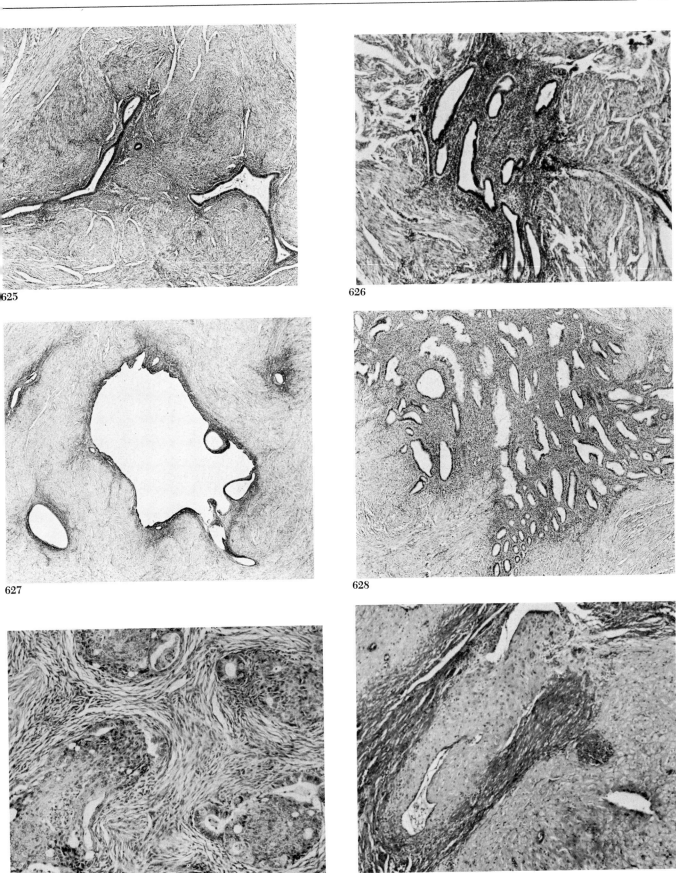

625

626

627

628

629

630

631   Adenomyosis of the myometrium treated with Enovid
High magnification of Fig. 630. Note the atrophy of the glandular epithelium. There is a pronounced pseudodecidual reaction of endometrial stromal cells. Enovid (norethynodrel [17 alpha-ethynyl-17 beta-hydroxy-5(10)-estrene-3-one] with added estrogen in the form of the 3-methyl ether of ethynylestradiol) is a progestational agent. (H&E. ×150)

632   Lymphangioma of the myometrium
The cystic tumor is composed of lymph vessels with flat endothelial lining. (H&E. ×40)

633   Hemangioma of the myometrium
The tumor is formed by numerous small vessels and intervening connective tissue stroma. (H&E. ×50)

634   Pericytoma of the myometrium
The tumor is composed of numerous capillaries surrounded by masses of pericytic cells. Reticulum stain will be helpful in demonstrating the position of tumor cells outside the reticulin sheath of the capillaries. (H&E. ×125)

635   Pericytoma of the myometrium
Different area of the tumor shown in Fig. 634. Tumor cells are arranged concentrically around small vessels and capillaries. They are ovoid or spindle shaped and have prominent dark nuclei. (H&E. ×125)

636   Adenomyoma of the myometrium
This condition should be differentiated from adenomyosis. Glandular elements of mesonephric or paramesonephric origin are surrounded by coats of fibrous connective tissue and smooth muscle fibers in an organoid pattern. Endometrial stromal cells are absent. The tumor is benign. (H&E. ×50)

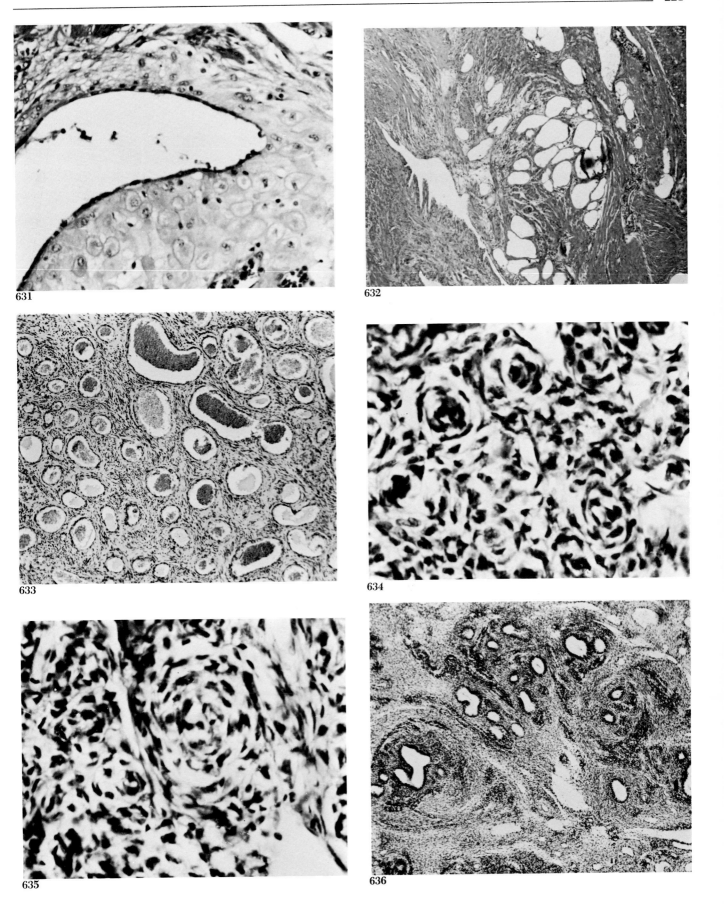

631

632

633

634

635

636

637 Dysontogenetic epidermal inclusions of the myometrium
Numerous epidermal cysts are scattered throughout the myometrium. They are filled with keratin material. Most probably they represent dysontogenetic rests from urogenital sinus epithelium. (H&E. ×20)

638 Dysontogenetic epidermal inclusions of the myometrium
High magnification of Fig. 637. The epidermal cyst in the myometrium is lined by well-differentiated squamous epithelium and contains keratin. (H&E. ×50)

639 Dysontogenetic epidermal inclusions of the myometrium
The wall of the cyst is destroyed by a granulomatous inflammatory process. The remaining keratin masses are surrounded by numerous foreign-body giant cells. (H&E. ×80)

640 Dysontogenetic epidermal inclusions of the myometrium
High magnification of Fig. 639. A minute island of squamous epithelium is surrounded by acute and chronic inflammatory cells and numerous foreign-body giant cells. (H&E. ×100)

641 Lipoma of the myometrium
The tumor is composed of mature fat cells arranged in irregular lobules. The intervening myometrial connective tissue shows hyalinization. (H&E. ×120)

642 Fibroma of the myometrium
The tumor consists of relatively densely packed fibrous connective tissue cells. Some tumor cells are cut transversely and some longitudinally. The neoplastic cells are uniform in size and shape and have elongated dark nuclei. There is no evidence of mitoses. (H&E. ×70)

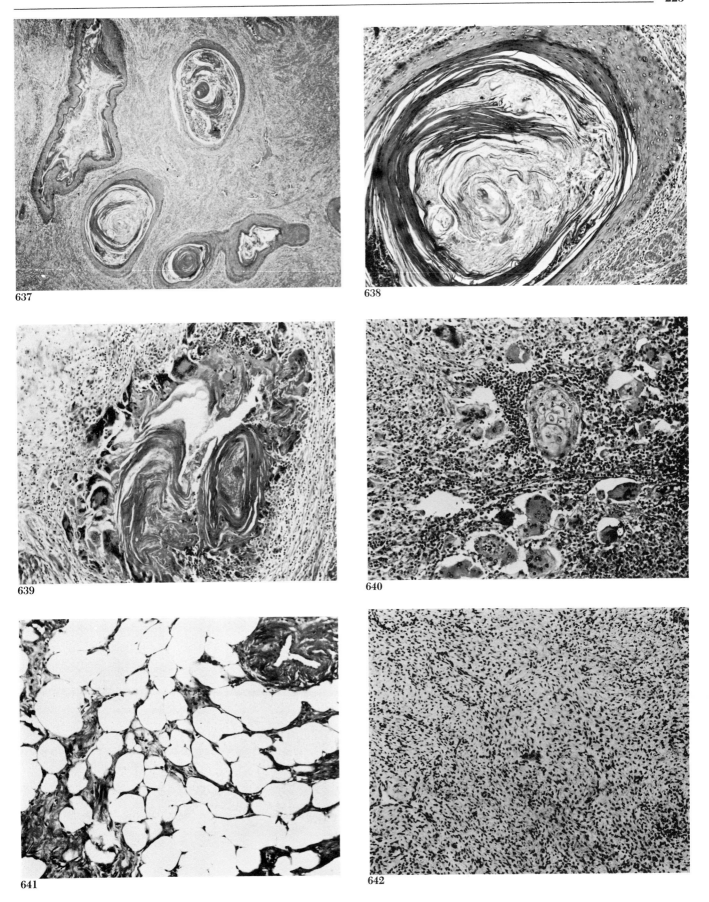

637

638

639

640

641

642

643 Lymphangiocystic fibroma of the myometrium

The tumor in the myometrium is composed of connective tissue stroma, cystically dilated vessels and capillaries. There is no sharp demarcation between the uterine wall and the tumor. This neoplasm is benign. (H&E. ×10)

644 Lymphangiocystic fibroma of the myometrium

High magnification of Fig. 643. The elongated lymphatic vessel is lined by flat endothelial cells and surrounded by tumor cells. Elongated cells of fibrous connective tissue with an irregular growth pattern are seen. The nuclei are hyperchromatic, and there is absence of mitotic activity. (H&E. ×60)

645 Lymphangiocystic fibroma of the myometrium

Another variety of lymphangiocystic fibroma is composed of several large, some cystically dilated, lymphatic vessels surrounded by myriads of small spaces containing irregular cells. The intervening connective tissue stroma shows hyalinization. (H&E. ×50)

646 Lymphangiocystic fibroma of the myometrium

High magnification of Fig. 645. Numerous small spaces reminiscent of vascular structures containing cells with irregular hyperchromatic nuclei surround a lymphatic vessel. The intervening connective tissue stroma is hyalinized. (H&E. ×180)

647 Lymphangiocystic fibroma of the myometrium

This is a third variety of lymphangiocystic fibroma with extensive hyalinization of intervening connective tissue stroma. Occasionally interspersed giant cells may be encountered. (H&E. ×50)

648 Lymphangiocystic fibroma of the myometrium

High magnification of Fig. 647. (H&E. ×150)

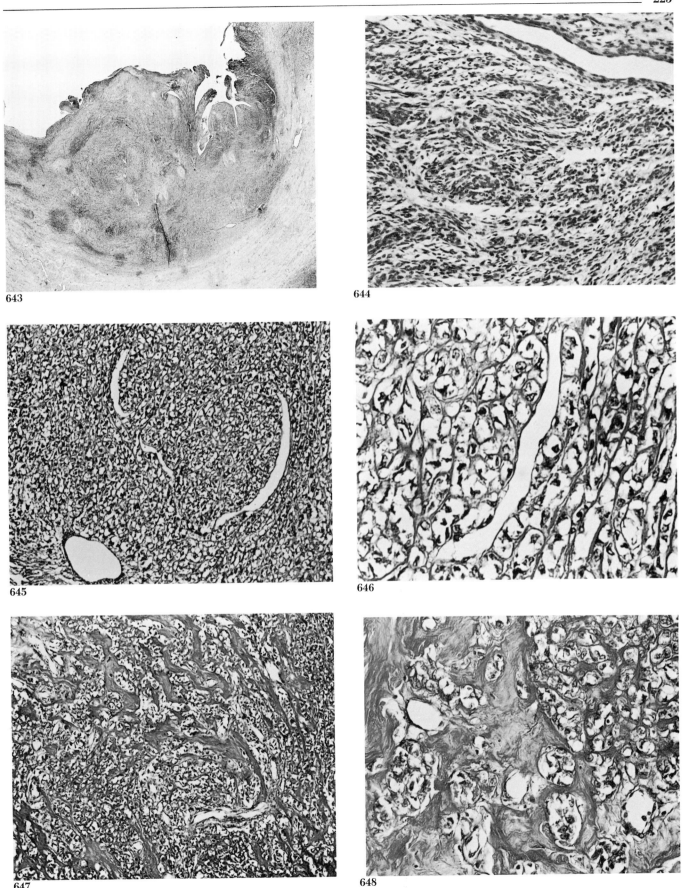

643

644

645

646

647

648

649   Adenomatoid tumor of the uterus
The tumor is developing in the subserosa and extending into the myometrium. Glandlike structures are numerous, and the stroma is fibromuscular. (H&E. ×30)

650   Adenomatoid tumor of the uterus
High magnification of Fig. 649. Numerous glandlike spaces lined by cuboidal epithelial cells have a pronounced eosinophilic cytoplasm and prominent round-to-ovoid hyperchromatic nuclei. Mucin-positive material may be encountered in the glandlike spaces. Intervening fibromuscular stroma is infiltrated with lymphocytes. (H&E. ×120)

651   Adenomatoid tumor of the uterus
High magnification of Fig. 650. This benign tumor arises from Müllerian vestiges. (H&E. ×220)

652   Stromal endometriosis
An island of endometrial stromal cells is seen within the myometrium. Claud W. Taylor's definition of this condition is the best contemporary view. Stromal endometriosis is like adenomyosis in that "it probably arises and grows out from the stroma of the endometrium. It is unlike adenomyosis in its method of propagation because it grows in solid cords beside or within the vessels throughout the uterus and into the surrounding structures and is therefore more like a neoplasm." (Magnus Haimes and Claud W. Taylor, Nature of Stromal Endometriosis in "Gynaecological Pathology," p. 169, Little, Brown and Company, Boston, 1962.) (H&E. ×50)

653   Stromal endometriosis
In 80 per cent of cases the clinical course of stromal endometriosis is benign. In 20 per cent there are recurrences. Even visible spread at operation does not necessarily mean a hopeless prognosis. Here, endometrial stromal cells infiltrate the myometrium and propagate along elongated lymphatic channels. (H&E. ×50)

654   Stromal endometriosis
High magnification of Fig. 653. Spindle-shaped endometrial stromal cells with oval hyperchromatic nuclei, in part, infiltrate myometrial connective tissue and, in part, merge with muscle fibers. (H&E. ×100)

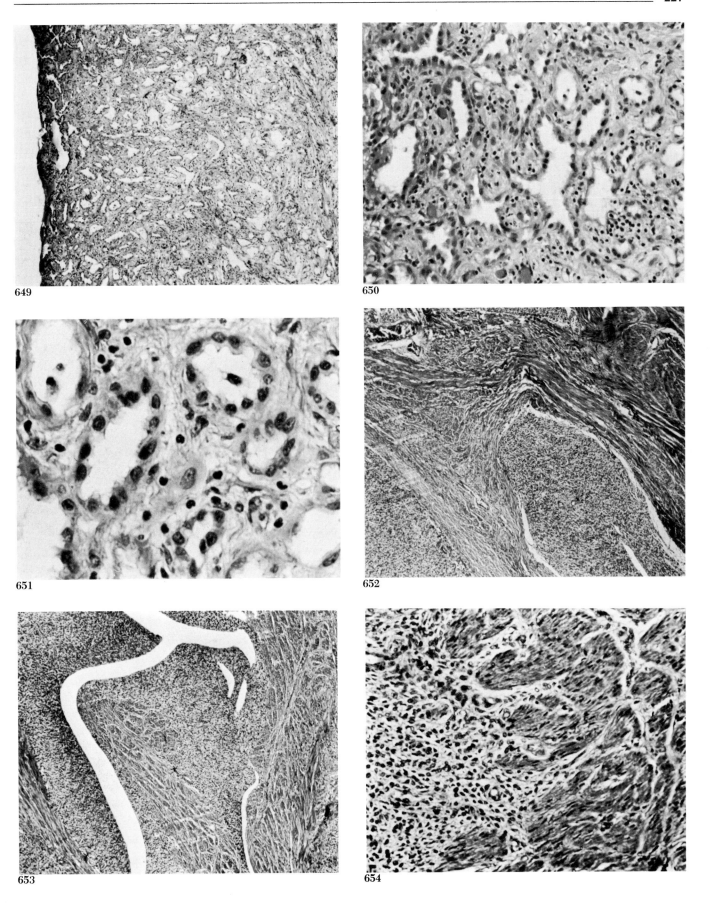

649

650

651

652

653

654

655   Stromal endometriosis
High magnification of Fig. 653. There is relative uniformity of the cellular and nuclear pattern. Mitoses are absent or exceedingly rare. (H&E. ×100)

656   Stromal endometriosis
There is perivascular growth of endometrial stromal cells with a tumor island within the lymphatic lumen and profound infiltration of the myometrium by tumor cells. (H&E. ×120)

657   Submucous leiomyoma of the uterus
The endometrial mucosa is encroached upon by a solid tumor composed of smooth muscle fibers arranged in whorls and interlacing bundles. The endometrial glands appear compressed. (H&E. ×40)

658   Submucous leiomyoma of the uterus
High magnification of Fig. 657. The tumor is formed by elongated smooth muscle cells which are uniform in size and shape. Cut across longitudinally the nuclei appear long and slender, with prominent nucleoli. No abnormal mitotic figures are seen. (H&E. ×150)

659   Cellular leiomyoma of the myometrium
The tumor is formed by a dense aggregation of smooth muscle fibers with a conspicuous decrease of connective tissue elements. The nuclei appear round in cross section. The cells are elongated and fusiform. (H&E. ×90)

660   Cellular leiomyoma of the myometrium
High magnification of Fig. 659. The tumor cells are uniform in size and shape, and mitotic figures are absent. Nuclear hyperchromatism is marked. Dense cellularity is the striking picture of this benign tumor. The fascicular structure is preserved. Such tumors are occasionally misinterpreted as sarcoma. (H&E. ×180)

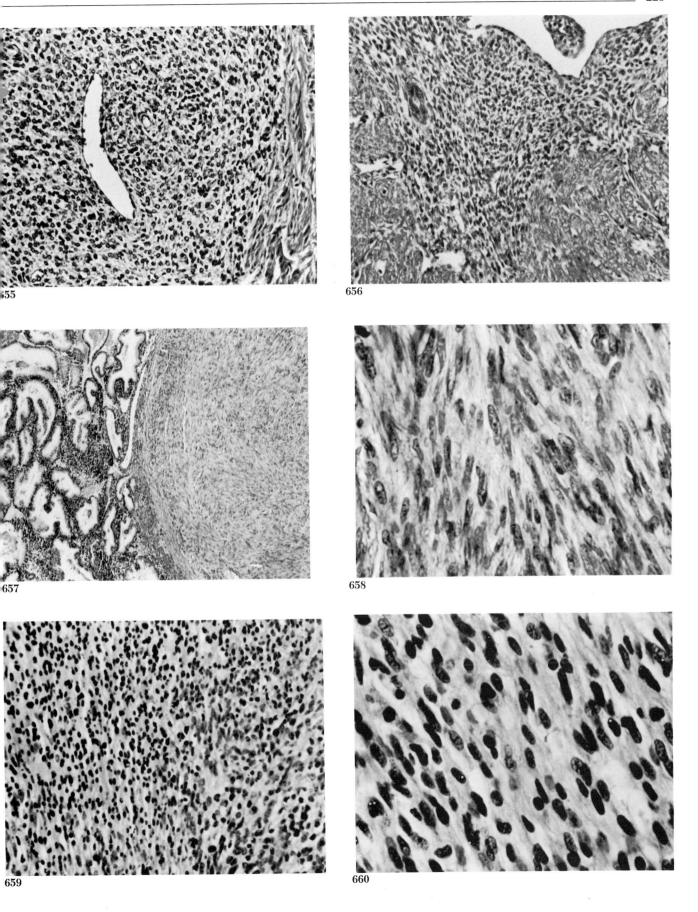

655

656

657

658

659

660

661 Rhythmic nuclear pattern in leiomyoma of the uterus
The leiomyoma is formed by parallel dark and light bands of muscle fibers. (H&E. ×50)

662 Rhythmic nuclear pattern in leiomyoma of the uterus
High magnification of Fig. 661. The dark bands are formed by palisading of the nuclei. (H&E. ×150)

663 Serpentinous leiomyoma of the myometrium
The leiomyoma of the uterus shows a serpentinous arrangement of nuclei of smooth muscle fibers. The nuclei have assumed a snake-like configuration forming giant rosettes. (H&E. ×50)

664 Serpentinous leiomyoma of the myometrium
High magnification of Fig. 663. (H&E. ×140)

665 Intravascular leiomyoma (intravenous leiomyomatosis) of the uterus
The lumen of the dilated myometrial vein contains a tumor formed by smooth muscle fibers. This benign neoplasm either may originate within the blood vessel or it may represent intravascular extension of a myometrial leiomyoma. (H&E. ×15)

666 Intravascular leiomyoma (intravenous leiomyomatosis) of the uterus
High magnification of Fig. 665. Verhoeff's elastic stain outlines the vessel and intravascular position of the leiomyoma. (×25)

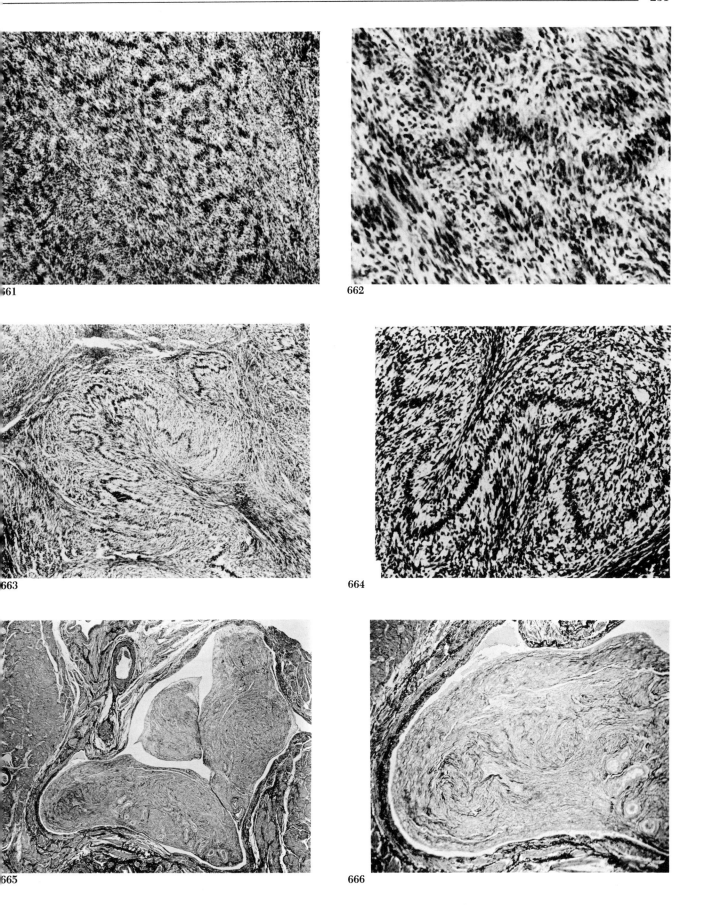

561

662

663

664

665

666

667 Angiomyoma of the myometrium
The tumor is formed by whorls of smooth muscle fibers concentrically arranged around small and large vascular channels. (H&E. ×100)

668 Leiomyoma of the myometrium with early hyaline degeneration
There is hyaline degeneration of tumorous muscle fibers. (H&E. ×50)

669 Leiomyoma of the myometrium with advanced hyaline degeneration
The structureless hyaline tissue is seen replacing tumorous muscle bundles and whorls. (H&E. ×150)

670 Leiomyoma of the myometrium with hyaline degeneration
Note the massive hyaline degeneration with scattered residual islands of smooth muscle cells. (H&E. ×50)

671 Leiomyoma of the myometrium with hyaline degeneration
Here predominantly perivascular hyaline degeneration is seen with atrophic changes of leiomyoma. (H&E. ×120)

672 Leiomyoma of the myometrium with edema
Note the interstitial edema occurring in leiomyoma. (H&E. ×90)

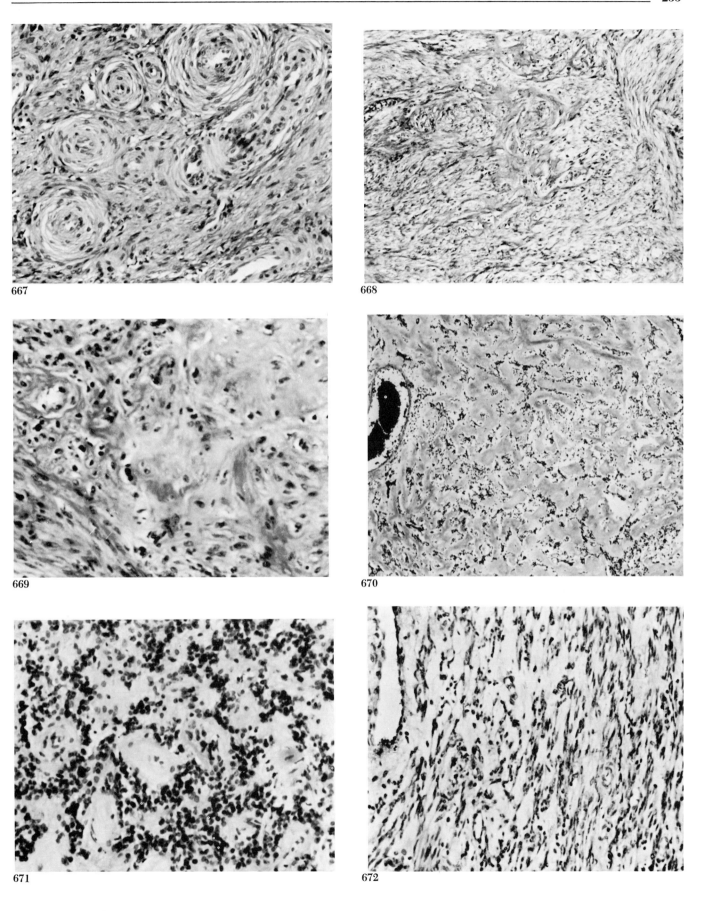

667

668

669

670

671

672

673 Leiomyoma of the myometrium with extensive edema

There is separation of tumorous muscle bundles by extensive interstitial edema. (H&E. ×65)

674 Leiomyoma of the myometrium with cystic degeneration

Cystic spaces are seen occurring in a degenerating leiomyoma. The cyst wall shows either hyaline degeneration or liquefaction necrosis. No epithelial lining is encountered. (H&E. ×50)

675 Leiomyoma of the myometrium with fatty degeneration

Single and clusters of mature fat cells are seen in the areas of antecedent degeneration of leiomyoma. (H&E. ×50)

676 Leiomyoma of the myometrium with necrosis

The area of extensive necrosis lacks stained nuclei. The margin of necrotic area shows proliferation of capillaries and fibroblasts. (H&E. ×120)

677 Leiomyoma of the myometrium with calcification

Areas of extensive hyaline degeneration are intermingled with areas of necrosis. There is scattered deposition of calcium. Ossification may occur in calcified areas. (H&E. ×50)

678 Atypical myometrial cells in early degeneration of leiomyoma

Degenerative changes in leiomyoma may precede nuclear enlargement, clumping, and hyperchromatism. (H&E. ×100)

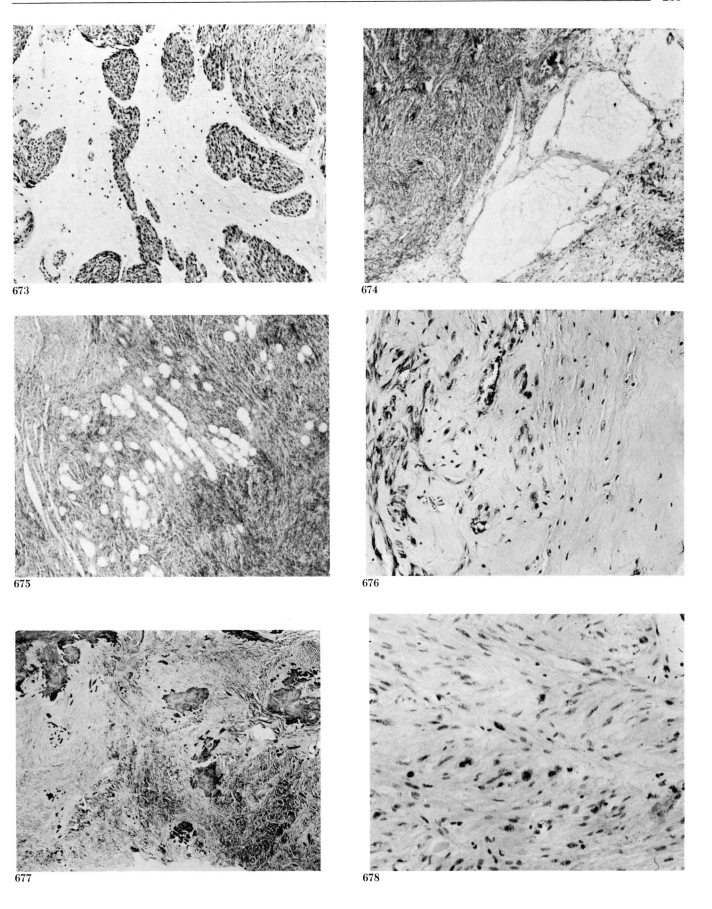

673

674

675

676

677

678

679 Degeneration and clumping of nuclei in leiomyoma simulating leiomyosarcoma
Nuclear degeneration and clumping surrounded by focal hyaline degeneration of muscle fibers is frequently misinterpreted as leiomyosarcoma. Note the absence of mitoses. (H&E. ×120)

680 Degeneration and clumping of nuclei in leiomyoma simulating leiomyosarcoma
Clumping of nuclei is occasionally misinterpreted as sarcomatous giant cells. Bizarre hyperchromatic nuclei, nuclear clumping, and variation in the size of nuclei are sometimes encountered with various degenerative changes in leiomyomas. (H&E. ×120)

681 Pseudosarcoma or pseudopregnancy changes in leiomyoma following norethindrone therapy
This pseudosarcomatous alteration was seen in the uterine leiomyoma of a 49-year-old patient treated with norethindrone in doses ranging from 30 to 60 mg a day over a period of 14 months. Norethindrone (Norlutin, norethisterone, 17 alpha-ethinyl-19-nortestosterone) is a progestational agent. (H&E. ×120)

682 Pseudosarcoma or pseudopregnancy changes in leiomyoma following norethindrone therapy
High magnification of Fig. 681. This excessively cellular tumor has large, bizarre, and hyperchromatic nuclei and rare mitoses. Caution is stressed in the interpretation of such findings to avoid possible confusion with a malignant tumor. (H&E. ×450)

683 Leiomyosarcoma developing in a leiomyoma of the myometrium
There is persistence of some muscle bundle pattern. The pleomorphic character of the cells is striking. Nuclear hyperchromatism, numerous atypical mitoses, and absence of intervening connective tissue stroma are important criteria in establishing a diagnosis. (H&E. ×90)

684 Leiomyosarcoma developing in a leiomyoma of the myometrium
High magnification of Fig. 683. This tumor is highly cellular. There is decrease or absence of intervening connective tissue and pronounced cellular pleomorphism. Masson's trichrome stain is very useful in demonstrating the smooth muscle origin of the tumor. (H&E. ×360)

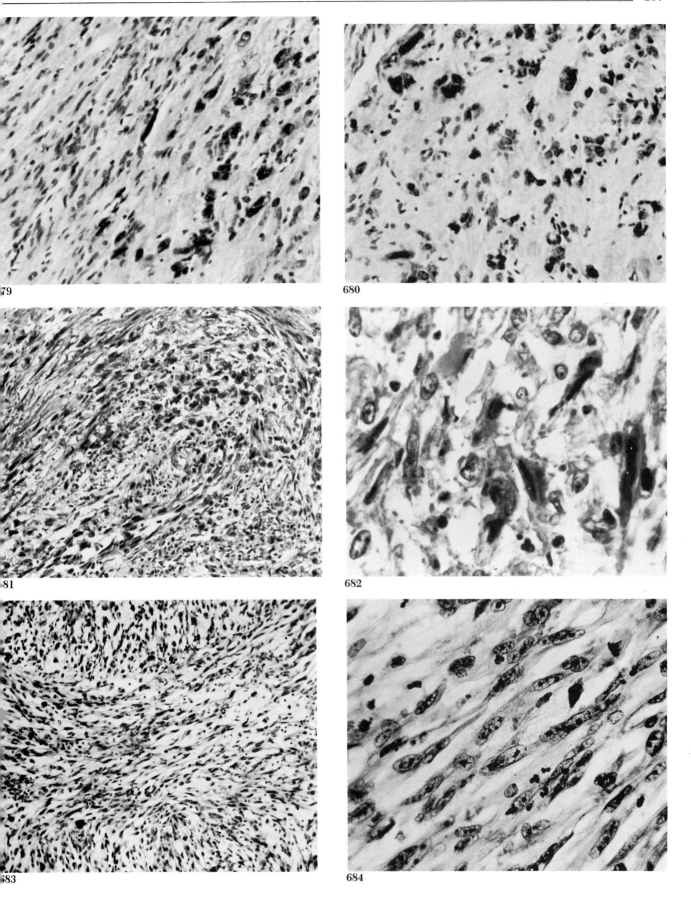

679

680

681

682

683

684

685 Leiomyosarcoma developing in a leiomyoma of the myometrium

Pleomorphism of the cells is striking. Atypical mitoses are frequent. Some preservation of muscle bundles indicates development in an antecedent leiomyoma. Differential diagnostic difficulties arise usually between leiomyosarcoma and cellular leiomyoma and between leiomyosarcoma and degenerative changes taking place in a leiomyoma. Examination of many blocks of tissue is mandatory. (H&E. ×100)

686 Leiomyosarcoma (mural sarcoma) of the myometrium

The leiomyosarcoma is developing in the myometrium without demonstrable origin from a leiomyoma. There is no evidence of a fascicular pattern. Diffuse overgrowth by pleomorphic neoplastic cells is seen. (H&E. ×180)

687 Fibrosarcoma (mural sarcoma) of the myometrium

The fibrosarcoma is developing from fibrous connective tissue elements of the myometrium without an antecedent leiomyoma. The tumor is composed of spindle cells with slight pleomorphism of nuclei. Atypical mitotic figures are interspersed. (H&E. ×100)

688 Pleomorphic sarcoma (mural sarcoma) of the myometrium

The tumor is formed by anaplastic, pleomorphic giant cells. Atypical mitoses are frequent. (H&E ×80)

689 Hemangioendotheliosarcoma of the myometrium

The tumor is formed by large and small vascular spaces and areas of hemorrhages. (H&E. ×20)

690 Hemangioendotheliosarcoma of the myometrium

High magnification of Fig. 689. The tumor is formed by atypical vascular channels and capillaries with a tendency to anastomosis. The vascular spaces are lined by irregular neoplastic endothelial cells (endothelioblasts) with elongated hyperchromatic nuclei. (H&E. ×50)

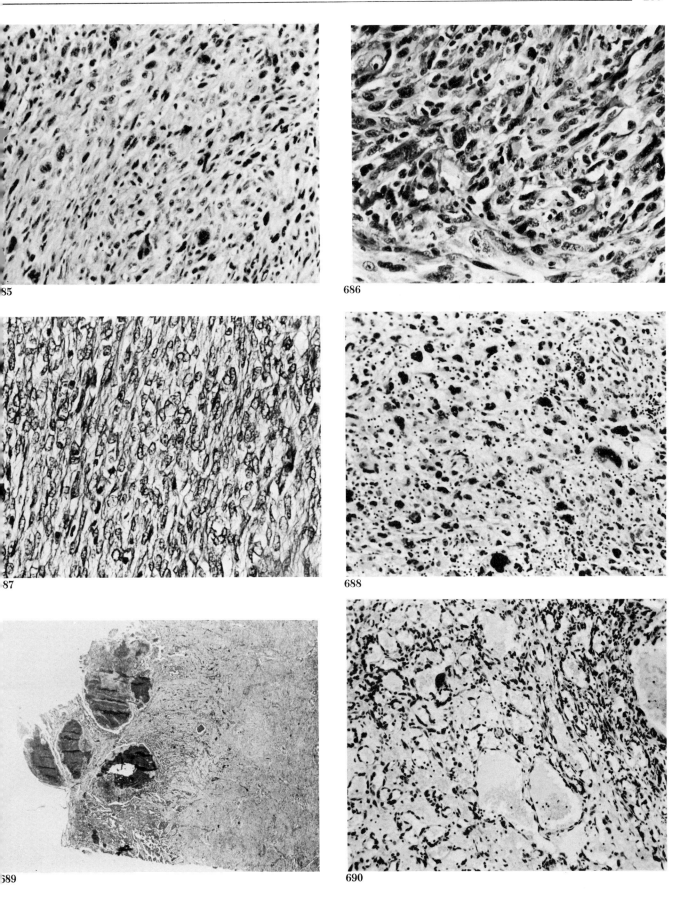

685

686

687

688

689

690

691 Hemangioendotheliosarcoma of the myometrium
The proliferation of neoplastic endothelial cells causes filling of the vascular lumens. (H&E. ×50)

692 Endometrial stromal sarcoma developing in a heterotopic endometrial island of adenomyosis (adenomyosis sarcomatosa)
To the right, an area of adenomyosis with development of an endometrial stromal sarcoma is seen. To the left, several islands of adenomyosis are seen. (H&E. ×25)

693 Adenocarcinoma arising in a heterotopic endometrial island of adenomyosis (adenomyosis carcinomatosa)
The carcinoma is developing in the epithelium of several areas of adenomyosis. Remnants of endometrial stromal cells are seen. (H&E. ×65)

694 Adenocarcinoma arising in a heterotopic endometrial island of adenomyosis (adenomyosis carcinomatosa)
High magnification of Fig. 693. (H&E. ×150)

695 Mesonephric carcinoma of the myometrium
The tumor is developing from vestiges of mesonephric duct. The ductal structure is lined by cuboidal epithelium with cytoplasmic vacuolization. (H&E. ×200)

696 Mesonephric carcinoma of the myometrium
There is diffuse infiltration of the lateral uterine wall by a tumor composed of clear cells. The neoplastic cells show marked vacuolization of cytoplasm and large ovoid hyperchromatic nuclei. Connective tissue stroma is scant. (H&E. ×150)

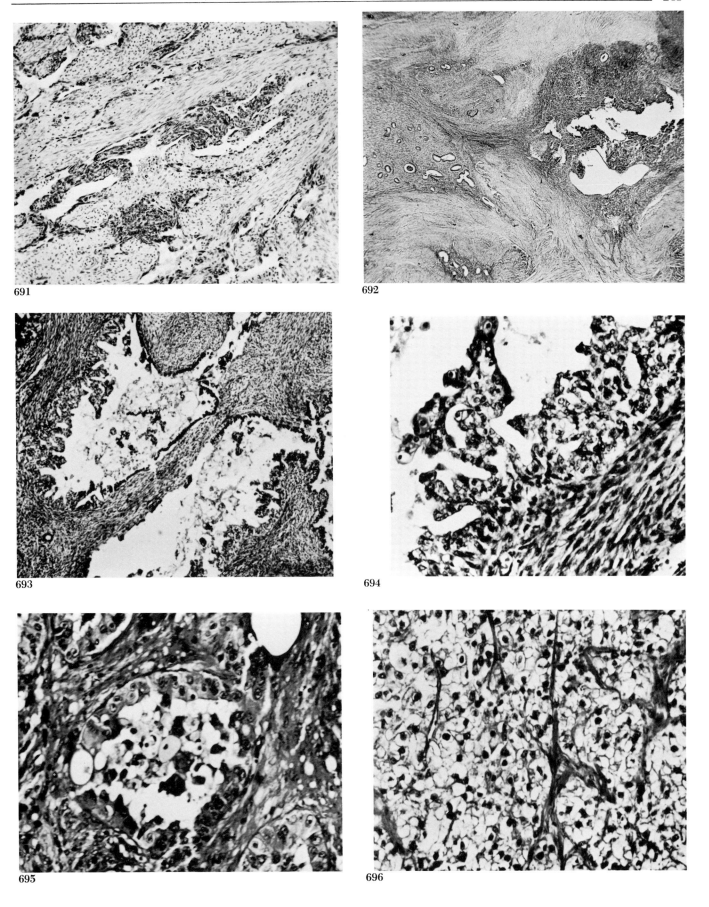

691

692

693

694

695

696

697 Mesonephric tumor of the myometrium
There is a circumscribed aggregation of tubular structures, originating from mesonephric duct rests, in the myometrium. The finding of a tumor 3 mm in diameter in the lateral uterine wall was incidental. (H&E. ×80)

698 Mesonephric tumor of the myometrium
High magnification of Fig. 697. Tubular structures with a prominent basement membrane are lined by columnar epithelium with elongated hyperchromatic nuclei. (H&E. ×150)

699 Mesonephric tumor of the myometrium
The lymphatic vessel in the vicinity of the tumor shown in Figs. 697 and 698 exhibits a tumor island in its lumen. (H&E. ×200)

700 Squamous cell carcinoma of the cervix metastatic to the myometrium
The lymphatic channels of the myometrium are filled with aggregates of exocervical squamous cell carcinoma. (H&E. ×90)

701 Carcinoma of the ovary metastatic to the myometrium
Retrograde lymphatic metastases are seen in the uterine wall. The dilated lymphatic channels of the myometrium contain cells of ovarian carcinoma. (H&E. ×65)

702 Malignant melanoma of the skin metastatic to the myometrium
Metastatic, pigment-containing malignant melanoma cells form an island in the myometrium. (H&E. ×50)

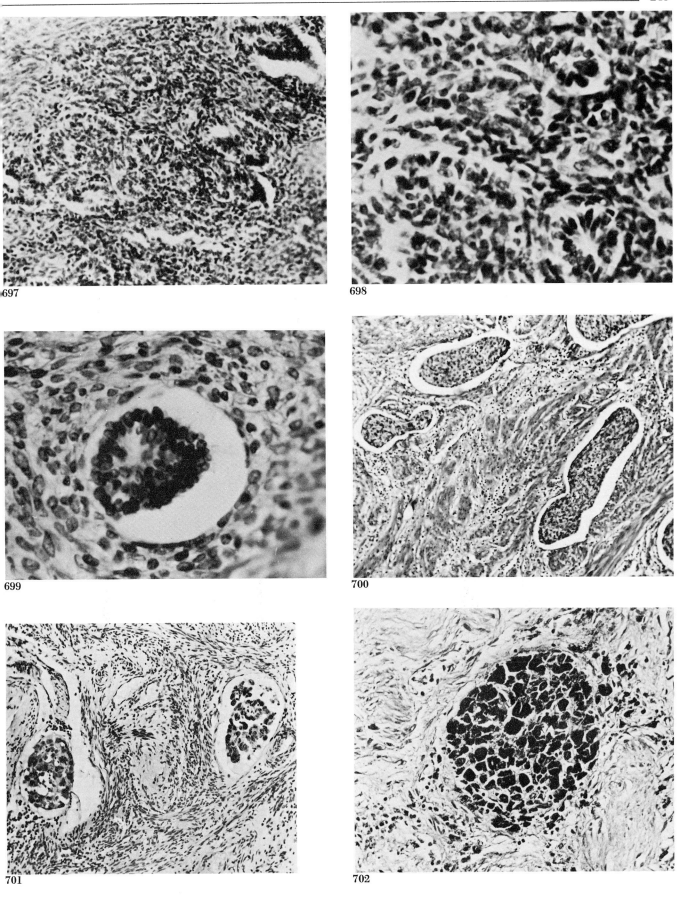

697

698

699

700

701

702

COLOR PLATES
Chapter 5
Diseases of the Myometrium
Plates 10 and 11

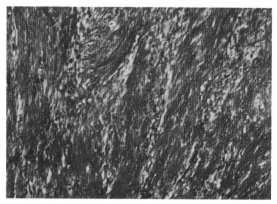

55 Myometrium during the reproductive age During reproductive age, 27.9 ± 3.7 per cent of the corpus uteri consists of smooth muscle fibers. The remainder consists of connective tissue and vessels. (Specht's trichrome stain. ×120)

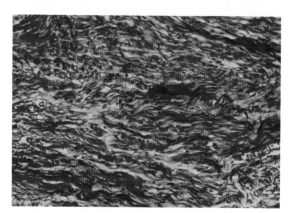

56 Myometrium after the menopause After the menopause, on the average 11.0 ± 1.5 per cent of the corpus uteri consists of smooth muscle fibers. (Specht's trichrome stain. ×120)

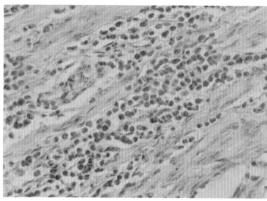

57 Eosinophilia of the myometrium Diffuse infiltration of the myometrium with eosinophilic leukocytes is seen. The cause is undetermined. (H&E. ×100)

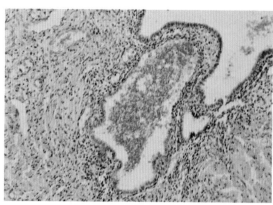

58 Adenomyosis during menstruation Glands of a heterotopic endometrial island in adenomyosis are filled with erythrocytes. The surrounding connective tissue stroma shows focal areas of recent hemorrhages. (H&E. ×50)

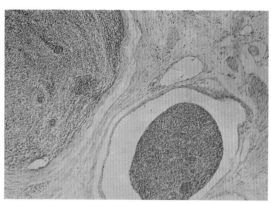

59 Stromal endometriosis Islands of endometrial stromal cells without glands permeate the myometrium and appear within lymphatic channels. (H&E. ×80)

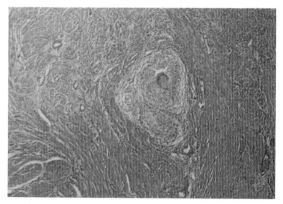

60 Tuberculous myometritis The myometrium contains a granuloma formed by epithelioid cells and a Langhans' giant cell. There is mild peripheral infiltration with lymphocytes. Sources of myometrial infection can be from endometrium and oviduct or hematogenous spread from an extragenital focus. (H&E. ×50)

Plate 10

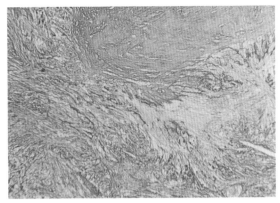

61 Leiomyoma with hyaline degeneration Hyaline is a translucent, homogeneous, structureless protein formed from connective tissue. (Mallory's connective tissue stain. ×50)

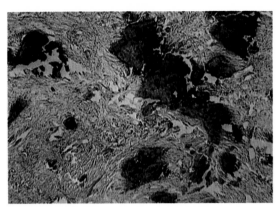

62 Leiomyoma with calcification (H&E. ×50)

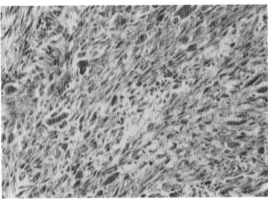

63 Leiomyosarcoma developing in a preexisting leiomyoma Smooth muscle cells show fasciculation and the presence of numerous pleomorphic cells. Mitotic activity is increased, an important diagnostic finding. Muscle fibers are red, collagen is blue. (Masson's trichrome stain. ×62)

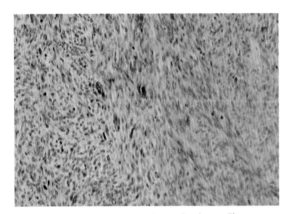

64 Leiomyosarcoma metastatic to the lung Three years prior the patient underwent hysterectomy for multiple uterine cellular leiomyomas, and a leiomyosarcoma was missed. The metastatic tumor shows distinct fasciculation. Atypical cells with hyperchromatic nuclei are present. Excessive cellularity and the absence of connective tissue stroma are characteristic findings. (H&E. ×50)

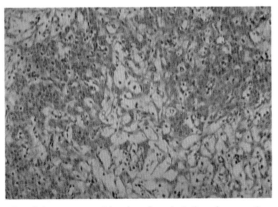

65 Leiomyoma with lymphangiectatic degeneration Marked teleangiectasia and lymphangiectasia are seen. The cystic spaces are lined by endothelium. Some vascular channels contain erythrocytes. Muscle fibers are clearly seen in a diffuse distribution between vascular channels. (H&E. ×100)

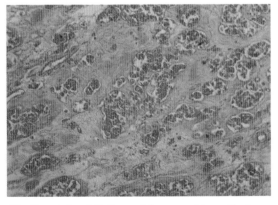

66 Hemangioendothelioma of the myometrium The tumor is formed by proliferating endothelioblasts lining and filling the vascular spaces. (H&E. ×120)

Plate 11

6
Diseases of the Oviduct

703 Cross section of the oviduct, mesosalpinx, and ovary in a 5-month-old fetus
The arrow indicates development of Walthard's cell rest from tubal serosa. Invagination of peritoneum is evident. (High magnification in right lower quadrant.) Mesonephric tubules are well developed in the mesosalpinx. (H&E. ×12 and ×120)

704 Endosalpinx of a 10-year-old girl
There is marked cellular crowding. Differentiation of cells is rather poor. Nonciliated or secretory cells are sparse but evident. (H&E. ×150)

705 Normal oviduct: (a) isthmic portion, (b) uterine interstitial portion
(H&E. ×8)

706 Ampullary portion of a normal oviduct with folds of endosalpinx
(H&E. ×8)

707 Resting epithelium of the endosalpinx in a woman of reproductive age
There are numerous columnar ciliated cells with pale-staining cytoplasm and round nuclei in the midcell position. The cilia project from free cellular borders. This is the estrogenic phase of the cycle. (H&E. ×125)

708 Secreting epithelium of the endosalpinx in a woman of reproductive age
There is an increased number of columnar, secretory, nonciliated cells with extrusion of secretions. Conglomeration of cilia. Slender, intercalated (peg) cells are seen extruding nuclei. Secretory cells have clear cytoplasm and round, dark-staining nuclei. This is the progestational phase of cycle. (H&E. ×125)

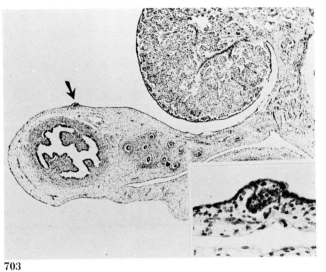

703

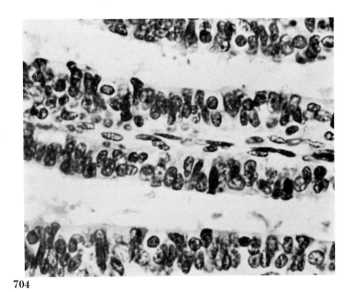

704

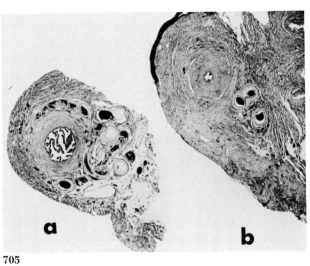

705

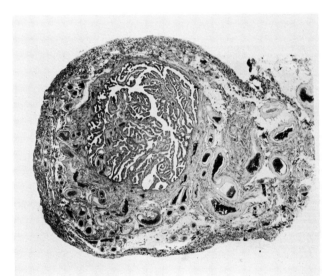

706

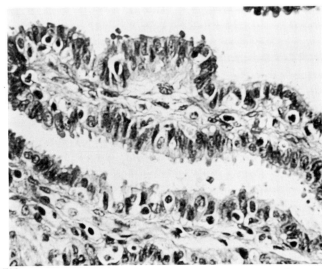

707

708

709 Hypoplasia of the endosalpinx in Turner's syndrome
Poorly developed, thin, slender folds of endosalpinx with inactive epithelium composed of
cuboidal cells are visible. Two types of cells are
present. (H&E. ×75)

710 Postmenopausal subatrophy of the endo-salpinx
The epithelial cells are cuboidal to flat. There is
disappearance of cilia. The epithelium is inactive. (H&E. ×125)

711 Senile atrophy of the endosalpinx
Flat, atrophic epithelial cells line the hyalinized
connective tissue stroma. (H&E. ×100)

712 Squamous metaplasia of the endosalpinx
Columnar epithelium is replaced by stratified
squamous epithelium. (H&E. ×50)

713 Squamous metaplasia in the fimbriated folds of the infundibulum of the endosal-pinx
(H&E. ×60)

714 Thrombosis of the myosalpinx with organi-zation
Partial thrombosis of a vein in the outer longitudinal muscle layer is seen. (H&E. ×50)

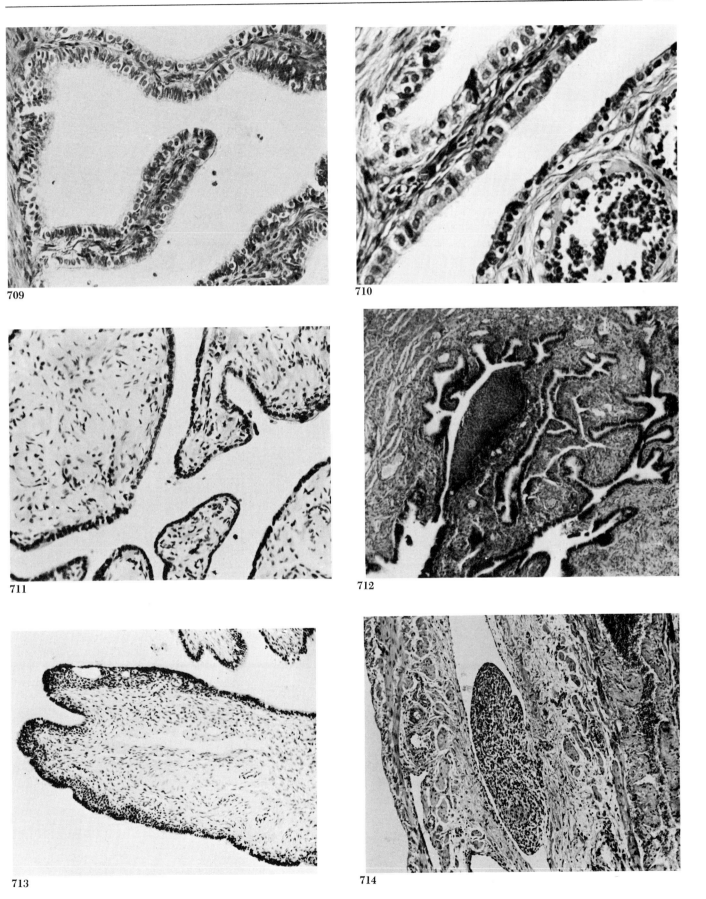

709

710

711

712

713

714

715   Marked ectasia of the interstitial vessels of the endosalpinx
Marked telangiectasis of the interstitial vessels of the endosalpinx is seen. This is observed in ectopic tubal pregnancy or in neoplasms of the oviduct. (H&E. ×50)

716   Peritoneal inclusion cyst of the oviduct
The cyst is lined by mesothelial cells. A small amount of serous transudate is present within the cyst. The cyst is located within the wall of the oviduct. It is necessary to differentiate this cyst from a mesonephric cyst. (H&E. ×80)

717   Accessory oviduct
This is a developmental anomaly of Müllerian duct system. (H&E. ×10)

718   Walthard cell rest in subserosa of an oviduct in a 9-month-old fetus
There is an accumulation of cuboidal cells with prominent round nuclei in the subserosa of the oviduct. (H&E. ×100)

719   Walthard cell rest in subserosa of an oviduct in a 14-year-old girl
The origin of the Walthard cell rest is most likely from invagination of tubal peritoneum. This is an endophytic type of growth. There is early cystic alteration of the central area. (H&E. ×70)

720   Walthard cell rest of the endosalpinx in a 38-year-old woman
A solid Walthard cell rest is present in the connective tissue stroma of the endosalpinx. (H&E. ×80)

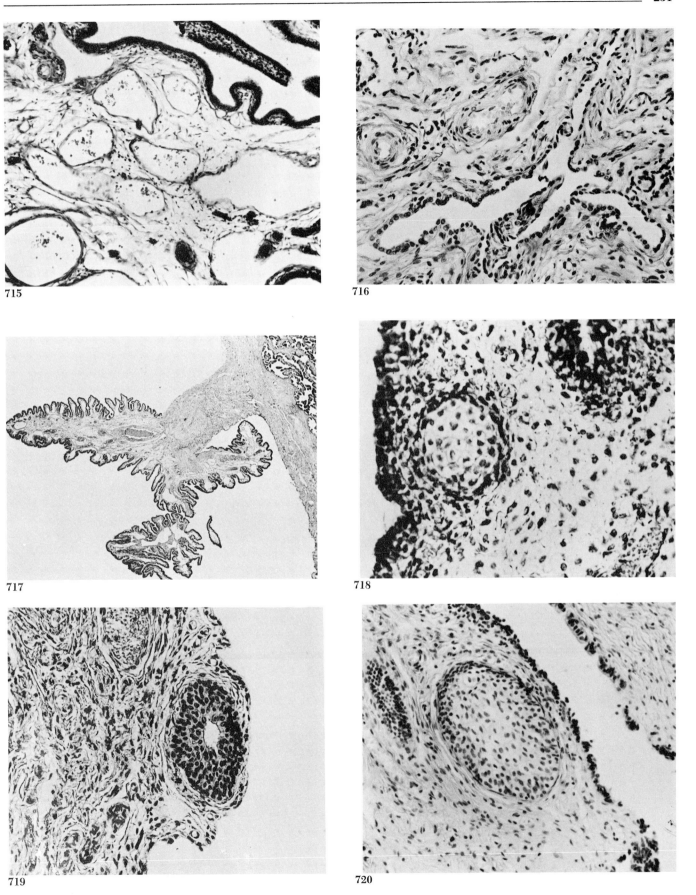

715

716

717

718

719

720

721 Walthard cell rests in subserosa of an oviduct of a 42-year-old woman
Cystic and solid Walthard cell rests are present in the subserosa of the oviduct. (H&E. ×150)

722 Cystic Walthard cell rest in subserosa of an oviduct in a woman of reproductive age
Exophytic type of growth of a subserosal cystic Walthard cell rest is seen. (H&E. ×20)

723 Early lipid storage of the endosalpinx
Clusters of epithelial cells are markedly enlarged by stored lipid material. Apparently the epithelial cells of the endosalpinx have the ability of phagocytizing and storing lipid. The connective tissue stroma is free of inflammatory cells. (H&E. ×180)

724 Advanced lipid storage of the endosalpinx
The lipid stored in columnar epithelial cells of the endosalpinx is probably derived from tubal lumen. Such storage activity or phagocytosis is not associated, as a rule, with inflammatory processes of the endosalpinx. (H&E. ×180)

725 Acute endosalpingitis
There is marked hyperemia and acute inflammatory exudate in the connective tissue stroma of the endosalpinx. Inflammatory cells and desquamated epithelial cells are present in the lumen of the endosalpinx. (H&E. ×125)

726 Pyosalpinx
Destruction of endosalpinx is seen. There is diffuse infiltration of the oviductal wall with acute and chronic inflammatory cells. The lumen of the oviduct is dilated and filled with pus. (H&E. ×25)

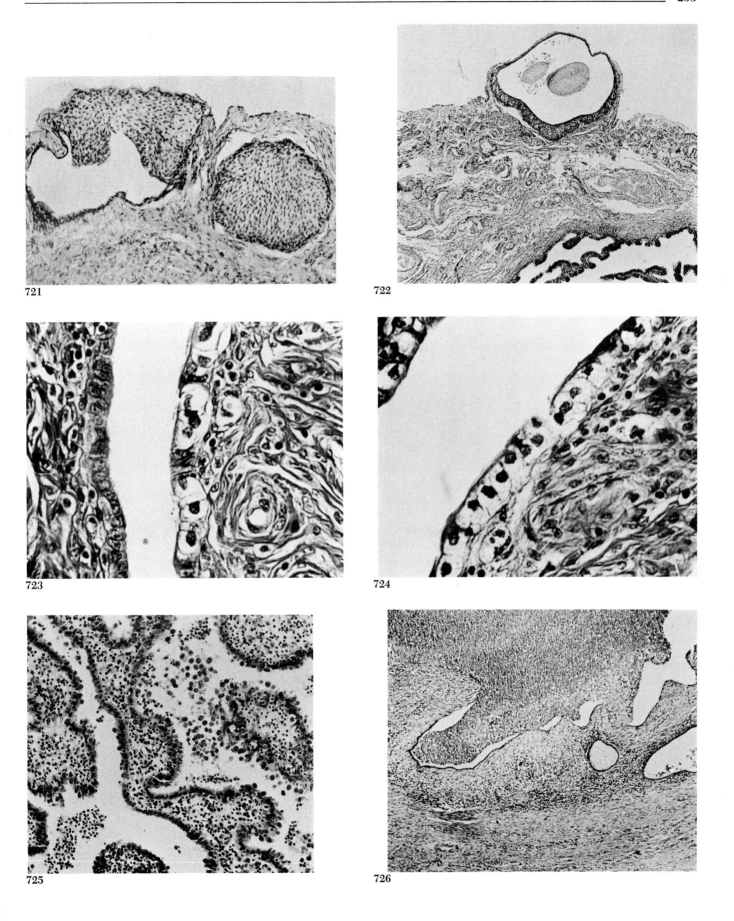

721

722

723

724

725

726

727 Chronic salpingitis
The mucosal folds are adherent, one to the other, forming glandlike spaces. Connective tissue stroma is heavily infiltrated with chronic inflammatory cells. (H&E. ×50)

728 Chronic salpingitis with hemosiderin macrophages
Connective tissue stroma shows large macrophages containing hemosiderin. This is a common finding in hematosalpinx. (H&E. ×200)

729 Granulomatous salpingitis, cause undetermined
The tubal wall shows a granulomatous inflammatory process with numerous foreign-body giant cells, lymphocytes, plasma cells, and polymorphonuclear leukocytes. The cause is undetermined. (H&E. ×125)

730 Healed salpingitis (so-called pseudofollicular salpingitis)
There is complete resolution of inflammatory exudate. The remaining mucosal adhesions form a pseudoglandular or follicular pattern. Such oviductal alterations predispose to ectopic tubal pregnancy. (H&E. ×15)

731 Interstitial and epithelial calcification of the endosalpinx
This condition is occasionally seen in healed salpingitis or in a normal oviduct attached or in proximity to a papillary serous cystadenocarcinoma of the ovary. (H&E. ×50)

732 Hydrosalpinx
There is extensive dilatation of the oviductal lumen. The endosalpinx is distended and atrophic, showing minute residual mucosal folds. The wall of the oviduct is thin and overstretched. (H&E. ×5)

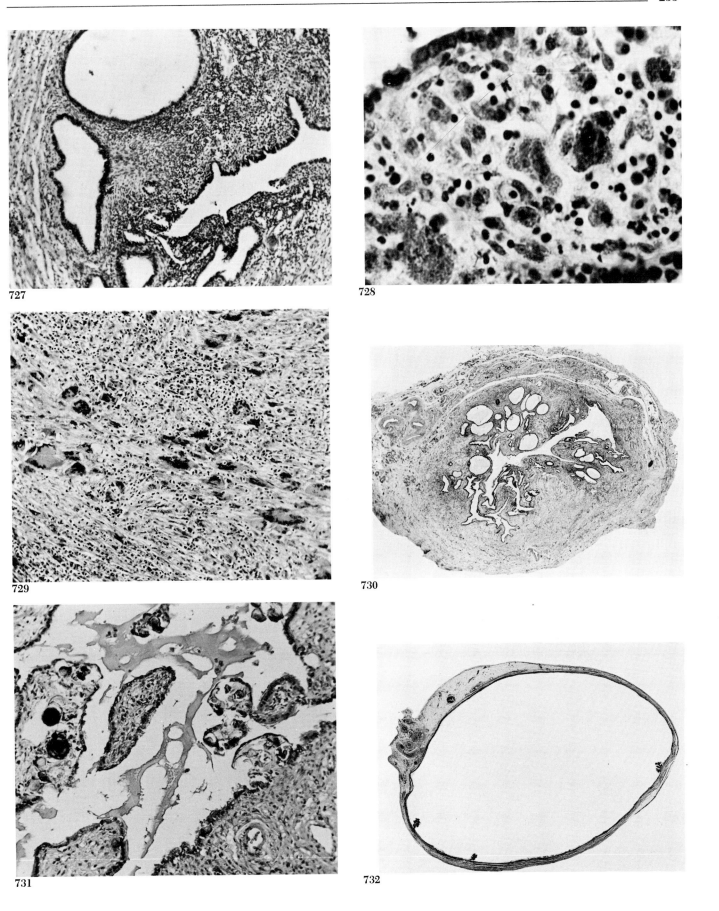

727

728

729

730

731

732

733 Hydrosalpinx with residual mucosal folds
(H&E. ×25)

734 Pseudoxanthomatous salpingitis following Lipiodol salpingography
The adherent mucosal folds form pseudocysts. The interstitial connective tissue stroma is infiltrated with acute and chronic inflammatory cells and numerous lipid macrophages. Lipiodol radiopaque contrast medium is used for hysterosalpingography. Lipiodol is a fatty acid of poppy seed oil containing organically bound iodine. (H&E. ×75)

735 Pseudoxanthomatous salpingitis following Lipiodol salpingography
Numerous histiocytic macrophages, lymphocytes, and plasma cells are seen infiltrating the endosalpinx and oviductal wall. (H&E. ×100)

736 Pseudoxanthomatous salpingitis following Lipiodol salpingography
The cystic spaces contain lipid material and are surrounded by foreign-body giant cells. Note the phagocytized lipid material within the cytoplasm of the giant cells. (H&E. ×180)

737 Chronic perisalpingitis
The peritoneal lining of the oviduct is covered by fibrin and subserosal connective tissue infiltrated by lymphocytes. (H&E. ×62)

738 Histiocytes (macrophages) in the endosalpinx
There is an accumulation of histiocytes in the connective tissue stroma of the oviductal mucosa. Similar cells are observed in endometriosis and endosalpingiosis. The mucosal projections are distended, and the overlying epithelium is flattened. Neutral fatty acids and cholesterol are frequently demonstrable in those macrophages. (H&E. ×125)

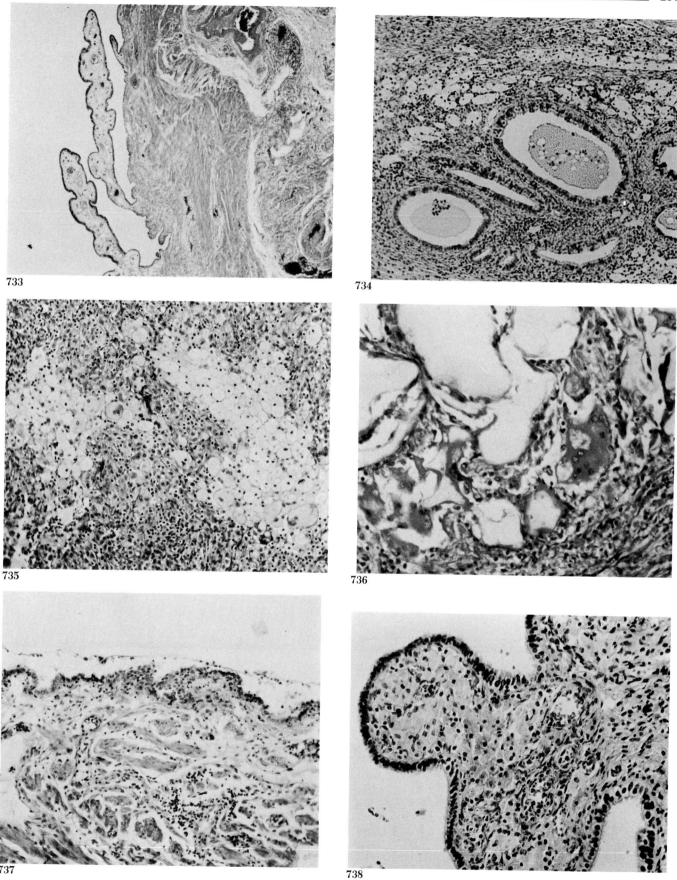

733

734

735

736

737

738

739 Histiocytes (macrophages) in the endosalpinx, forming an interstitial nodule
There is an accumulation of large histiocytes in the connective tissue stroma of the endosalpinx. These cells contain brown pigment granules and are slightly sudanophilic. As a rule, hemosiderin is absent. PAS and Alcian blue substances are detected in the cytoplasm. Chronic inflammation is frequently present. (H&E. ×200)

740 Tuberculous salpingitis
Discrete tuberculous granulomas are seen involving the interstitial stroma of the endosalpinx. (H&E. ×50)

741 Tuberculous salpingitis
The conglomeration of tubercles is formed by epithelioid cells and typical Langhans type of giant cells. There is diffuse infiltration by lymphocytes and plasma cells. Agglutination and adhesions of mucosal folds produce a pseudo-adenomatous pattern, occasionally mistaken for adenocarcinoma. (H&E. ×90)

742 Caseating tuberculous salpingitis
There is extensive caseation necrosis of the endosalpinx and oviductal wall. Ghost tubercles and occasional well-preserved giant cells are noted. Numerous tubercle bacilli are seen in sections stained with Ziehl-Neelsen stain. (H&E. ×18)

743 Enterobius (Oxyuris) vermicularis in the oviduct
The endosalpinx is destroyed by the inflammatory process which forms an abscess around the female pinworm. The oviductal wall is infiltrated by chronic inflammatory cells and shows proliferation of fibroblasts. (H&E. ×50)

744 Enterobius (Oxyuris) vermicularis in the oviduct
High magnification of Fig. 743. A cross section of a gravid female pinworm is seen. The migration of the gravid female worm was from the anus via the vagina and uterine cavity to the oviduct. There is an acute inflammatory reaction around the worm with numerous eggs. (H&E. ×200)

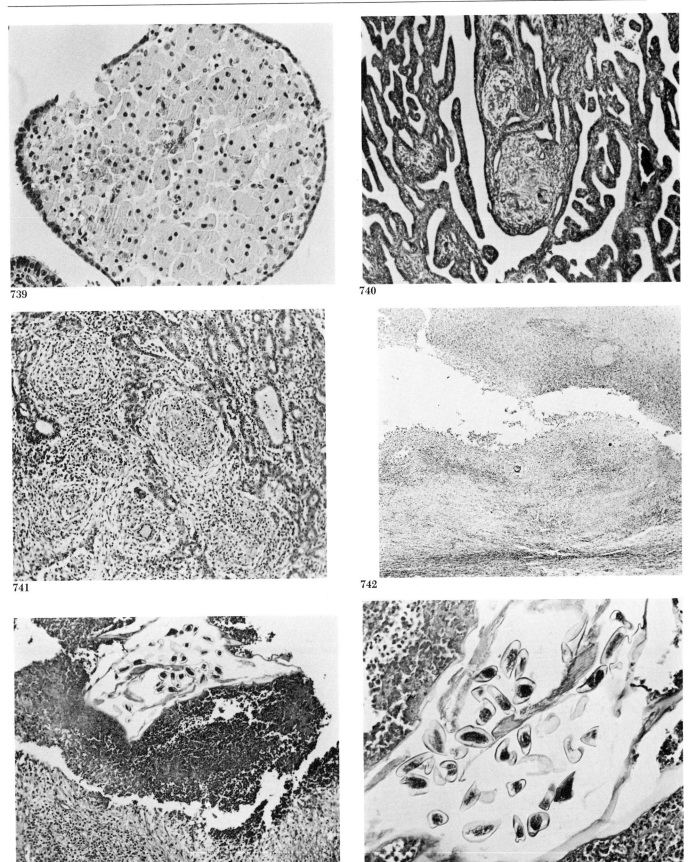

739

740

741

742

743

744

745   Endometrial extension into the interstitial portion of the oviduct
(H&E. ×35)

746   Endometriosis of the endosalpinx
The oviductal mucosa is replaced by islands of endometrium composed of glands and endometrial stromal cells. (H&E. ×20)

747   Endosalpingiosis of the oviduct
The wall of the isthmic portion of an oviduct is infiltrated with cystlike structures lined by a tubal type of epithelium. (H&E. ×8)

748   Endosalpingiosis of the oviduct
Vestigial remains of tubal lumen are seen. The wall of the oviduct contains numerous foci of misplaced tubal mucosa forming glandlike structures. Some are cystically dilated. Serial sections demonstrate continuity between the lumen of the endosalpinx and glandlike structures in the oviductal wall. (H&E. ×15)

749   Endosalpingiosis of the oviduct, longitudinal section
The wall of an enlarged oviduct is diffusely infiltrated with glandlike structures lined by typical tubal mucosa. The inflammatory origin of so-called salpingitis isthmica nodosa is untenable in the light of present knowledge. Consequently, the term "salpingitis isthmica nodosa" is inappropriate and this morphological alteration should be called endosalpingiosis. (H&E. ×10)

750   Endosalpingiosis of the oviduct
High magnification of Fig. 749. Glandlike structures are lined by columnar epithelium with three types of cells, namely: ciliated, nonciliated or secretory, and intercalated (peg) cells. (H&E. ×50 and ×120)

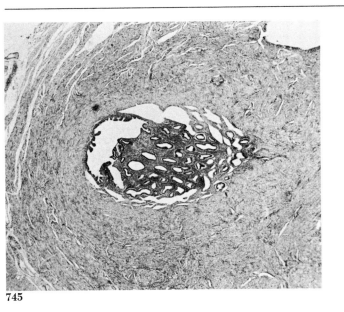

745

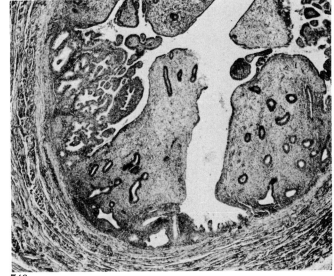

746

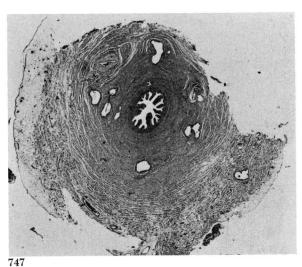

747

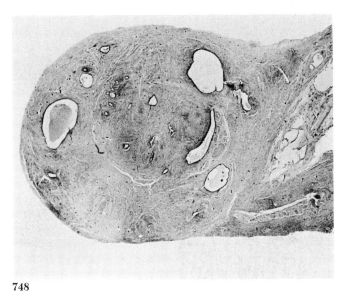

748

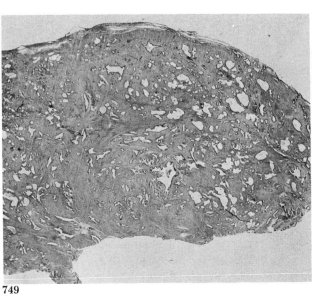

749

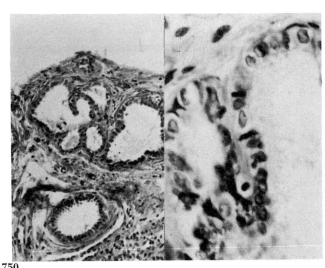

750

751   Intraluminal papilloma of the oviduct
The papilloma is formed by proliferated connective tissue stroma and is lined by flattened epithelium. (H&E. ×20)

752   Intramural lipoma of the oviduct
There is infiltration of the tubal muscularis by mature fat cells. No distinct encapsulation is seen. This tumor of the oviduct is rare. (H&E. ×50)

753   Adenomatoid tumor of the oviduct
The circumscribed tumor is localized in the muscularis of the oviduct. The upper and lower poles of tumor show massive accumulation of lymphocytes. This tumor usually is small and is found incidentally. (H&E. ×8)

754   Adenomatoid tumor of the oviduct
High magnification of Fig. 753. The tumor shows cystic spaces lined by flattened cells. The fibromuscular connective tissue stroma is moderately developed. Neutral mucopolysaccharides are present in cystic structures and in the cytoplasm of lining cells. (H&E. ×160)

755   Adenomatoid tumor of the oviduct
The tumor is formed by cystic spaces of varied size lined by flattened cells with dark prominent nuclei. Such tumors have been diagnosed as lymphangiomas, mesotheliomas, or adenomas. Müllerian epithelial rests are most likely the origin of these tumors. In females the tumors are observed in the uterus, oviduct, and ovary. In males, they are found in the epididymis. (H&E. ×180)

756   Adenomatous hyperplasia (dysplasia) of the endosalpinx
The endosalpinx is lined by stratified epithelium. The cells are relatively small with elongated dark-stained nuclei. Mitoses are seen in the basal layer. (H&E. ×150)

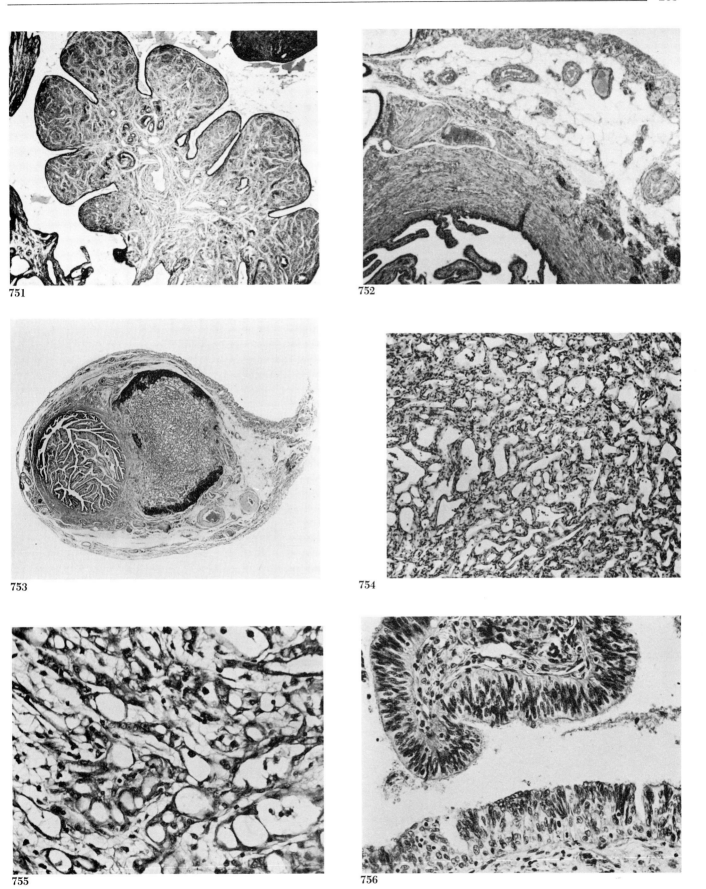

751

752

753

754

755

756

757   Adenomatous hyperplasia (dysplasia) of the endosalpinx
High magnification of Fig. 756. Note the focal preservation of the cilia. There is marked crowding and piling of epithelial cells. (H&E. ×220)

758   Adenomatous hyperplasia (dysplasia) of the endosalpinx
The focal area of adenomatous hyperplasia shows contrast with the normal lining epithelium of the endosalpinx. (H&E. ×125)

759   Adenomatous hyperplasia (dysplasia) of the endosalpinx
High magnification of Fig. 758. There is crowding of small cells with round to elongated hyperchromatic nuclei. Note the areas showing preservation of normal differentiation of nonciliated secretory cells. Occasional mitoses are seen. (H&E. ×180)

760   Intraepithelial carcinoma (carcinoma in situ) of the endosalpinx
The fold of endosalpinx is lined by highly atypical immature cells with irregular hyperchromatic nuclei. (H&E. ×90)

761   Intraepithelial carcinoma (carcinoma in situ) of the endosalpinx
High magnification of Fig. 760. The cells show scant cytoplasm and large hyperchromatic nuclei. Highly abnormal cell proliferation is seen. There is absence of cilia with lack of differentiation. (H&E. ×150)

762   Intraepithelial carcinoma (carcinoma in situ) of the endosalpinx
High magnification of Fig. 760. The highly immature cells show irregular large hyperchromatic nuclei. The basement membrane is intact. (H&E. ×220)

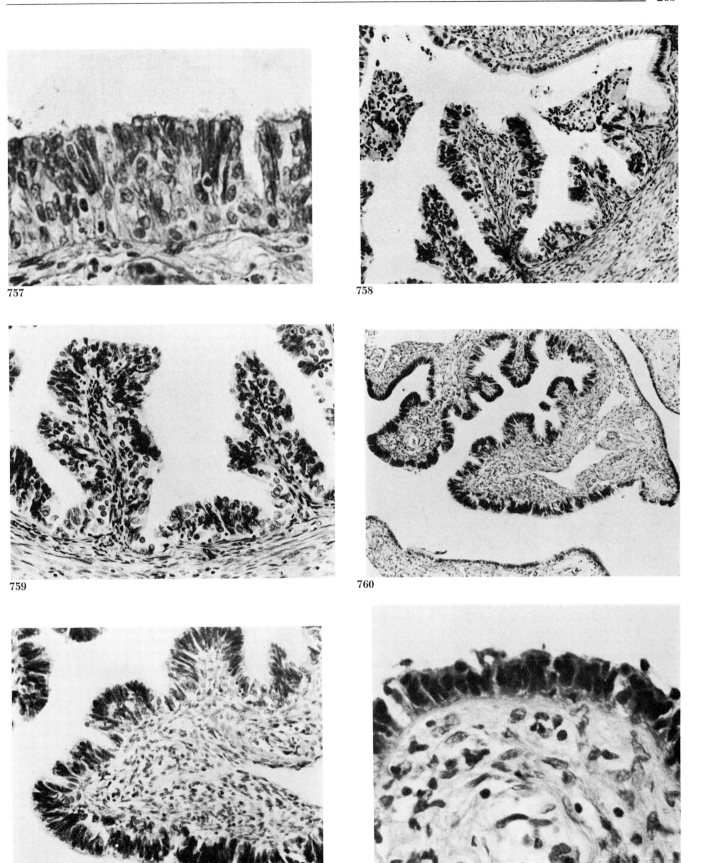

757

758

759

760

761

762

763   Early carcinoma of the oviduct
An epithelial fold of the endosalpinx is seen undergoing malignant changes. (H&E. ×50)

764   Early carcinoma of the oviduct
High magnification of Fig. 763. There is proliferation of malignant neoplastic cells. Some are being exfoliated into the tubal lumen; others are invading the connective tissue stroma of the endosalpinx. (H&E. ×125)

765   Early polypoid carcinoma of the oviduct
This intraluminal polypoid growth is composed of abortive papillary and glandular structures. These are lined by neoplastic epithelium. There is beginning invasion of tubal wall at the base of the polypoid structure. (H&E. ×25)

766   Early polypoid carcinoma of the oviduct
High magnification of Fig. 765. Superficial neoplastic papillary projections are seen. There is invasion of connective tissue stroma and the formation of glandlike structures by neoplastic epithelium. Mitoses are infrequent. The connective tissue stroma is heavily infiltrated with lymphocytes. (H&E. ×70)

767   "Inflammatory" carcinoma of the oviduct
The tumor is formed by neoplastic glands and connective tissue stroma with heavy inflammatory infiltration. The tumor replaces the endosalpinx and invades the tubal wall. (H&E. ×80)

768   Early polypoid carcinoma of the oviduct
High magnification of Fig. 765. (H&E. ×125)

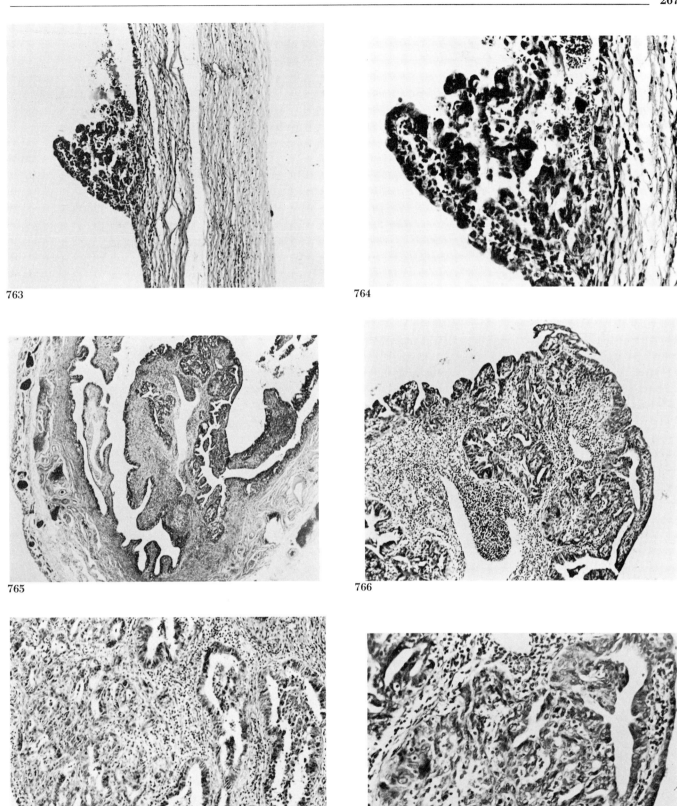

763

764

765

766

767

768

769 Papillary endometrioid type adenocarcinoma of the oviduct
This papillary adenocarcinoma with neoplastic cells resembles an endometrial carcinoma. (H&E. ×100)

770 Papillary endometrioid type adenocarcinoma of the oviduct
High magnification of Fig. 769. This well-differentiated carcinoma of the endosalpinx shows moderate mitotic activity. (H&E. ×200)

771 Coarse papillary adenocarcinoma of the oviduct
The tumor is formed by numerous papillary projections lined by several layers of neoplastic cells. (H&E. ×125)

772 Papillary adenocarcinoma of the oviduct
The papillary structure of the tumor is partly preserved. Neoplastic cells are arranged in solid cords. Mitotic figures are frequent. (H&E. ×50)

773 Adenocarcinoma of the oviduct
The tumor is formed by glandular structures with no papillary projections. The tumor is confined to the endosalpinx. (H&E. ×125)

774 Squamous cell carcinoma of the oviduct
The endosalpinx and oviductal wall are invaded by a tumor composed of squamous neoplastic cells. This form of tubal carcinoma is rare. (H&E. ×180)

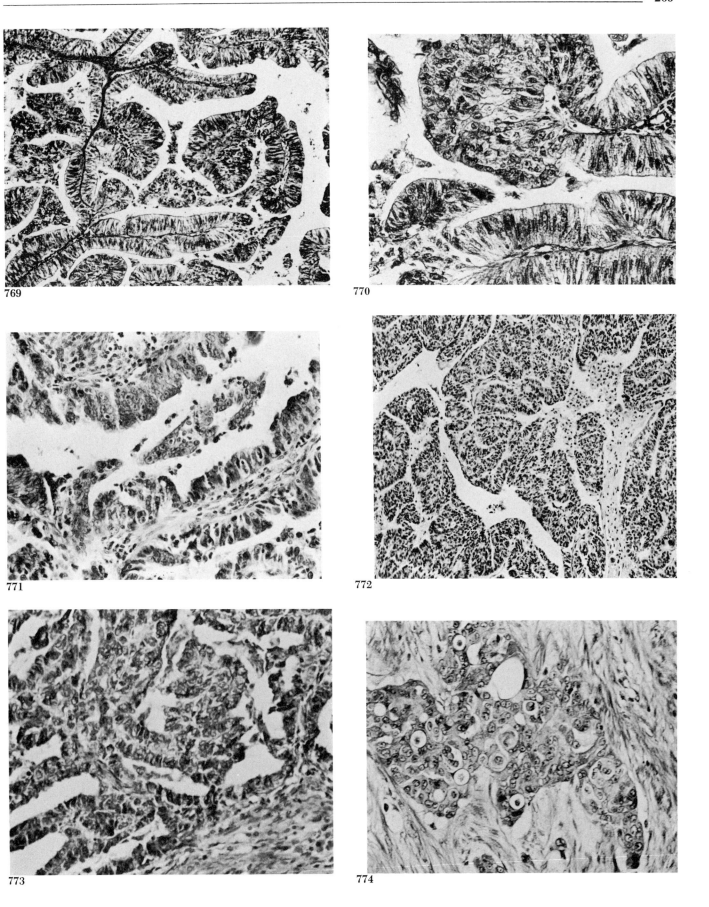

769

770

771

772

773

774

775   Squamous cell carcinoma of the oviduct
Neoplastic squamous cells are arranged in an alveolar pattern. Primary tumors in the cervix, uterus, and ovary have been excluded. (H&E. ×180)

776   Anaplastic carcinoma of the oviduct with pseudoxanthomatous cells
This highly undifferentiated carcinoma is composed of pleomorphic cells with large hyperchromatic nuclei. Interspersed are numerous lipid macrophages. (H&E. ×150)

777   Carcinosarcoma of the oviduct
This tumor is composed of a papillary carcinoma of the endosalpinx and a sarcoma of the intervening connective tissue stroma and/or oviductal wall. (H&E. ×80)

778   Carcinosarcoma of the oviduct
High magnification of Fig. 777. The tumor is most likely arising from Müllerian mesoderm. This tumor is highly malignant. (H&E. ×180)

779   Reticulum cell sarcoma of the oviduct
The connective tissue stroma of the endosalpinx is diffusely infiltrated with pleomorphic cells. Note the preservation of the mucosal lining epithelium. (H&E. ×80)

780   Reticulum cell sarcoma of the oviduct
High magnification of Fig. 779. The tumor is formed by pleomorphic reticulum cells. The cytoplasm is eosinophilic, and nucleoli are prominent. Phagocytosis by reticulum cells may be observed. (H&E. ×180)

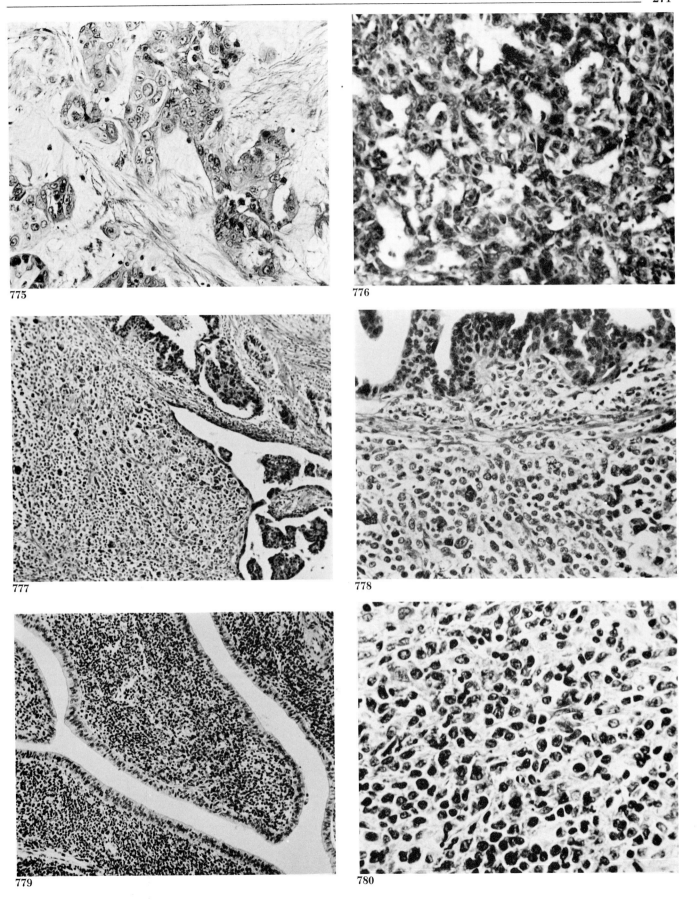

775

776

777

778

779

780

781   Reticulum cell sarcoma of the oviduct
Formation of reticulum fibers (reticulin) is seen between individual neoplastic cells. (Wilder's reticulum stain. ×180)

782   Malignant lymphoma (lymphoblastic lymphosarcoma) of the oviduct
There is diffuse infiltration of the connective tissue stroma of the endosalpinx with relatively uniform lymphoblasts. (H&E. ×35)

783   Malignant lymphoma (lymphoblastic lymphosarcoma) of the oviduct
High magnification of Fig. 782. The infiltrating neoplastic cells are larger than lymphocytes. Differentiation from lymphatic leukemia is extremely difficult. (H&E. ×180)

784   Carcinoma of the ovary metastatic to the oviduct
Islands of metastatic ovarian carcinoma are seen in the connective tissue stroma and lymphatics of the mucous membrane of the oviduct. (H&E. ×80)

785   Endosalpingiosis of the vermiform appendix
The muscle layer of the vermiform appendix contains numerous cystically dilated glandular structures. Note the absence of endometrial stromal cells. (H&E. ×5)

786   Endosalpingiosis of the vermiform appendix
High magnification of Fig. 785. The cyst is lined by a tubal type of epithelium located subperitoneally in the vermiform appendix. (H&E. ×100 and ×180)

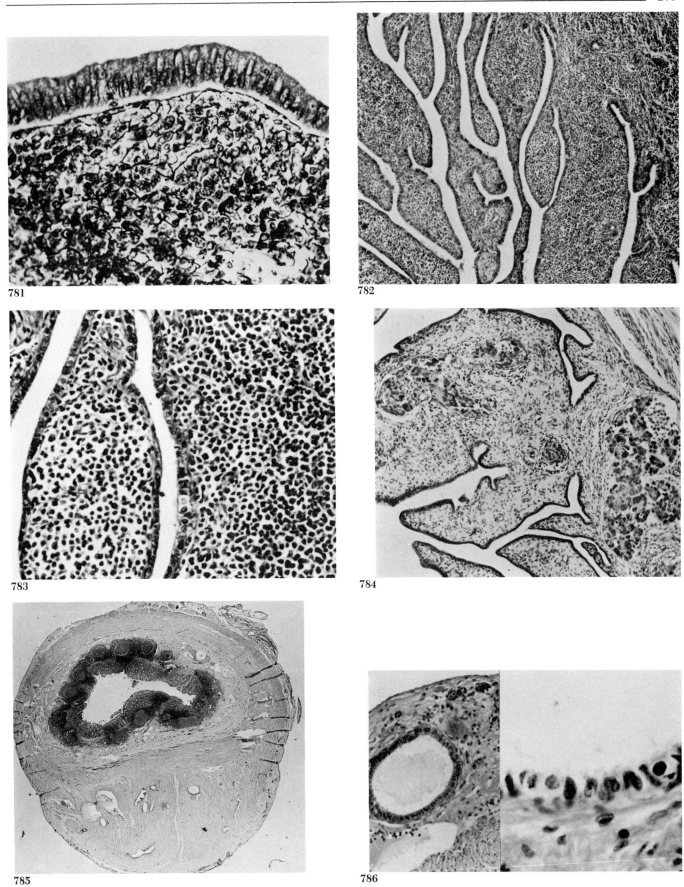

781

782

783

784

785

786

COLOR PLATES
Chapter 6
Diseases of the Oviduct
Plate 12

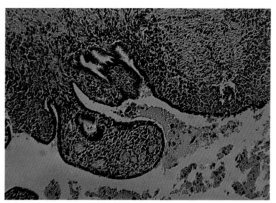

67 Intraluminal endometriosis with hematosalpinx An intraluminal island of endometrial tissue is seen with massive deposition of hemosiderin. (H&E. ×100)

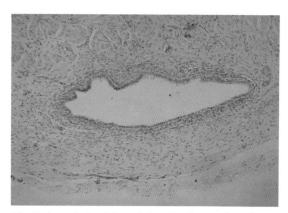

68 Endometriosis of the tubal wall The muscle wall contains heterotopic endometrial gland which is surrounded by endometrial stromal cells. There is no inflammatory reaction. (H&E. ×52)

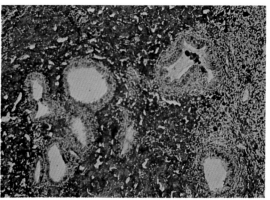

69 Pseudoxanthomatous salpingitis following Lipiodol salpingography There are numerous lipid containing macrophages and pseudo-glandular formations in the endosalpinx. (Sudan III. ×65)

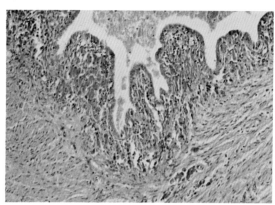

70 Histiocytes (macrophages) of the endosalpinx The interstitial connective tissue of the endosalpinx contains large macrophages. Neutral mucopolysaccharides present in macrophages. (PAS stain. ×62)

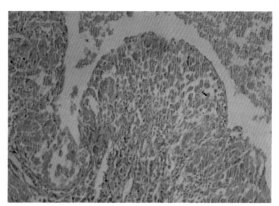

71 Histiocytes (macrophages) of the endosalpinx Acid mucopolysaccharides are present in macrophages. (Alcian blue. ×50)

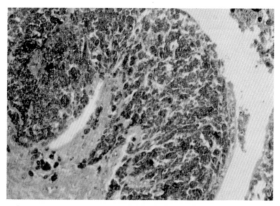

72 Histiocytes (macrophages) of the endosalpinx Considerable lipid is detected in the macrophages. (Sudan black B. ×100)

Plate 12

7

Diseases of the Ovary

787 Frontal section of the female reproductive organs in a 3-month-old fetus
(H&E. ×9)

788 Cortex of the ovary in a 3-month-old fetus
High magnification of Fig. 787. There is absence of the tunica albuginea. Numerous primordial germ cells are surrounded by undifferentiated ovarian parenchyme. (H&E. ×80)

789 Neonatal ovary
Numerous follicles of varying sizes are seen. Follicles are found through the prepubertal period. (H&E. ×17)

790 Cortex of a neonatal ovary
High magnification of Fig. 789. The ovarian surface is covered by columnar peritoneal (serosal) epithelium. Numerous primordial follicles are formed by ova surrounded by elongated connective tissue cells. (H&E. ×180)

791 Cortex of the ovary at the prepubertal period (13-year-old girl)
Note the numerous primordial follicles, several maturing follicles, and two atretic follicles with luteinization of theca cells. (H&E. ×15)

792 Cortex of the ovary at the prepubertal period (13-year-old girl)
High magnification of Fig. 791. The ovarian surface is covered by flattened serosal (germinal) cells. There is a marked decrease in the number of primordial follicles. Young cortical connective tissue stroma is increased. (H&E. ×80)

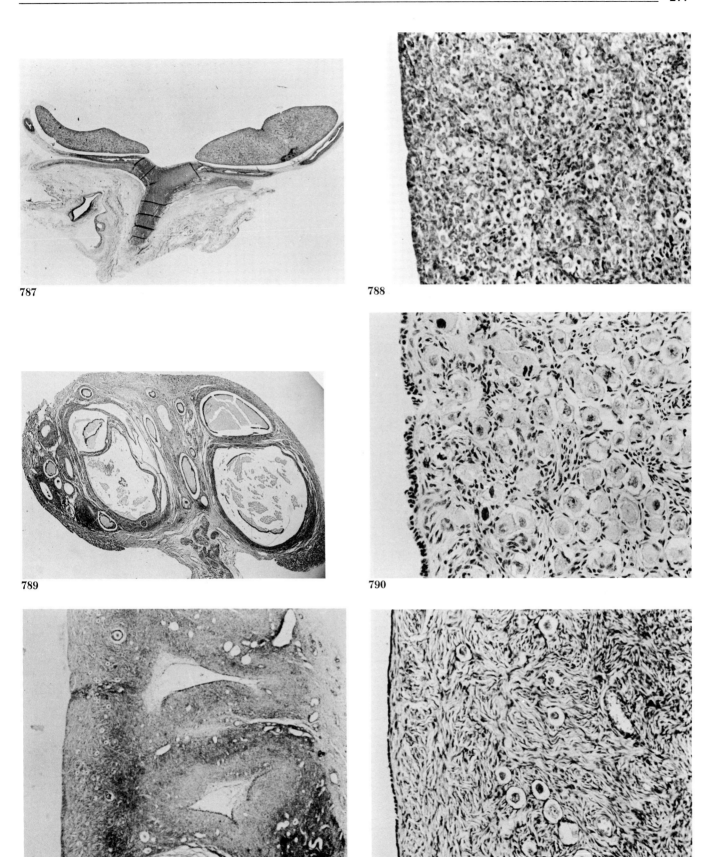

787

788

789

790

791

792

793   Cortex of the ovary in a woman of reproductive age (30 years of age)
Occasional primordial follicles are seen. The large graafian follicle is adjacent to two atretic follicles. (H&E. ×30)

794   Cortex of the ovary in a woman of reproductive age (30 years of age)
High magnification of Fig. 793. Germinal epithelium is absent. Dense connective tissue forms the tunica albuginea. Scattered primordial follicles are seen beneath the tunica albuginea. The cortical connective tissue stroma is increased. (H&E. ×50)

795   Cortex of the ovary in a woman after the menopause (55 years of age)
Germinal epithelium is absent. The condensation of the cortical stroma is due to atrophy. There are numerous corpora albicantia in the subcortical area. (H&E. ×30)

796   Cortex of the ovary in a woman after the menopause (55 years of age)
High magnification of Fig. 795. There is cortical atrophy and fibrosis. A degenerating single primordial follicle is seen. (H&E. ×50)

797   Ovarium gyratum
The senile ovary shows a gyrate appearance of the fibrosed cortex. (H&E. ×6)

798   Bony metaplasia in the cortex of an atrophic ovary
(H&E. ×50)

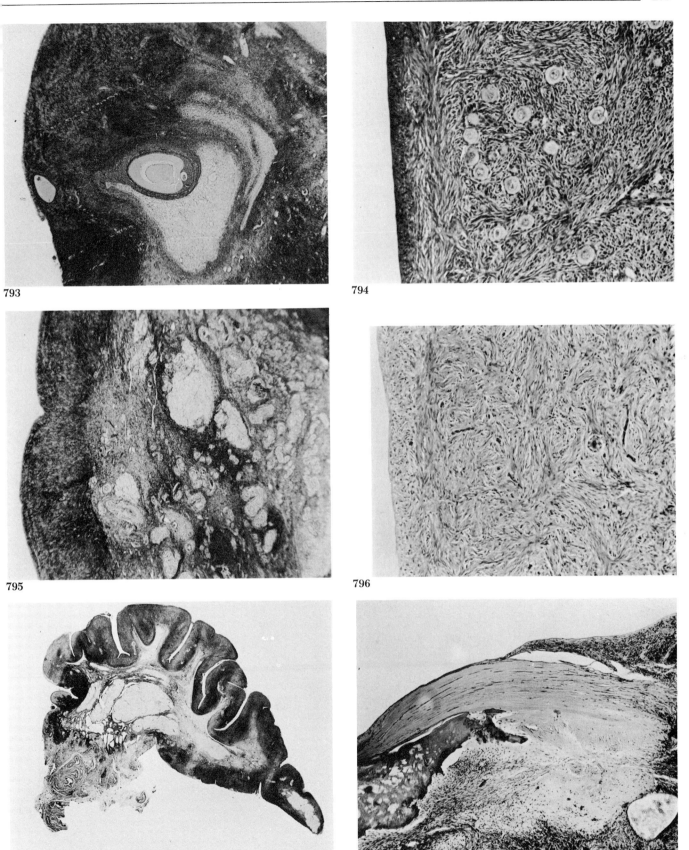

793

794

795

796

797

798

799   Primordial follicles of the ovary
The primordial follicles, 42 to 45 μ in diameter, have a round ovum and an excentric nucleus. They are surrounded by a layer of flattened follicular cells. (H&E. ×150)

800   Graafian follicle of the ovary
The graafian follicle is lined by several layers of follicular (granulosa) cells forming a prominent cumulus oophorus. The theca interna is composed of lipid-containing polyhedral cells, and the theca externa is formed by concentrically arranged fusiform cells. The theca cone, in juxtaposition to the cumulus oophorus, is seen with the apex directed toward the ovarian surface. (H&E. ×62)

801   Primordial follicle with a polynuclear ovum
As many as eight nuclei in one ovum have been described. (H&E. ×200)

802   Dystrophic calcification of a growing follicle
(H&E. ×280)

803   Perifollicular hyalinization
There is hyalinization of the basement membrane of a follicle. This is probably an early stage of follicular atresia. (H&E. ×50)

804   Wall of an early luteinized mature graafian follicle prior to rupture
Note the well-developed lipid-containing theca interna cells. (H&E. ×70)

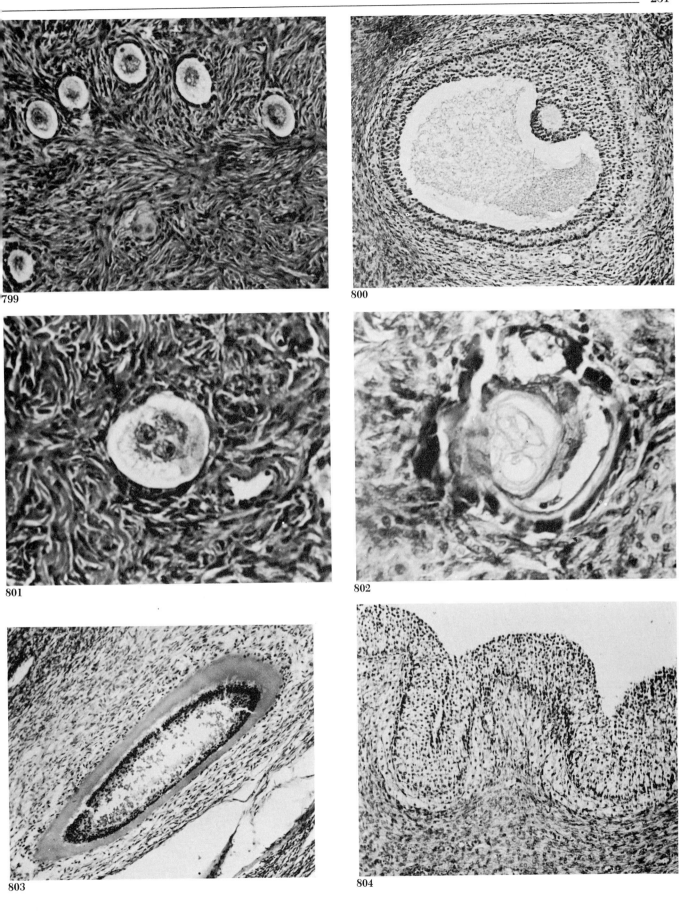

799

800

801

802

803

804

805 Proliferative stage of the corpus luteum of menstruation
There is hypertrophy and proliferation of granulosa cells with the formation of granulosa lutein cells. (H&E. ×65)

806 Vascularization stage of the corpus luteum of menstruation
Capillary sprouts extend radially from the theca interna layer between columns of granulosa lutein cells. (H&E. ×65)

807 Vascularization stage of the corpus luteum of menstruation
High magnification of Fig. 806. Well-developed capillaries are surrounded by columns of granulosa lutein cells. (H&E. ×125)

808 Maturity or bloom stage of the corpus luteum of menstruation
Large granulosa lutein cells are surrounded by a narrow rim of cuboidal luteinized theca interna cells, the so-called theca lutein cells or paralutein cells. There is no transition between these two types of lutein cells. Approximately twenty-fifth day of the cycle. (H&E. ×160)

809 Regression stage of the corpus luteum of menstruation
Granulosa lutein cells are small having lost their trabecular arrangement. The nuclei are pyknotic. There is diffuse infiltration with acute and chronic inflammatory cells. Disappearance of theca lutein cells. The corpus luteum is approximately 8 weeks old. (H&E. ×50)

810 Regression stage of the corpus luteum of menstruation
High magnification of Fig. 809. There is degeneration and regression of granulosa lutein cells and replacement by fibrous connective tissue cells with the ultimate formation of the corpus albicans. (H&E. ×100)

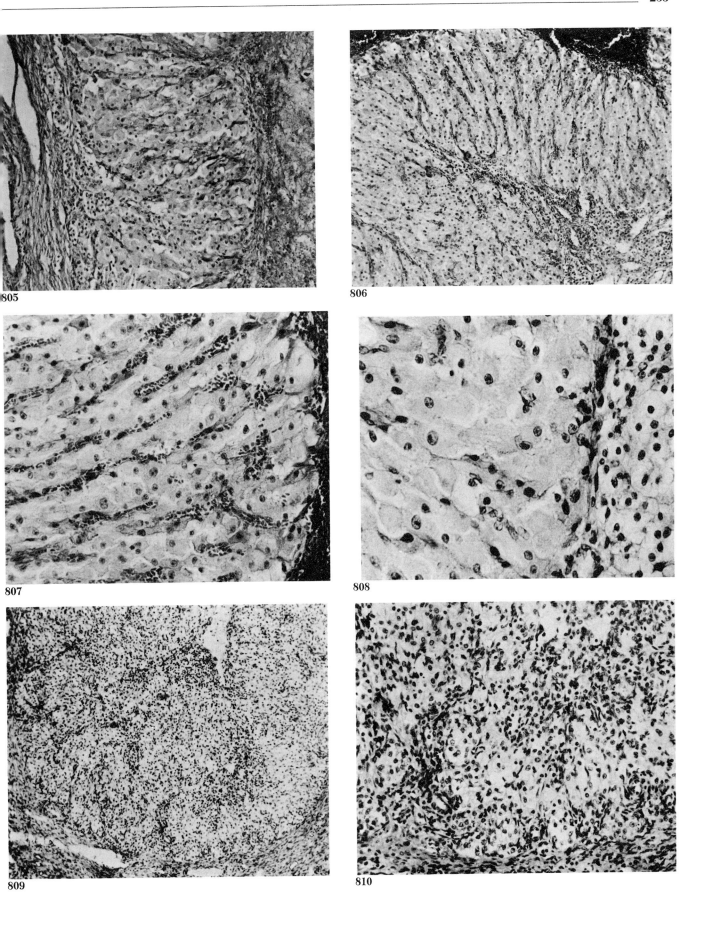

805

806

807

808

809

810

811   Rupturing corpus luteum of menstruation
Incipient rupture of a mature corpus luteum of menstruation is seen. (H&E. ×12) AFIP Acc No. 512572

812   Atretic follicle
The follicular cavity is filled with fibroblasts. The basement membrane is increased in thickness. Radial arrangement of theca interna cells is beginning. Note the absence of hyalinization of the basement membrane (glassy membrane) and lack of luteinization of theca interna cells. (H&E. ×80)

813   Atretic follicle with cystic change
The follicular cavity is partially filled with edematous connective tissue stroma with preservation of a cystic central area. Remnants of follicular epithelium are scattered on the basement membrane. Theca interna cells are prominent. Note the absence of hyalinization of the basement membrane (glassy membrane) and lack of luteinization of the theca interna cells. (H&E. ×25)

814   Atretic follicle with degeneration of ovum and luteinization of theca interna cells
The degenerating ovum, lacking a corona radiata, is floating freely in follicular fluid. There is early hyalinization of the basement membrane. Theca interna cells are luteinized. (H&E. ×100)

815   Early stage of luteinized atretic follicle
There is marked luteinization of follicular epithelium and theca interna cells. (H&E. ×85)

816   End stage of luteinized atretic follicle
The residue of the ovum is surrounded by fibrous connective tissue. The wavy basement membrane is hyalinized (glassy membrane). The theca cells are in regression. (H&E. ×65)

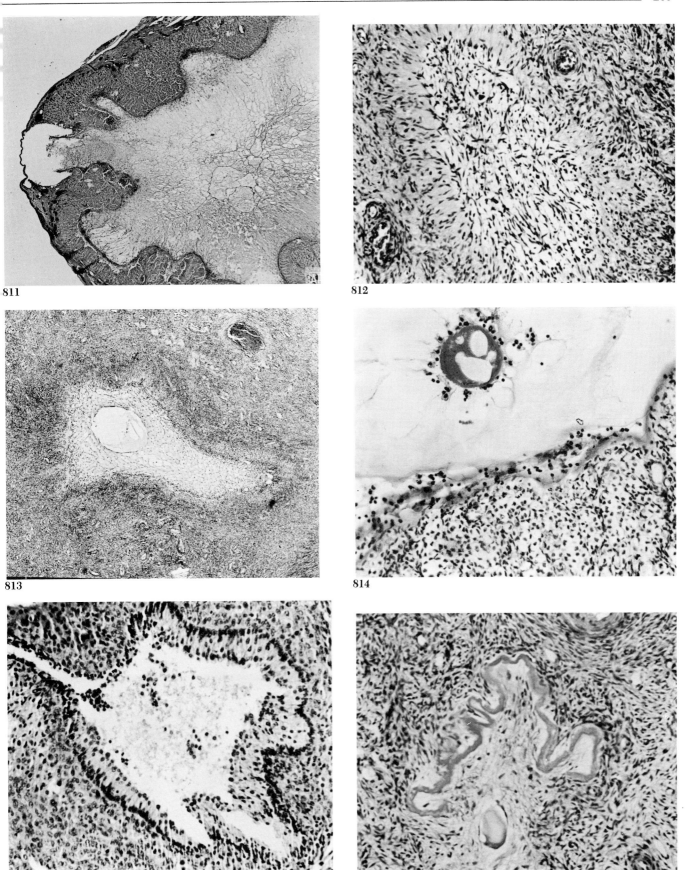

811

812

813

814

815

816

817 End stage of luteinized atretic follicle with cystic change

The follicular cavity is partly filled with fibroblasts and edematous matrix, leaving a central cystic space. There is marked hyalinization of the basement membrane. The theca interna cells show regression. The glassy membrane is also known as Grohe-Slavjansky membrane. (H&E. ×150)

818 Corpora albicantia of the ovary

Multiple fibrosed and hyalinized rests of corpora lutea are seen. (H&E. ×25)

819 Calcification of a corpus albicans
(H&E. ×35)

820 Normal rete ovarii

The branching tubular structures are located in ovarian hilum. They represent rudimentary connections between the mesonephros and gonad. (H&E. ×35)

821 Normal rete ovarii

High magnification of Fig. 820. Glandlike structures, some with papillary projections, are lined by cuboidal epithelium with round prominent nuclei. Cilia are occasionally seen. (H&E. ×150)

822 Hilus cell of the ovary showing diffuse distribution

Irregular cords of large polyhedral cells are diffusely scattered in stroma. The cytoplasm contains lipochrome pigment granules and lipid. (H&E. ×180)

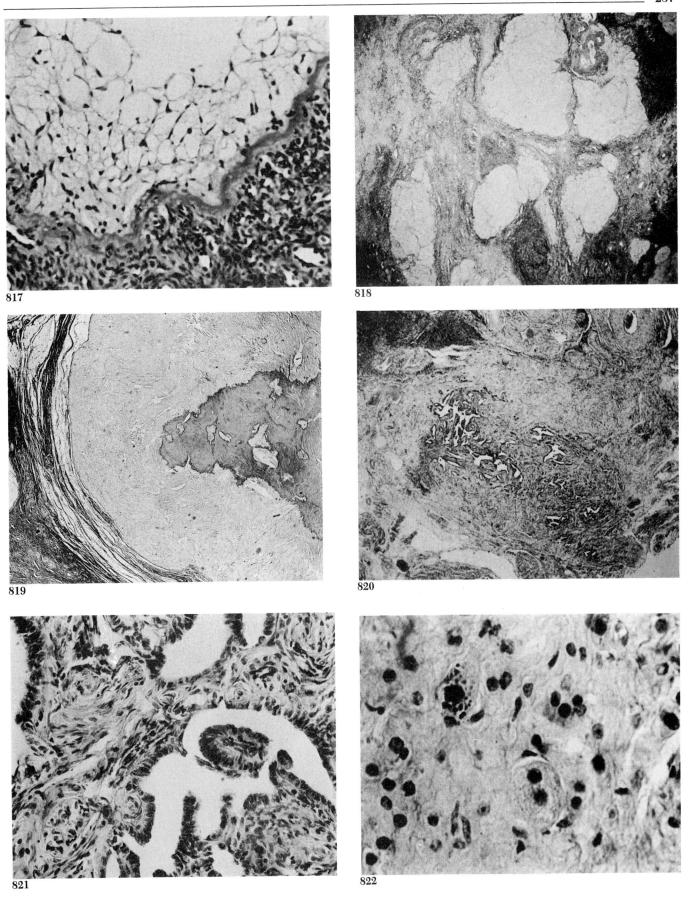

817

818

819

820

821

822

823 Diffuse distribution of hilus cells of the ovary
Epithelioid cells with prominent round nuclei are eccentrically placed. The cytoplasm is rich in lipid material. (Wilder's reticulum stain. ×150)

824 Perineural distribution of hilus cells of the ovary
Hilus (interstitial) cells surround nerve fibers. The cytoplasm is strongly eosinophilic and finely granular. Sometimes the cytoplasm is brown because of the high content of lipochrome pigment. The vitamin C content is high. Crystalloids of Reinke are occasionally seen. They are intracytoplasmic protein inclusions. (H&E. ×125)

825 Oophoritis associated with infectious parotitis
There is diffuse infiltration of the ovarian cortex by mononuclear inflammatory cells. The patient is a 12-year-old girl with mumps. (H&E. ×100)

826 Abscess of the ovary
Massive tissue necrosis is surrounded by inflammatory exudate composed of acute and chronic inflammatory cells. There is considerable fibrosis of underlying tissue. Ovarian components are obliterated. (H&E. ×24)

827 Tuberculous oophoritis
Scattered tubercles, within the ovarian cortex, consist of epithelioid cells and Langhans type of giant cells. There is diffuse lymphocytic infiltration. (H&E. ×50)

828 Caseating tuberculous oophoritis
The large caseous area in the ovary is surrounded by conglomerating tubercles. There is marked peripheral infiltration with lymphocytes. (H&E. ×25)

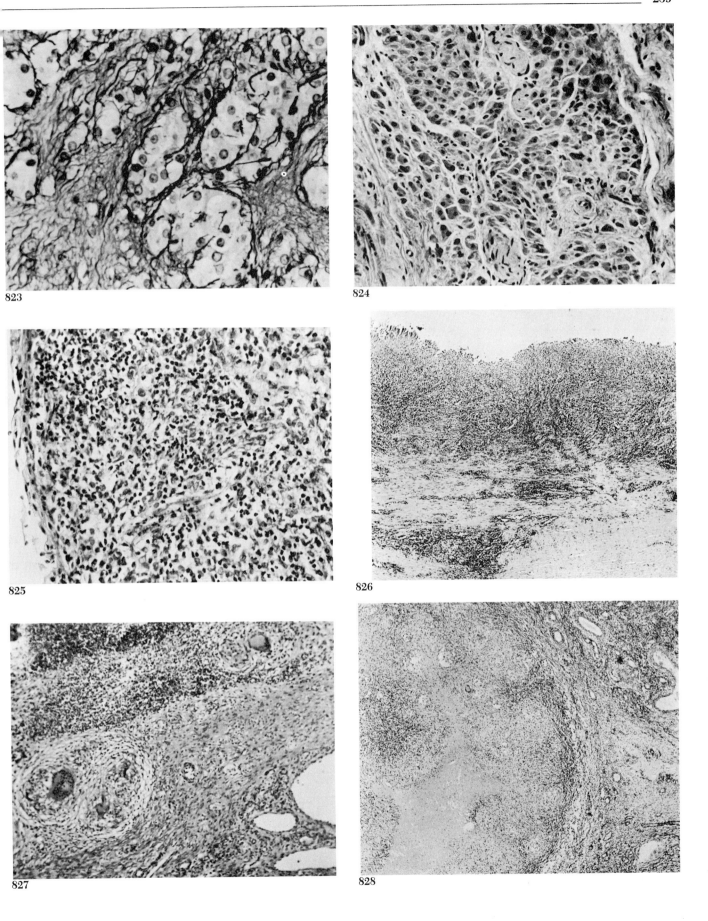

823

824

825

826

827

828

829 Enterobius (Oxyuris) vermicularis of the ovary
The ovarian abscess contains within the necrotic area a gravid adult female pinworm. (H&E. ×24)

830 Enterobius (Oxyuris) vermicularis of the ovary
High magnification of Fig. 829. The cross section shows the gravid female pinworm containing numerous ova. The gravid female pinworm migrated from the anus via the vagina, uterus, and oviduct to the ovary, producing an ovarian abscess. (H&E. ×125)

831 Syphilis of the ovary
The cortex and medulla of the ovary show numerous perivascular granulomas formed by plasma cells and lymphocytes. The lesion represents the late secondary stage. The right lower quadrant shows *Treponema pallidum* in the same ovary. (H&E. ×30. Horálek's silver impregnation. ×600)

832 Extensive necrosis of the corpus luteum in thrombotic thrombocytopenic purpura
Extensive areas of hemorrhagic necrosis are seen in the corpus luteum of menstruation. (H&E. ×12)

833 Necrosis of the corpus luteum in thrombotic thrombocytopenic purpura
High magnification of Fig. 832. Numerous capillary, arteriolar, and venular thromboses are associated with extensive areas of ischemic and hemorrhagic infarction of the corpus luteum of menstruation. (H&E. ×80)

834 Chronic organizing perioophoritis
The serosal lining of the ovary is replaced by a vascular and edematous connective tissue layer interspersed with chronic inflammatory cells. (H&E. ×50)

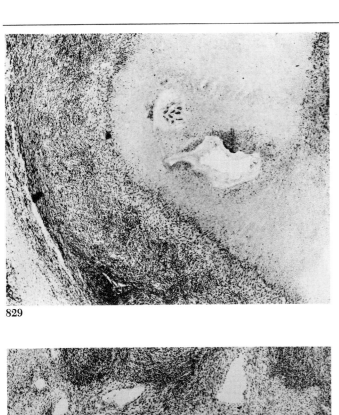

829

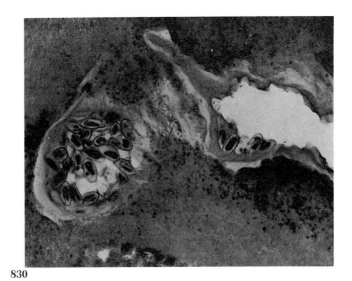

830

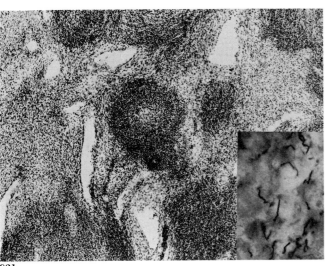

831

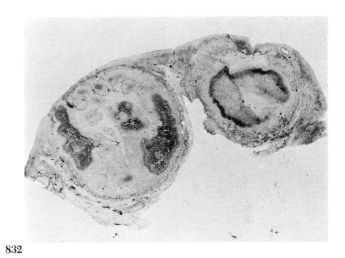

832

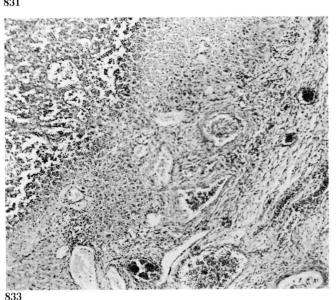

833

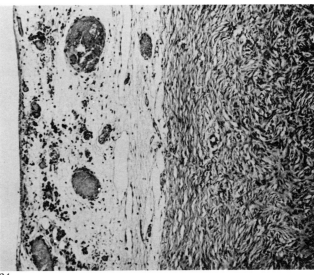

834

835 Tubo-ovarian adhesion
The mucosal folds of the oviduct are attached by old organized adhesions to the surface of the ovary. (H&E. ×27)

836 Healed perioophoritis with adhesions
Numerous fibrovascular adhesions are attached to the ovarian surface. Scattered inflammatory cells are seen in the adhesive connective tissue. (H&E. ×50)

837 Diffuse stromal luteinization of the ovary
Polyhedral lutein cells containing lipid are diffusely scattered throughout the cortical stroma. Stromal cell luteinization may be associated with ovarian stromal hyperplasia. Whether these lutein cells represent an integral part of stromal hyperplasia or are follicular residuals is highly debatable. (H&E. ×62)

838 Circumscribed stromal luteinization of the ovary
A focus of large lutein cells in partly hyalinized ovarian stroma is seen. (H&E. ×62)

839 Extrauterine decidual reaction (deciduosis) of the ovary not associated with pregnancy
These ovarian decidual changes are present in a nonpregnant woman. Such changes have been observed during the reproductive age and after the menopause. Proximity of an active corpus luteum and local progesterone activity has been suggested as the cause of deciduosis in some cases. (H&E. ×120)

840 Follicular cyst of the ovary
A unilocular cyst, usually over 2 cm in diameter. (H&E. ×4)

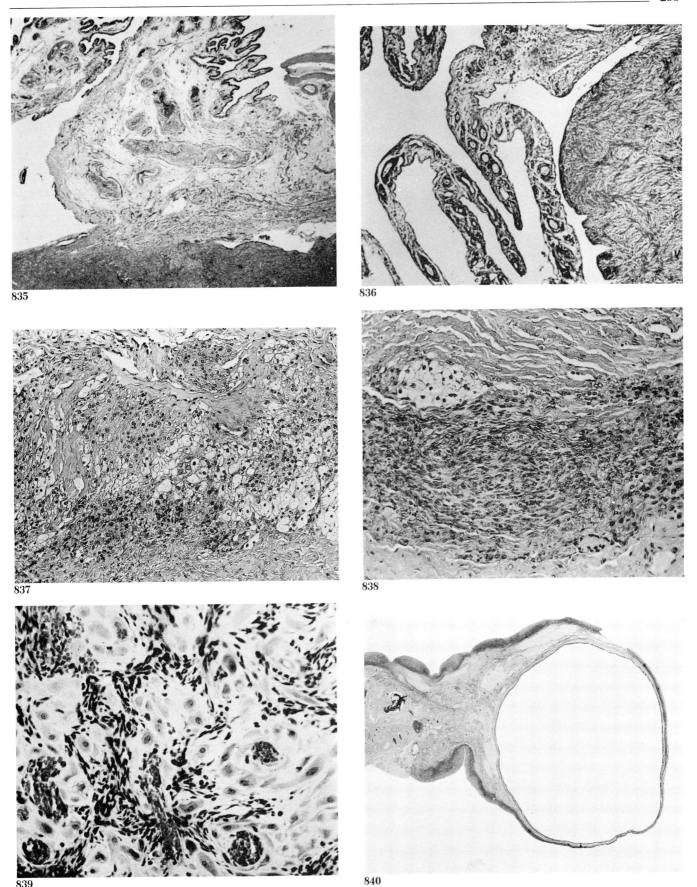

835

836

837

838

839

840

841 Follicular cyst of the ovary
High magnification of Fig. 840. The flattened granulosa and theca cell layers form the lining of a follicular cyst. (H&E. ×220)

842 Follicular cyst of the ovary with intracystic hemorrhage and partial luteinization (H&E. ×50)

843 Atretic luteinized follicle cyst of the ovary, end stage
Comp. with Figs. 815, 816 and 817. (H&E. ×20)

844 Corpus luteum cyst of the ovary
Regression of the corpus luteum shows arrest with subsequent formation of a cyst. The lining is formed by an inner zone of connective tissue and an outer zone of granulosa lutein cells. (H&E. ×6)

845 Theca lutein cyst of the ovary
The lining of the cyst is composed of luteinized theca interna cells. Such cysts are encountered after administration of gonadotropin or clomiphene citrate, with hydatidiform mole or choriocarcinoma, and occasionally in normal pregnancy. (H&E. ×150)

846 Cyst of the ovary, not otherwise specified
The cyst lining is not discernible. (H&E. ×35)

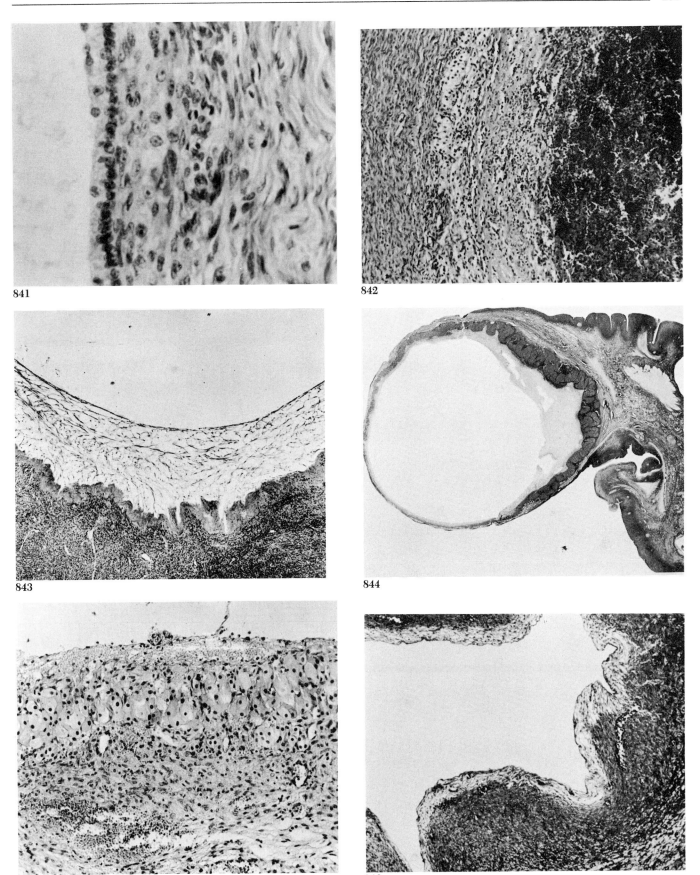

841

842

843

844

845

846

847 Polycystic ovary
Cortical sclerosis is absent. Multiple cysts of varying size with no evidence of perifollicular luteinization are seen. There is normal maturation of the corpus luteum and formation of the corpora albicantia. The menstrual cycle was normal. Such ovarian changes are frequently associated with uterine leiomyomas. (H&E. ×5)

848 Polycystic ovary
High magnification of Fig. 847. The cyst lining is formed by granulosa cells and flattened theca cells. (H&E. ×200)

849 Polycystic ovary with atrophic granulosa cell layer
The patient, 22 years old, had a unilateral polycystic ovary. There was no history of cyclic or hormonal aberration. Polycystic ovary may also occur with chronic pelvic inflammation. (H&E. ×4)

850 Polycystic ovary with atrophic granulosa cell layer
High magnification of Fig. 849. The cyst lining consists of flattened and atrophic granulosa and theca layers. (H&E. ×155)

852 Polycystic ovary with hyperplasia of granulosa cell layer (giant follicular hyperplasia)
High magnification of Fig. 851. There is marked hyperplasia of the granulosa cell lining of the ovarian cyst. The theca interna cells show minimal luteinization. Giant follicular hyperplasia is always associated with massive production of estrogen. (H&E. ×200)

851 Polycystic ovary with hyperplasia of granulosa cell layer (giant follicular hyperplasia)
The patient, 7 years of age, had precocious uterine bleeding and feminization. (H&E. ×3)

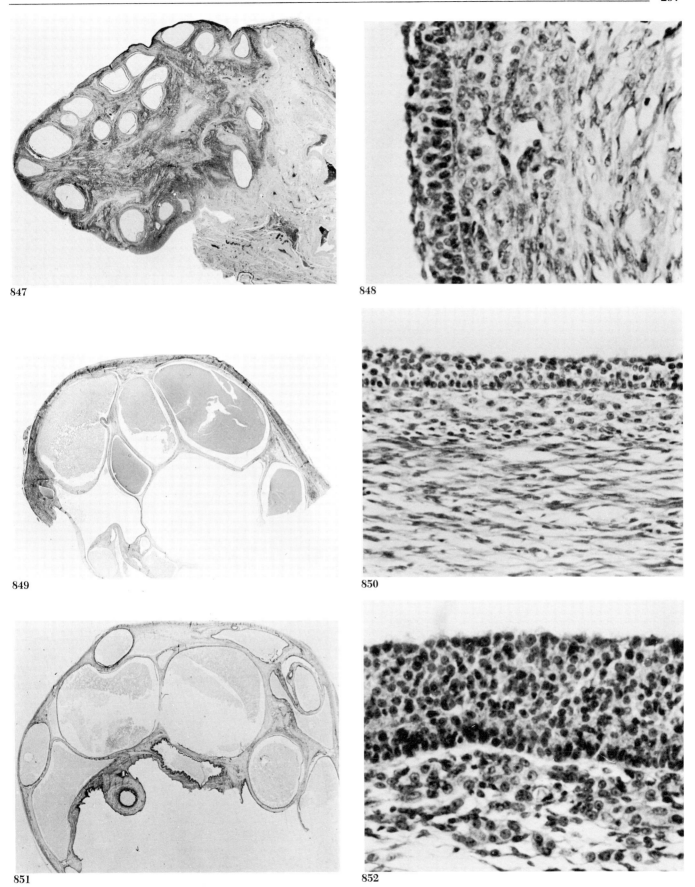

847

848

849

850

851

852

853 Micropolycystic ovary in Stein-Leventhal syndrome
Note the presence of multiple follicular cysts' with and without evidence of previous ovulation (presence of corpora lutea and corpora albicantia). There is pronounced thickening of the tunica albuginea and perifollicular luteinization of theca interna cells. (H&E. ×8)

854 Cortical fibrosis in micropolycystic ovary (Stein-Leventhal syndrome)
High magnification of Fig. 853. The patient, 22 years old, had oligomenorrhea, mild hirsutism, and enlarged clitoris and was obese. Note the cortical stromal condensation and fibrosis. (H&E. ×60)

855 Perifollicular hyperthecosis (hyperthecosis ovarii) in micropolycystic ovary (Stein-Leventhal syndrome)
The marked luteinization of theca interna cells extends into the theca externa. Perifollicular hyperthecosis can be observed in normal pregnancy, as a response to hormone therapy, in hydatidiform mole and choriocarcinoma. (H&E. ×120)

856 Micropolycystic ovary with early papillary serous cystadenocarcinoma
(H&E. ×8)

857 Germinal epithelium of the ovary
The epithelium covering the surface of the ovary is formed by a single row of cuboidal cells with prominent round nuclei. (H&E. ×180)

858 Squamous metaplasia of the germinal epithelium of the ovary
Cuboidal epithelium is replaced by stratified squamous epithelium. (H&E. ×125)

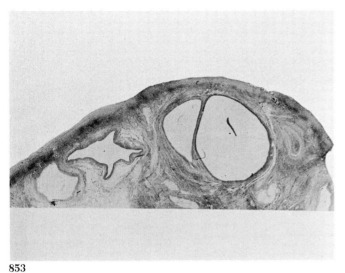

853

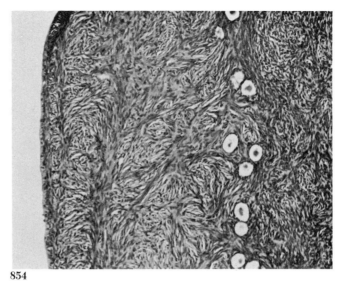

854

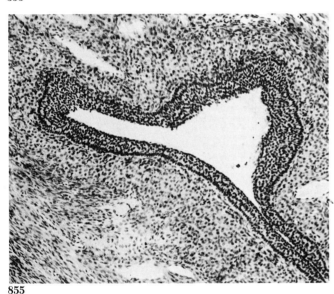

855

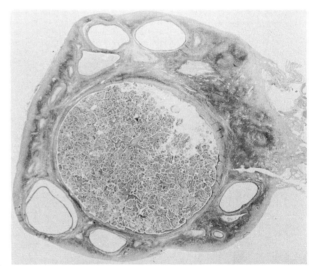

856

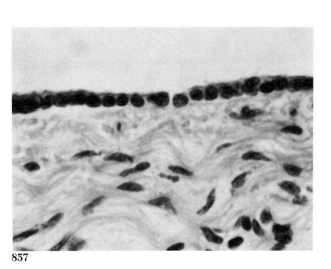

857

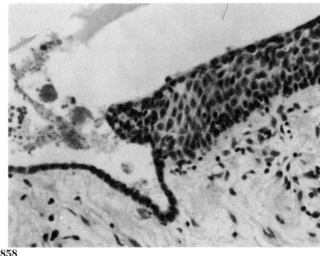

858

859 Mucinous epithelial metaplasia of the germinal epithelium of the ovary
Cuboidal epithelium is replaced by mucin-producing epithelium. (H&E. ×50)

860 Mucinous epithelial metaplasia of the germinal epithelium of the ovary
High magnification of Fig. 859. (H&E. ×125)

861 Endometriosis of the ovary with early secretory changes
The heterotopic endometrial island in the ovary is composed of secreting endometrial glands and relatively dense endometrial stroma. (H&E. ×62)

862 Endometriosis of the ovary (endometrial cyst, chocolate cyst), early stage
The cyst lining is formed by endometrial tissue. The endometrial glands and stroma are well developed. (H&E. ×50)

863 Endometriosis of the ovary with macrophages (endometrial cyst, chocolate cyst)
Endometrial epithelium forms the lining of the cyst. Numerous pigment-containing macrophages are present in the stroma. (H&E. ×120)

864 Endometriosis ovary (endometrial cyst, chocolate cyst), end stage
Recognizable endometrial tissue is absent. The cyst wall contains macrophages and shows considerable fibrosis. (H&E. ×24)

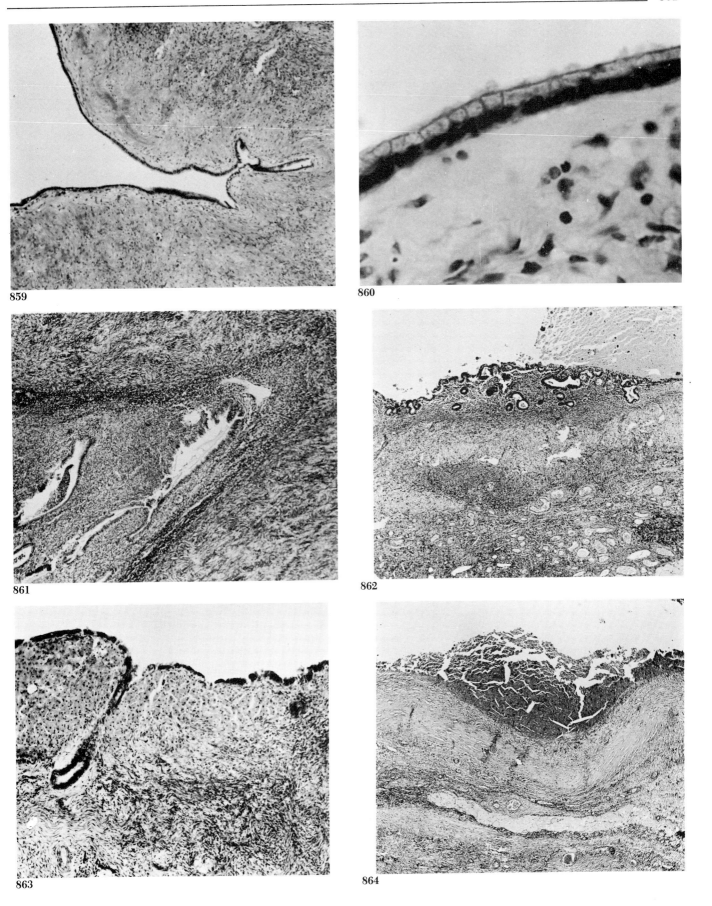

859

860

861

862

863

864

865 Endometriosis of the ovary with formation of an abortive endometrial cavity (H&E. ×25)

866 Papillary serous cystadenoma developing in an endometrial cyst
The arrow indicates a typical endometrial island in the wall of the cyst. (H&E. ×12)

867 Adenocarcinoma developing in endometriosis of the ovary
The arrow indicates an area of adenocarcinoma surrounded by endometrial tissue. Some endometrial glands are cystically dilated. The central area shows the formation of an abortive endometrial cavity. (H&E. ×18)

868 Adenocarcinoma developing in endometriosis of the ovary
High magnification of Fig. 867. The area indicated by the arrow in Fig. 867 is composed of neoplastic glandular and tubular structures lined by highly atypical epithelial cells. (H&E. ×75)

869 Endosalpingiosis of the ovary
Scattered glandular or tubular structures are seen in an ovarian cortex. They are lined by oviductlike epithelium and show secretory cells, ciliated cells, and intercalated (peg) cells. (H&E. ×80)

870 Endosalpingiosis of the ovary
The tubo-ovarian adhesion shows direct ingrowth of fimbriated tubal mucosa into the ovarian cortex. Note the cyst formation and focal calcification. (H&E. ×25)

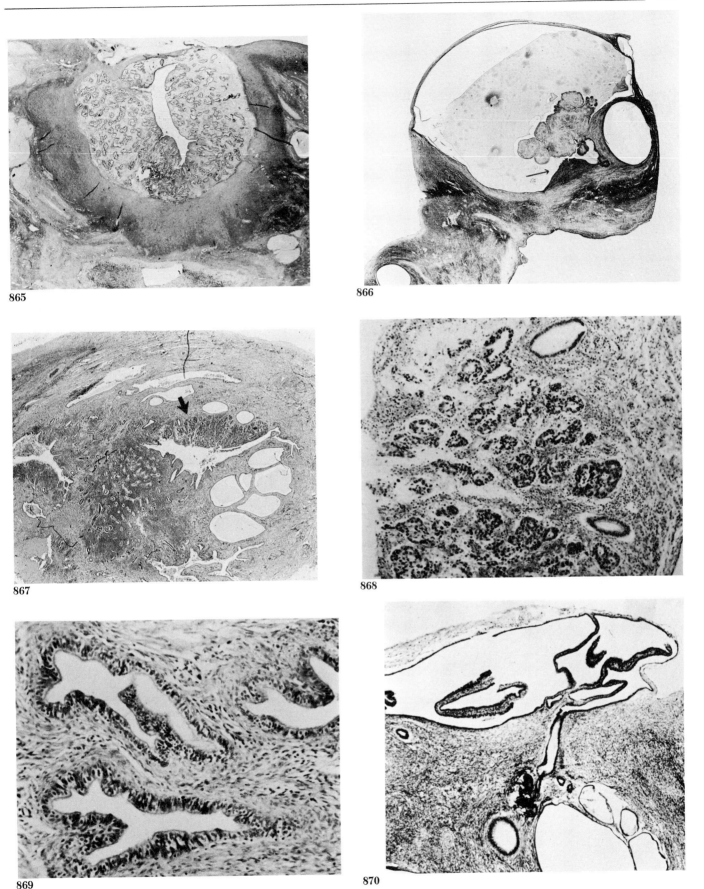

865

866

867

868

869

870

871 Endosalpingiosis of the ovary
The cystic structures located in an ovarian cortex result from ingrowth of tubal mucosal epithelium, subsequent to tubo-ovarian adhesion. (H&E. ×62)

872 Endosalpingiosis of the ovarian cortex with multiple cyst formations
Multiple cysts are lined by oviductal epithelium. Such cysts have been considered a result of invagination of serosal epithelium into cortical stroma and are called germinal inclusion cysts. (H&E. ×20)

873 Extensive endosalpingiosis of the ovary
The numerous glandular structures lined by epithelium are identical with those seen in the normal adult endosalpinx. Endosalpingiosis is a condition in which tissue characteristic of adult endosalpinx is found in abnormal sites. Theories applying to the histogenesis and cause of endometriosis are equally valid for endosalpingiosis. (H&E. ×50)

874 Extensive endosalpingiosis of the ovary
High magnification of Fig. 873. The cysts are lined by columnar epithelium, and there is a focal area of stromal calcification. (H&E. ×150)

875 Extensive endosalpingiosis of the ovary
The ovarian cortex exhibits branching glandlike structures. Stromal condensation may occur around these structures. The possibility is not excluded that some of these cysts developed from inclusion or invagination of germinal (serosal) epithelium which had undergone endosalpingeal metaplasia. (H&E. ×50)

876 Papillary cystadenoma developing in endosalpingiosis
(H&E. ×14)

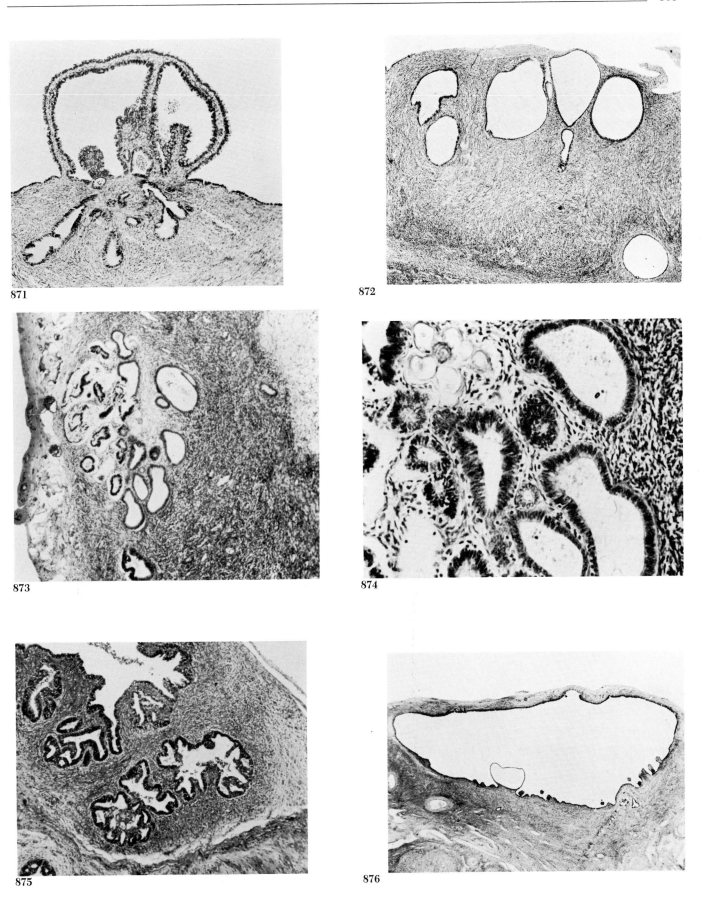

871

872

873

874

875

876

877 Surface papillomatous proliferation of an ovarian cortex without alteration of serosal epithelium
Numerous surface papillary projections are covered by cuboidal serosal (germinal) epithelium. (Wilder's reticulum stain; H&E. ×62)

878 Surface papillomatous proliferation of an ovarian cortex with alteration of serosal epithelium
The serosal (germinal) epithelium covering the surface of papillary projections shows crowding and microvilli formation. (H&E. ×35)

880 Hyperthecosis of the ovary
High magnification of Fig. 879. Stromal cells show delicate vacuolization of cytoplasm containing a moderate amount of lipid. Virilism, obesity, hypertension, and disturbance of glucose tolerance have been reported with hyperthecosis. (H&E. ×150)

879 Hyperthecosis of the ovary
The diffuse cortical stromal hyperplasia is frequently found in the menopause. (H&E. ×20)

881 Subcortical stromal hyperplasia in a polycystic ovary
The central portion of the ovary shows marked stromal hyperplasia. It may be associated with micropolycystic ovary in the Stein-Leventhal syndrome, or it may represent an isolated hyperthecosis with stromal luteinization. (H&E. ×15)

882 Diffuse cortical fibrosis of the ovary
Fibrosis of the cortical stroma shows no evidence of stromal luteinization. This condition is observed in the menopause. (H&E. ×45)

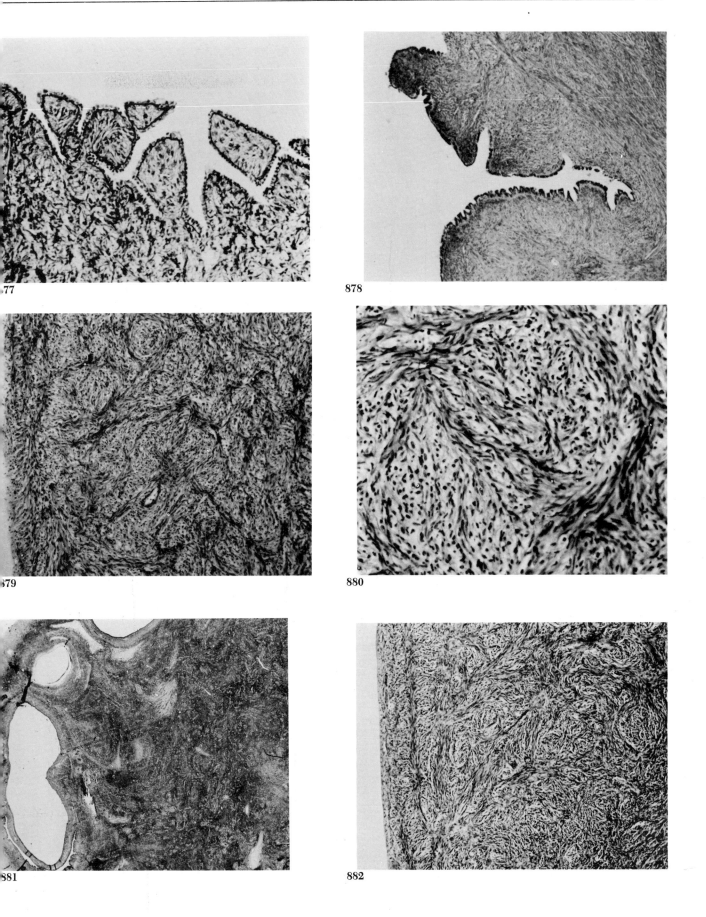

877

878

879

880

881

882

883 Nodular cortical fibrosis of the ovary
Cortical nodular fibrosis, as a rule, is not associated with stromal luteinization. This condition when observed before and during the menopause indicates failing ovarian function. (H&E. ×45)

884 Cortical hyalinization of the ovary
The massive hyalinization of the tunica albuginea is associated with cortical stromal fibrosis. This condition is observed with the Stein-Leventhal syndrome, long-standing chronic pelvic inflammatory diseases, and in the menopause. (H&E. ×100)

885 Cortical nodular fibrosis and advanced medullary arteriosclerosis of the ovary
This condition is frequently seen during the menopause. (H&E. ×24)

886 Calcific arteriosclerosis of the ovary
The mural calcification of an ovarian vessel shows partial thrombosis and organization. (H&E. ×60)

887 Isolated cortical calcification of the ovary
Foci of cortical calcification are of unknown origin. (H&E. ×110)

888 Cortical granuloma of the ovary
The small granuloma is composed of relatively large lipid-containing cells. Cortical granulomas may be encountered with cortical stromal hyperplasia. The cause is undetermined. (H&E. ×160)

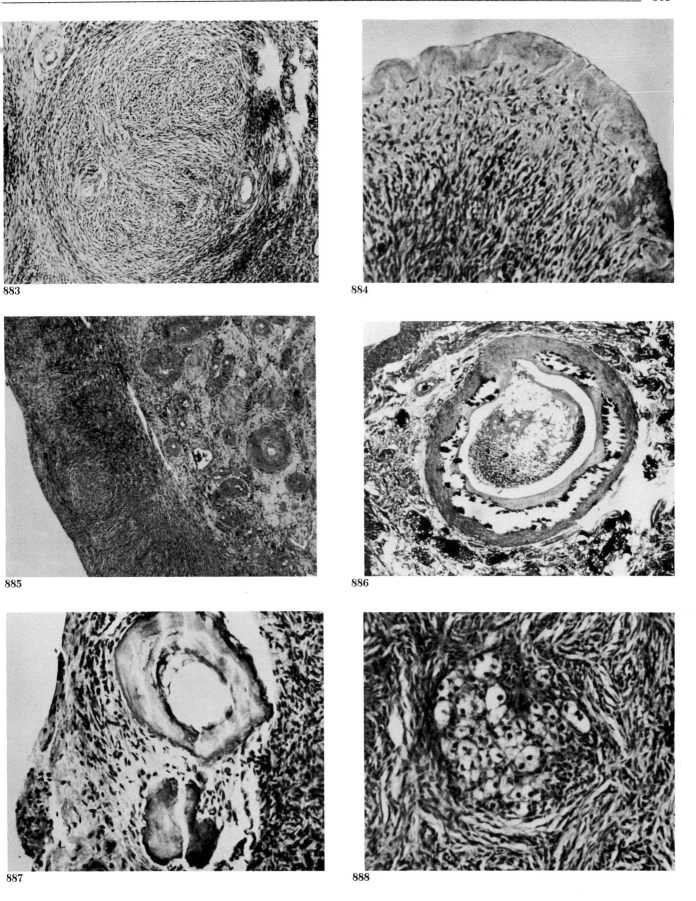

883

884

885

886

887

888

889   Cortical granuloma of the ovary
This cortical granuloma is formed by large lipid containing cells. (H&E. ×150)

890   Cortical granuloma of the ovary, probably an end stage
This cortical granuloma is formed by mature fat cells simulating a microlipoma. (H&E. ×100)

891   Cortical granuloma of the ovary
Perivascular accumulation of chronic inflammatory cells is seen in a hyalinized stroma. (H&E. ×125)

892   Cortical granuloma of the ovary
This cortical granuloma is composed of epithelioid cells, giant cells, lymphocytes, and plasma cells. The cause is undetermined. (H&E. ×180)

893   Amyloidosis of the ovary
Secondary amyloidosis is seen involving the ovarian cortex and medulla. There is perivascular and stromal deposition of amyloid. Amyloid can be demonstrated with iodine, Congo red, and by metachromatic dyes. (H&E. ×80)

894   Stromal hemosiderin deposition of the ovary
Hemorrhages occurring in different ovarian structures may lead to stromal hemosiderin deposition and/or phagocytosis by macrophages. (H&E. ×90)

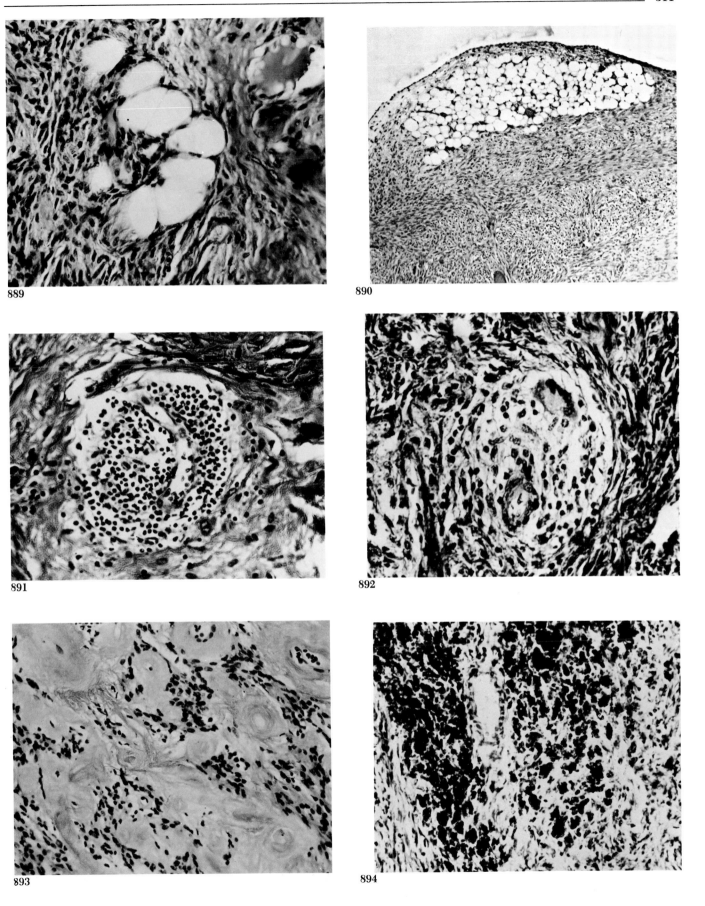

889

890

891

892

893

894

895 Splenogonadal fusion (descended para-gonadal spleen)
Discontinuous splenogonadal fusion is seen in which accessory splenic tissue is attached to the ovary. The paragonadal spleen is well encapsulated and surrounded by ovarian stromal tissue. (H&E. ×18)

896 Autograft ovary in the abdominal wall
Autotransplantation of a resected fragment of ovary into the rectus muscle of the abdominal wall has been performed. A biopsy then taken 6 months later shows marked hyalinization of surrounding striated muscle fibers. Condensation and atrophy of ovarian stroma with an abortive maturation of a follicle is seen. (H&E. ×80)

897 Ovary in adrenogenital syndrome in a 10-day-old infant
Numerous primordial follicles and developing follicles are present. (H&E. ×55)

898 Ovary in adrenogenital syndrome in a 10-day-old infant
High magnification of Fig. 897. There is no alteration in the cortical stroma. (H&E. ×75)

899 Ovary in adrenogenital syndrome in a 5-year-old child
There is a decreased number of developing and atretic graafian follicles. Note the absence of perifollicular luteinization. The medullary portion may show an increase in hilus (interstitial) cells. (H&E. ×10)

900 Ovary in adrenogenital syndrome in a 5-year-old child
High magnification of Fig. 899. There is a decreased number of primordial follicles with an increase and maturation of cortical stromal cells. (H&E. ×75)

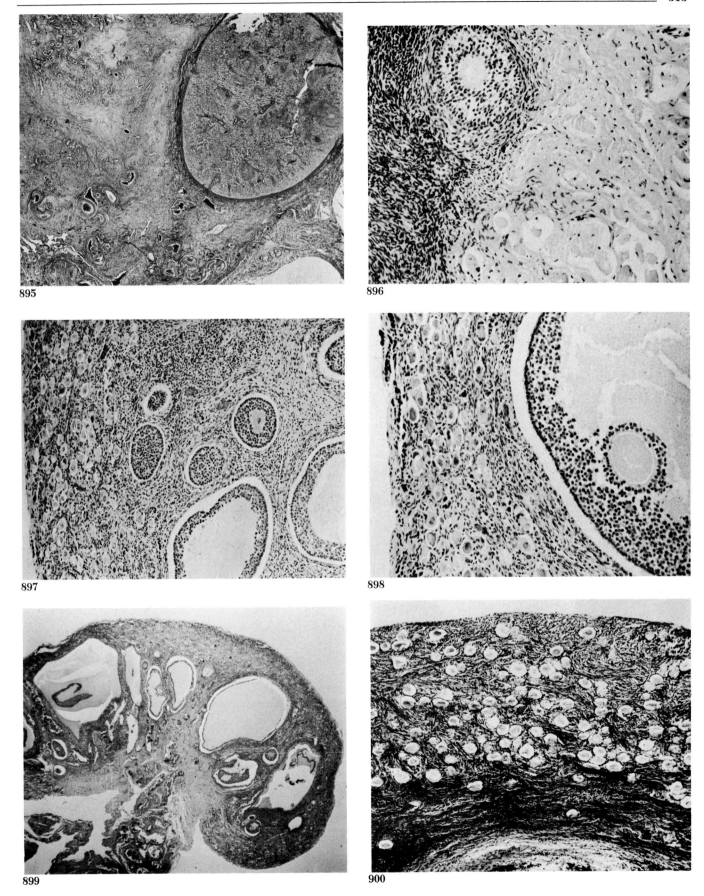

895

896

897

898

899

900

901 Gonadal dysgenesis
Preservation of germinal epithelium and scattered germ cells are noted. There is no evidence of primordial or any other variety of follicles. (H&E. ×60)

902 Gonadal dysgenesis
High magnification of Fig. 901. Considerable stromal fibrosis and hyalinization are seen. Germ cells arranged in cordlike pattern are present. The patient, 19 years old, had primary amenorrhea and a nuclear sex chromatin pattern of a male. (H&E. ×180)

903 Hypoplasia of the ovary
The patient, 18 years old, is a genetic female with a history of primary amenorrhea. Cortical fibrosis and atrophy are seen. All varieties of follicles are absent. (H&E. ×50)

904 Hypoplasia of the ovary, with hilus cells
The same patient as in Fig. 903. The medulla shows an increased number of hilus cells. (H&E. ×60)

905 Hypoplasia of the ovary
The patient, 35 years old, is a genetic female with a history of primary amenorrhea. The germinal epithelium is attenuated. There is marked cortical fibrosis. All varieties of follicles are absent. (H&E. ×62)

906 Radiation effect of the ovary
These changes occurred 2 years after administration of x-ray castration doses to the ovary. There is marked cortical fibrosis with scattered areas of hyalinization. Pronounced telangiectasis is seen. (H&E. ×50)

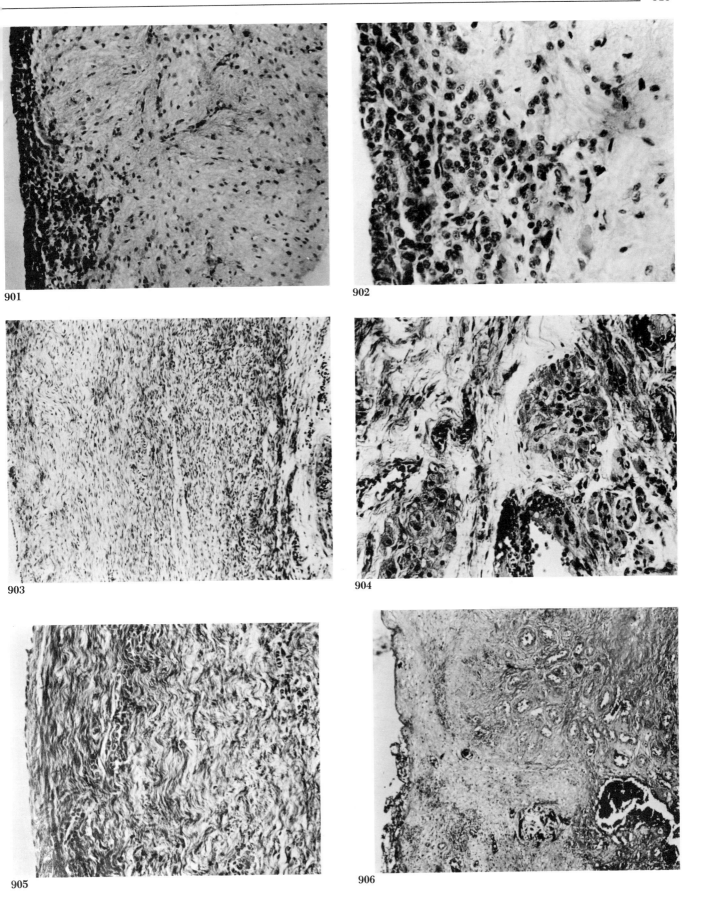

901

902

903

904

905

906

907 Ovary in induced ovulation with clomiphene citrate
The patient, 18 years old, received 100 mg of clomiphene citrate daily for 14 days. The multicystic ovary shows stromal edema. The predominantly follicular cysts show marked luteinization of the theca interna. Clomiphene citrate (1-[P-(B-diethylaminoethoxyl) phenyl]-1, 2-diphenyl-2-chloroethylene) is an analogue of the synthetic nonsteroid estrogen chlorotrianisene. (H&E. ×24)

908 Ovary in induced ovulation with clomiphene citrate
Note the formation of a theca lutein cyst. (H&E. ×60)

910 Ovary in induced ovulation with clomiphene citrate
An extreme degree of stromal edema with proliferation of capillaries and vascular hyperemia is seen. There is a tendency for massive intracystic and stromal hemorrhage and eventual rupture of the ovary. The morphologic and clinical picture is similar to that reported with hyperstimulation produced by gonadotropins. Clomiphene citrate is a potential cause of ovarian enlargement. Patients receiving this compound should be observed closely. (H&E. ×50)

909 Ovary in induced ovulation with clomiphene citrate
Corpus luteum is seen in the stage of vascularization. (H&E. ×35)

911 Ovotestis
The gonad is composed of ovarian cortical stroma with primordial follicles and seminiferous tubules. A skin biopsy showed that only 15 per cent of the 6,000 cells contained the sex chromatin body. (H&E. ×62)

912 Ovotestis
High magnification of Fig. 911. The oocyte in the seminiferous tubule is without sustentacular cells. Such an intratubular oocyte, in an unfavorable environment, may become a psammoma body. (H&E. ×320)

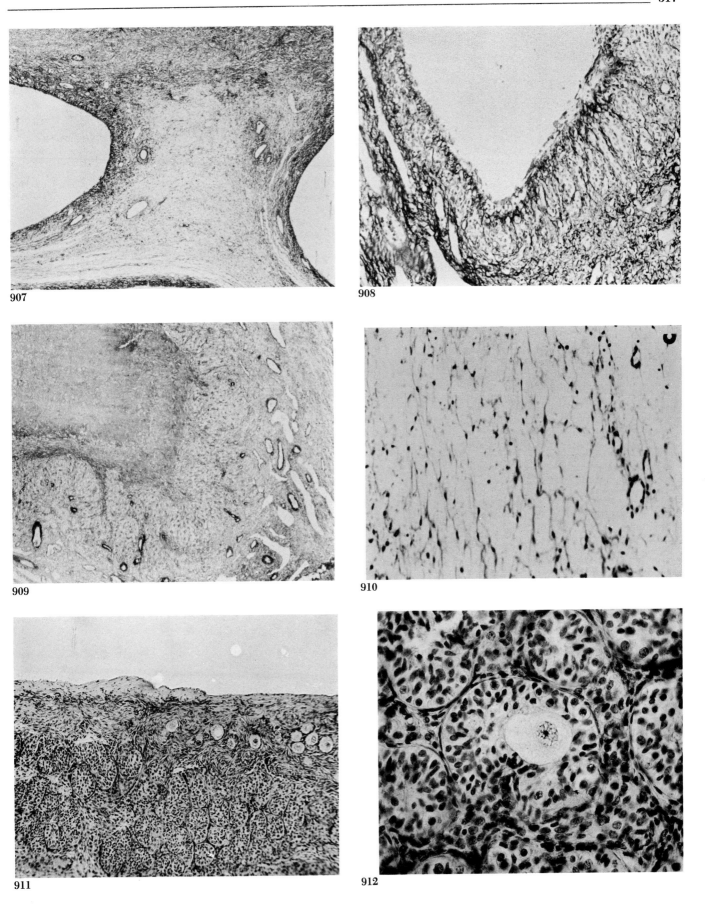

907

908

909

910

911

912

913   Agenesis of the ovary, rudimentary epididymis, and infundibular portion of the oviduct

The patient, 22 years old, is a female pseudo-hemaphrodite with the nuclear sex chromatin pattern of a female. (H&E. ×24)

914   Testicular feminization syndrome

The patient, 20 years old, has primary amenorrhea, a chromatin-negative sex pattern, and an XY chromosomal pattern. Examination disclosed the absence of axillary and pubic hair, normal vulva, vagina 8 cm deep, and absence of internal reproductive organs. Bilateral inguinal hernias with gonads were present. There was marked fibrosis of the tunica albuginea of the testis. Fibrosis of the seminiferous tubules and interstitial connective tissue was present. Several tubular adenomas were present (Pick). (H&E. ×18)

915   Testicular feminization syndrome

There is marked interstitial fibrosis, peritubular fibrosis, and atrophy of tubular epithelium. Formation of microadenomas is seen to the left. (H&E. ×60)

916   Testicular feminization syndrome

Hyperplastic islands of interstitial Leydig cells are present. The seminiferous tubules show atrophy with preservation of Sertoli cells. There is complete germinal cell aplasia. (H&E. ×200)

917   Testicular feminization syndrome

Hyperplasia of interstitial cells and Sertoli cells is seen. This syndrome is hereditary, with transmission through the maternal line. (H&E. ×200)

918   Testicular feminization syndrome

Formation of tubular adenoma (Pick) or andro-blastoma in feminizing testis is seen. The tumor is composed of tubular structures lined by vacuolated primitive Sertoli cells. Tubular adenoma or multiple adenomas are constantly found in association with feminizing testis, and they are usually of a well-differentiated variety. (H&E. ×180)

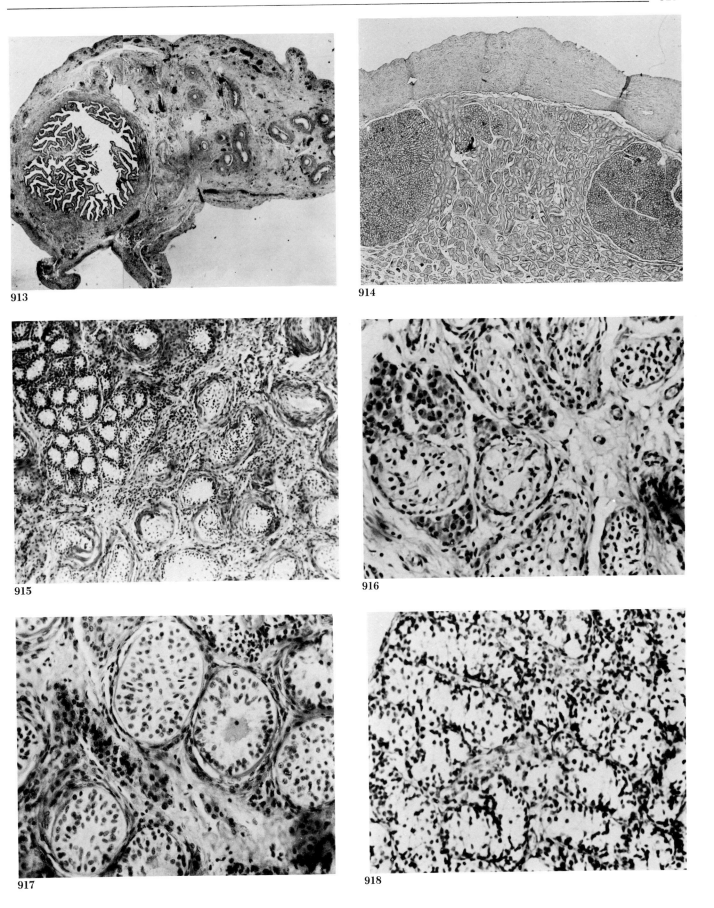

913

914

915

916

917

918

919   Serous cystadenoma of the ovary
Note the lining epithelium. (H&E. ×500)

920   Unilocular serous cystadenoma of the ovary
The lining of an unilocular ovarian serous cystadenoma is seen. (H&E. ×24)

921   Coarse papillary serous cystadenoma of the ovary
Coarse, warty, papillae are lined by a single layer of low cuboidal epithelium. There is predominance of connective tissue stroma. (H&E. ×35)

922   Fine papillary serous cystadenoma of the ovary
Papillary projections are lined by columnar epithelium. (H&E. ×50)

923   Fine papillary serous cystadenoma of the ovary
Papillary projections are lined by tall columnar epithelium with distinct ciliated brush borders. There is predominance of epithelial elements. (H&E. ×50)

924   Fine papillary serous cystadenoma with edematous stroma of the ovary
(H&E. ×50)

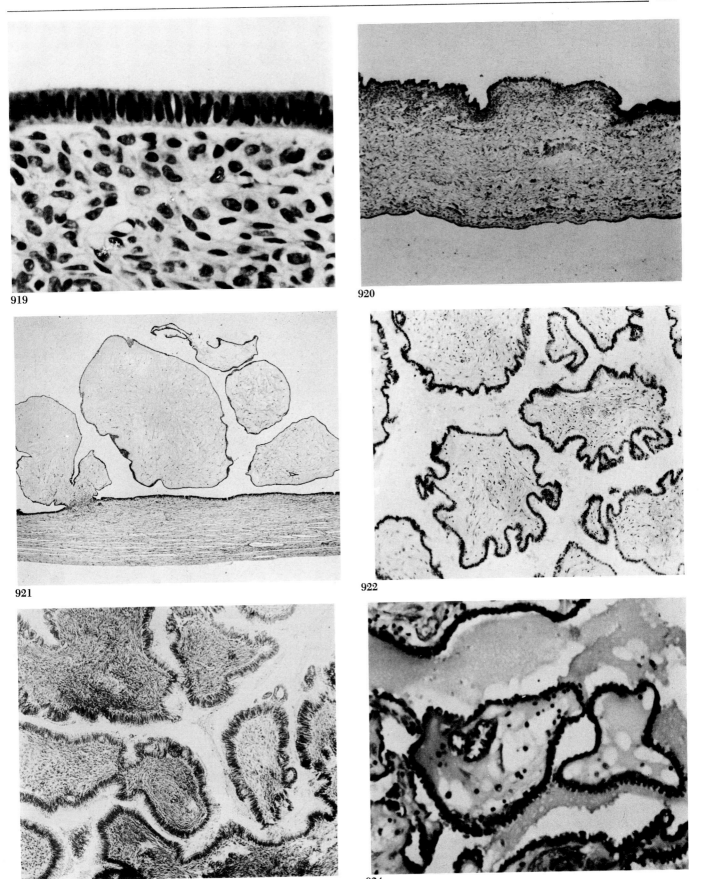

919

920

921

922

923

924

**925 Serous papillary cystadenoma of the ovary
with psammoma bodies**
There is deposition of laminated calcific structures in the connective tissue stroma of papillary projections. (H&E. ×50)

**926 Proliferating serous papillary cystadenoma
without stromal invasion of the ovary**
Such a morphologic picture is encountered in borderline or possibly malignant tumors. Occasionally such a growth has been termed a low grade carcinoma. (H&E. ×50)

**927 Proliferating serous papillary cystadenoma
without stromal invasion of the ovary**
Well-differentiated columnar epithelium is seen lining papillary projections and cystic spaces. Note the presence of psammoma bodies in connective tissue stroma. (H&E. ×125)

**928 Proliferating serous papillary cystadenoma
of the ovary without stromal invasion**
There is no visible evidence of an infiltrative and/or destructive growth pattern. (H&E. ×50)

**929 Proliferating serous papillary cystadenoma
of the ovary without stromal invasion**
High magnification of Fig. 928. Slight piling up of epithelial cells is present. Cyst formation is seen in the stroma. (H&E. ×125)

**930 Proliferating serous papillary cystadenoma
of the ovary without stromal invasion**
High magnification of Fig. 928. The lining epithelium may show nuclear abnormalities. (H&E. ×125)

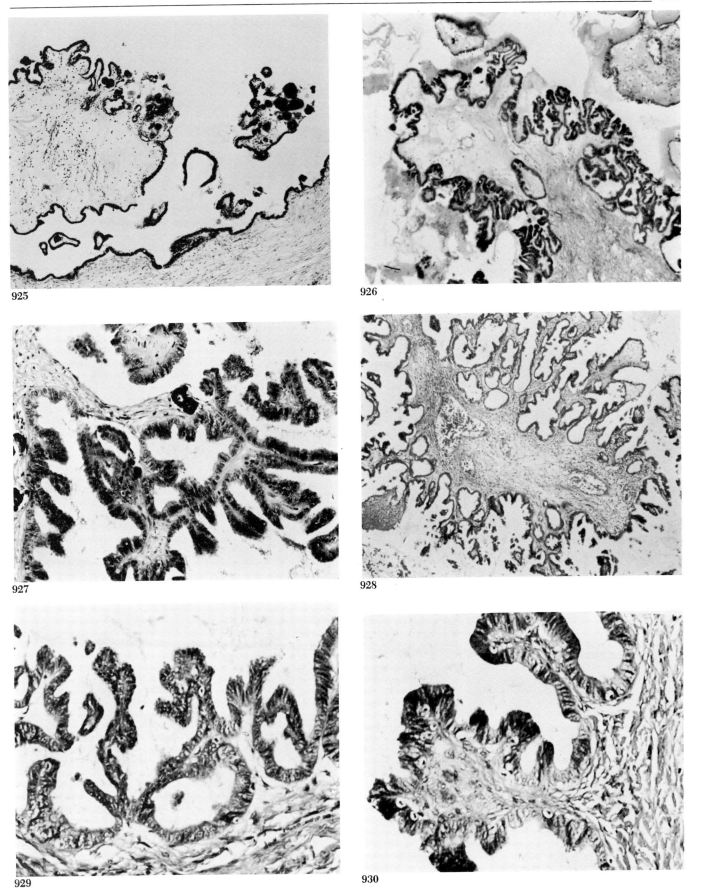

925

926

927

928

929

930

931   Malignant transformation of an unilocular serous cystadenoma of the ovary

Carcinomatous transformation of epithelium is seen lining an unilocular serous cystadenoma. (H&E. ×75)

932   Papillary serous cystadenocarcinoma of the ovary with a break through the capsule

The papillary serous cystadenocarcinoma is seen developing within the ovarian cortex and destroying the tunica albuginea. The corpus luteum is located beneath the tumor. (H&E. ×6)

933   Papillary serous cystadenocarcinoma of the ovary

High magnification of Fig. 932. This detail shows the neoplastic cells covering a papillary projection. (H&E. ×320)

934   Well-differentiated papillary serous cystadenocarcinoma of the ovary

Multiple papillary projections are covered by highly atypical epithelial cells. There is invasion of the stroma by malignant epithelial cells. (H&E. ×55)

935   Well-differentiated papillary serous cystadenocarcinoma of the ovary

The tumor is formed by papillary projections and cysts with a scant amount of connective tissue stroma. Piling up of neoplastic epithelial cells is prominent. The tumor cells vary in size and in the staining quality of their nuclei. (H&E. ×50)

936   Moderately well-differentiated serous papillary cystadenocarcinoma of the ovary

Note the irregular appearance of papillary structures. Epithelial cells are small and poorly differentiated. Mitotic figures are frequent. (H&E. ×125)

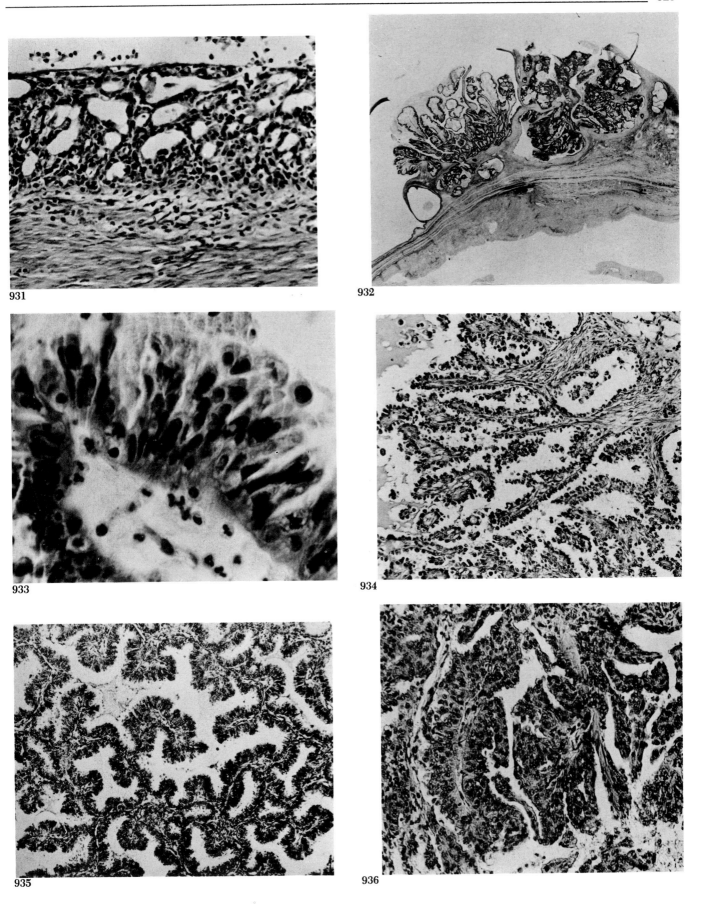

931

932

933

934

935

936

937 Moderately well-differentiated papillary serous cystadenocarcinoma of the ovary
The tumor cells are arranged in an alveolar pattern. They are columnar and show frequent mitotic figures. (H&E. ×150)

938 Moderately well-differentiated papillary serous cystadenocarcinoma of the ovary
Note the vacuolated, alveolar appearance of tumor masses covering the connective tissue stalk. (H&E. ×125)

939 Poorly differentiated papillary serous cystadenocarcinoma of the ovary
Papillary structures are absent. The tumor is composed of solid sheaths of neoplastic cells forming occasional glandlike structures. Neoplastic cells vary in size and shape. Nuclear hyperchromatism and pleomorphism are present. There is massive infiltration of connective tissue stroma by tumor cells. (H&E. ×150)

940 Anaplastic papillary serous cystadenocarcinoma of the ovary
The tumor cells are undifferentiated. Connective tissue stroma is almost completely absent. (H&E. ×125)

941 Serous cystadenocarcinoma of the ovary with acanthomatous changes (adenoacanthoma)
Note the appearance of neoplastic squamous epithelium in cysts of serous carcinoma. Two types of adenoacanthoma should be differentiated: one is a form of serous cystadenocarcinoma, and the second, a form of endometrioid cystadenocarcinoma. (H&E. ×50)

942 Papillary serous cystadenocarcinoma of the ovary with irradiation effects
The patient received cancerocidal doses of roentgen and radium therapy for inoperable papillary serous cystadenocarcinoma of the ovary with extensive abdominal spread. (H&E. ×50)

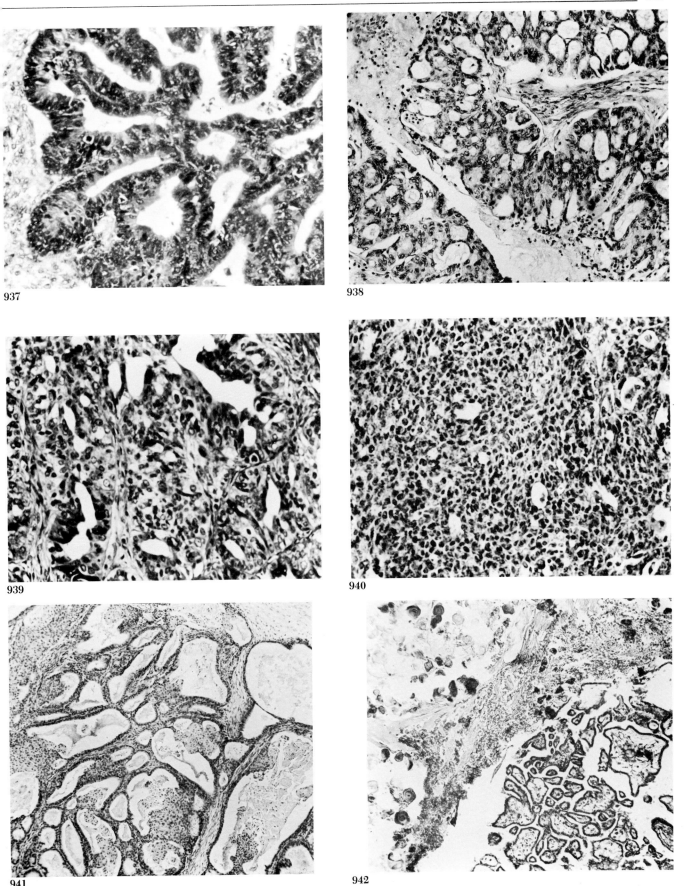

937

938

939

940

941

942

943 Mucinous cystadenoma of the ovary
Note the lining epithelium. (H&E. ×500)

944 Mucinous cystadenoma of the ovary
Interspersed goblet cells and characteristic mucinous tall columnar cells are seen. The latter are similar to mucinous cells of the endocervix and intestine. (Mayer's mucicarmine stain. ×260)

945 Simple mucinous cystadenoma of the ovary
The simple cyst is lined by tall columnar mucinous epithelium. (H&E. ×150)

946 Pseudoglandular type mucinous cystadenoma of the ovary
The tumor is composed of epithelial invaginations forming pseudoglandular structures. (H&E. ×150)

947 Pseudoglandular type mucinous cystadenoma (microcystic pattern) of the ovary
The tumor is formed by numerous cystic structures lined by tall columnar epithelium. The cystic spaces contain large amounts of secretion. The connective tissue stroma is scant and compressed. (H&E. ×50)

948 Papillary type mucinous cystadenoma of the ovary
Papillary projections are seen protruding into cystic spaces. (H&E. ×50)

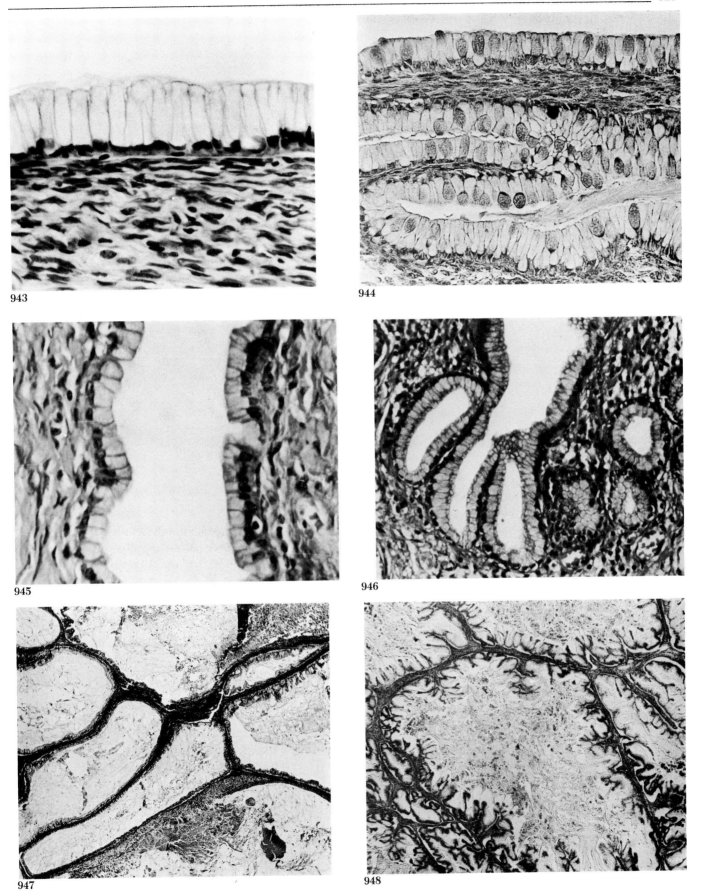

943

944

945

946

947

948

949 Papillary type mucinous cystadenoma of the ovary
(H&E. ×125)

950 Mucinous cystadenoma of the ovary (so-called pseudomyxoma ovarii)
Note the decrease of connective tissue stroma. Fusion of papillary projections is seen. Overproduction of thick mucinous substance penetrates the connective tissue stroma. Spilling of the content of this tumor into the peritoneal cavity results in peritoneal tumor implantation known as pseudomyxoma peritonei. (H&E. ×125)

951 Mucinous cystadenoma of the ovary (so-called pseudomyxoma ovarii)
Extremely thin connective tissue septums can be seen between cystic spaces. There is disruption of the cyst walls with cyst fusion. Thick mucinous material is present in the remaining connective tissue stroma. (H&E. ×50)

952 Tuberculosis in the wall of a unilocular simple mucinous cystadenoma of the ovary
Partial destruction of cyst lining by a tuberculous granuloma can be seen. (H&E. ×50)

953 Pseudoglandular proliferating mucinous cystadenoma of the ovary without stromal invasion
A so-called borderline or possibly malignant tumor is seen. Well-differentiated epithelial cells line glandlike spaces. There is, however, piling up of epithelial cells. No nuclear atypism is seen. (H&E. ×150)

954 Papillary type proliferating mucinous cystadenoma of the ovary without stromal invasion
Cystic spaces with papillary projections are lined by tall columnar epithelium. There is moderate nuclear atypism. Occasional piling up of epithelial cells and epithelial budding is seen. In the past, such tumors were designated as low grade carcinomas. (H&E. ×75)

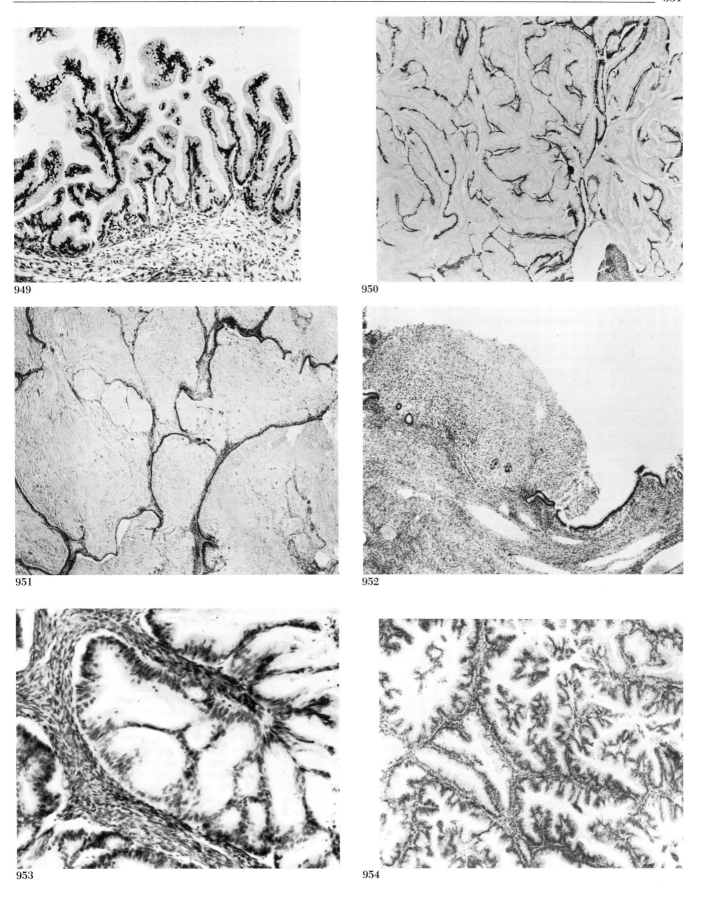

949

950

951

952

953

954

955 Carcinoma developing in a unilocular, simple mucinous cystadenoma of the ovary
To the right, a benign tumor area is seen; to the left, the malignant portion is shown. (H&E. ×50)

956 Carcinoma developing in unilocular, simple mucinous cystadenoma of the ovary
High magnification of Fig. 955. (H&E. ×125)

957 Well-differentiated mucinous cystadeno-carcinoma of the ovary
Numerous glandlike structures and scant connective tissue stroma are seen. These are lined by tall columnar mucinous epithelial cells with scattered mitotic figures. (H&E. ×150)

958 Well-differentiated mucinous cystadeno-carcinoma of the ovary
The crowded glandular structures are almost without intervening connective tissue stroma. The epithelial cells are differentiated and mucin-producing. (H&E. ×150)

960 Moderately well-differentiated mucinous cystadenocarcinoma of the ovary
The neoplastic epithelial cells are irregular in arrangement. There is marked epithelial piling up and budding. Pronounced infiltration with polymorphonuclear leukocytes is seen. (H&E. ×150)

959 Moderately well-differentiated mucinous cystadenocarcinoma of the ovary
Irregular glandlike structures are lined by atypical epithelial cells showing excessive piling up and frequent mitotic figures. (H&E. ×180)

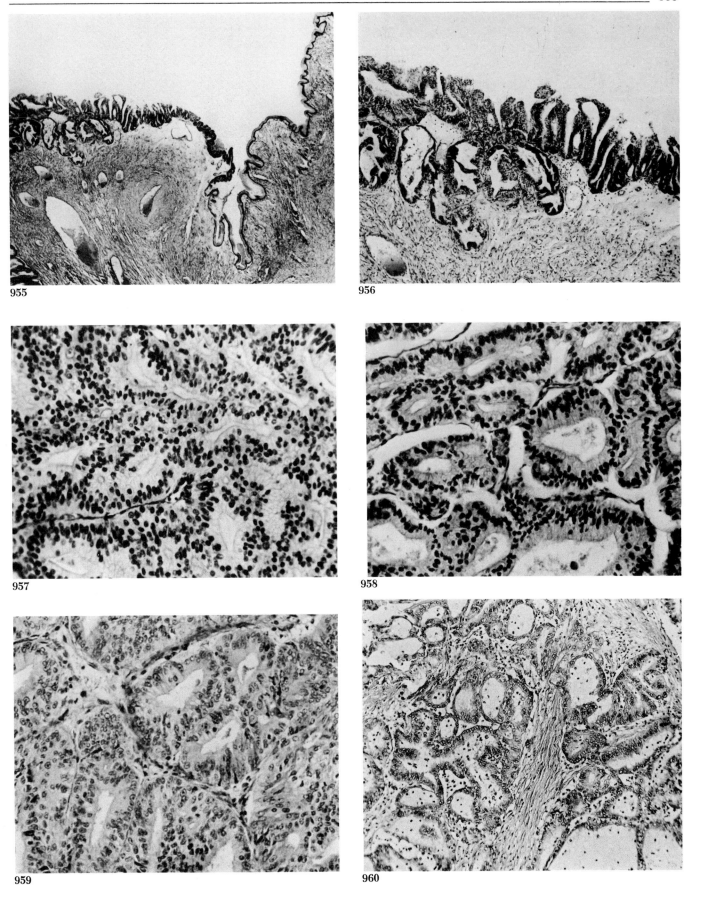

955

956

957

958

959

960

961   Moderately well-differentiated mucinous cystadenocarcinoma of the ovary
The epithelial lining is composed of columnar cells with hyperchromatic nuclei. Numerous tufts and fingerlike projections are present. (H&E. ×150)

962   Moderately well-differentiated mucinous cystadenocarcinoma of the ovary
Papillary projections are covered by irregular neoplastic epithelial cells with hyperchromatic nuclei. There is marked cellular pleomorphism. (H&E. ×200)

963   Poorly differentiated mucinous cystadenocarcinoma of the ovary
Poorly differentiated epithelial cells form tufts and glandlike structures. Nuclear pleomorphism is striking. The intervening connective tissue stroma is scant. (H&E. ×180)

964   Poorly differentiated mucinous cystadenocarcinoma of the ovary
Degenerative changes are seen occurring in relatively poorly differentiated neoplastic epithelium. Traces of mucinous secretion are present. (H&E. ×180)

965   Poorly differentiated mucinous cystadenocarcinoma of the ovary
There is piling up of poorly differentiated epithelial cells. Cytoplasmic vacuolization is present. The production of mucinous substance is considerably decreased. (H&E. ×320)

966   Anaplastic mucinous cystadenocarcinoma of the ovary
The tumor is formed by solid sheaths of undifferentiated cells. An occasional cell contains mucin. (H&E. ×125)

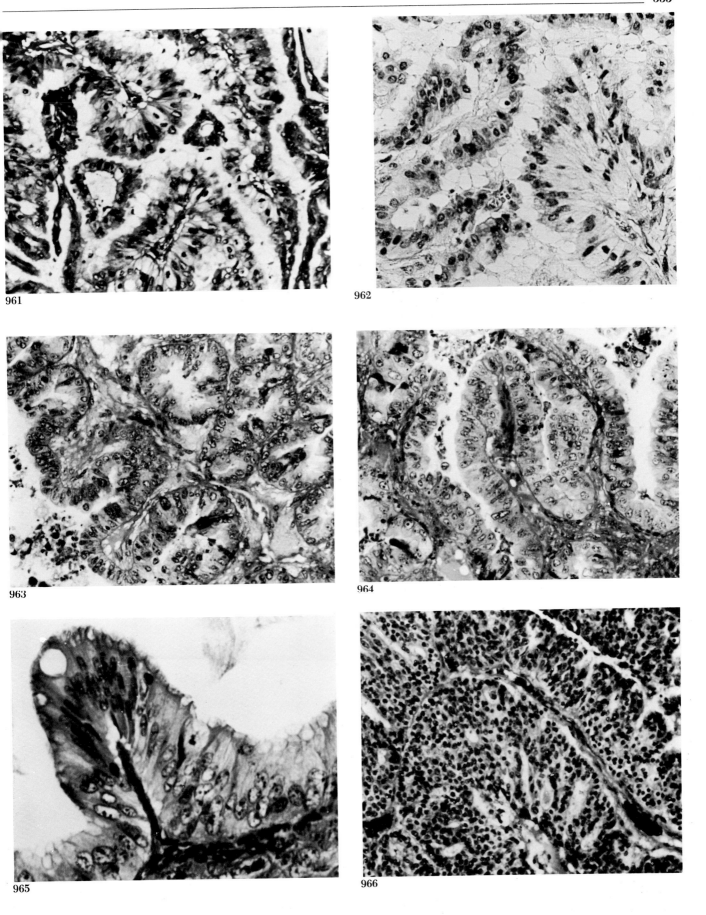

961

962

963

964

965

966

967 Proliferating endometrioid cystadenoma of the ovary without stromal invasion (Horalek-Santesson)

The origin of this tumor is debatable. Some have probably arisen in or from preexisting ovarian endometriosis. The term "endometrioid" implies the morphologic similarity of this ovarian neoplasm to the uterine endometrial neoplasms. (H&E. ×25)

968 Proliferating endometrioid cystadenoma of the ovary without stromal invasion (Horalek-Santesson)

The papillary projections are lined by tall columnar epithelial cells with elongated plump nuclei. There are foci of epithelial piling and some nuclear atypicalities. Occasional mitotic figures are seen. This tumor is possibly malignant. (H&E. ×80)

969 Well-differentiated endometrioid carcinoma of the ovary (Horalek-Santesson)

There is striking resemblance to an endometrial adenocarcinoma. This slow-growing ovarian tumor has a relatively better overall prognosis. Histogenesis: some originate from preexisting ovarian endometriosis, the majority from pluripotential Müllerian epithelium. (H&E. ×150)

970 Well-differentiated endometrioid carcinoma of the ovary (Horalek-Santesson)

Neoplastic glands, somewhat irregularly shaped, are lined by columnar cells with eosinophilic cytoplasm. An occasional mitotic figure is seen. (H&E. ×180)

971 Moderately well-differentiated endometrioid carcinoma of the ovary (Horalek-Santesson)

Glandular structures are lined by proliferating epithelial cells. The ovoid nuclei are rich in chromatin. (H&E. ×180)

972 Poorly differentiated endometrioid carcinoma of the ovary (Horalek-Santesson)

The tumor is composed of alveolar structures packed with cuboidal neoplastic cells. Atypical mitotic figures are frequent. The connective tissue stroma is scant. (H&E. ×180)

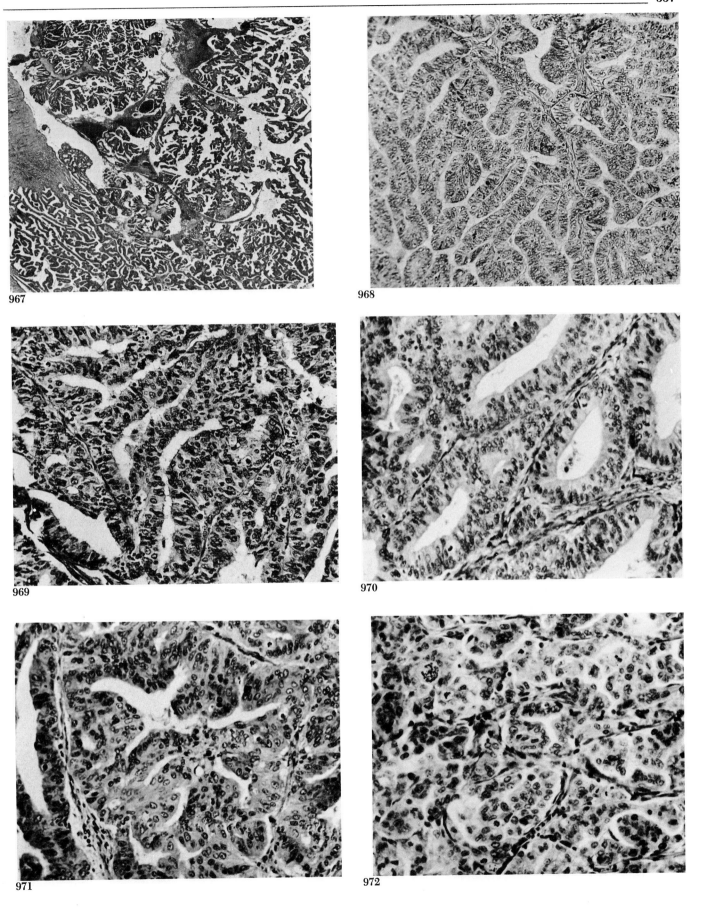

967

968

969

970

971

972

973 Endometrioid carcinoma of the ovary with acanthomatous changes (adenoacanthoma) (Horalek-Santesson)
Note the appearance of neoplastic squamous epithelium within the glandular structures of the tumor. Mucinous material is present in the cystically dilated glands. This tumor should be differentiated from adenoacanthoma developing from serous carcinoma of the ovary. (H&E. ×150)

974 Dimorphic mixed seromucinous cystadenoma of the ovary (Glasunow)
The glandlike structures are lined by tall columnar mucinous epithelium and in places by a typical serous type of epithelium. The distribution of mucinous and serous tumor elements varies within a dimorphic cystadenoma. (H&E. ×100)

975 Dimorphic mixed seromucinous cystadenoma of the ovary without stromal invasion (Glasunow)
Glandlike structures are lined partly by mucinous, partly by serous epithelium. Cyst formation is seen in the stroma. There is no evidence of nuclear abnormalities. (H&E. ×80)

976 Dimorphic mixed seromucinous cystadenoma of the ovary without stromal invasion (Glasunow)
High magnification of Fig. 975. An area of mucinous epithelium is surrounded by typical serous epithelium. (H&E. ×180)

977 Dimorphic, mixed seromucinous cystadenocarcinoma of the ovary (Glasunow)
Two morphologically distinct neoplastic areas are seen in an ovarian cystadenocarcinoma. Area *A* is formed by glandular structures which are filled with mucinous material. Area *B* is composed of glandular elements with epithelial cells resembling those in serous carcinoma. (H&E. ×80)

978 Dimorphic, mixed seromucinous cystadenocarcinoma of the ovary (Glasunow)
High magnification of Fig. 977A. (H&E. ×150)

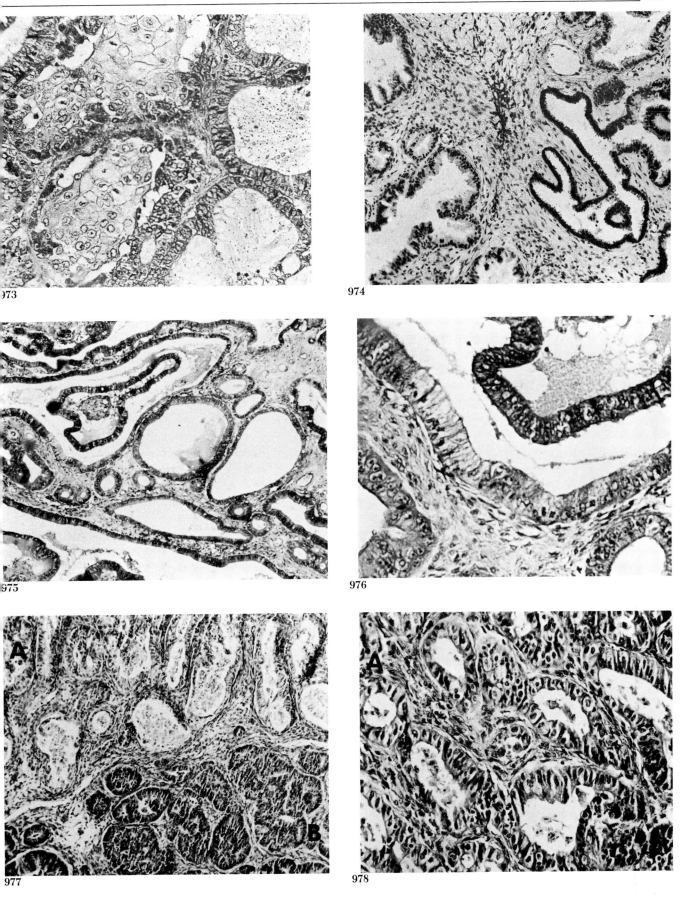

973

974

975

976

977

978

**979   Dimorphic, mixed seromucinous cystade-
nocarcinoma of the ovary (Glasunow)**
High magnification of Fig. 977B. (H&E. ×150)

**980   Dimorphic, mixed, poorly differentiated
carcinoma of the ovary**
This tumor is composed of two distinct types of
tumor cells. Tumor areas A and B both show
considerable cellular anaplasia. (H&E. ×80)

**981   Dimorphic, mixed, poorly differentiated
carcinoma of the ovary**
High magnification of Fig. 980A. (H&E. ×100)

**982   Dimorphic, mixed, poorly differentiated
carcinoma of the ovary**
High magnification of Fig. 980B. (H&E. ×100)

983   Cystadenofibroma of the ovary
The tumor is formed largely by proliferating neoplastic fibrous connective tissue in which are
embedded neoplastic cysts lined by cuboidal or
columnar epithelium. The lining epithelium of
the cysts may be ciliated, serous type or may be
mucus-secreting, resulting in two varieties of
tumor, namely, serous cystadenofibroma and
mucinous cystadenofibroma. Papillary structures
composed of dense fibrous tissue are frequently
encountered. (H&E. ×15)

984   Cystadenofibroma of the ovary
High magnification of Fig. 983. Typical ciliated
serous type epithelial cells are seen lining the
cyst. (H&E. ×220)

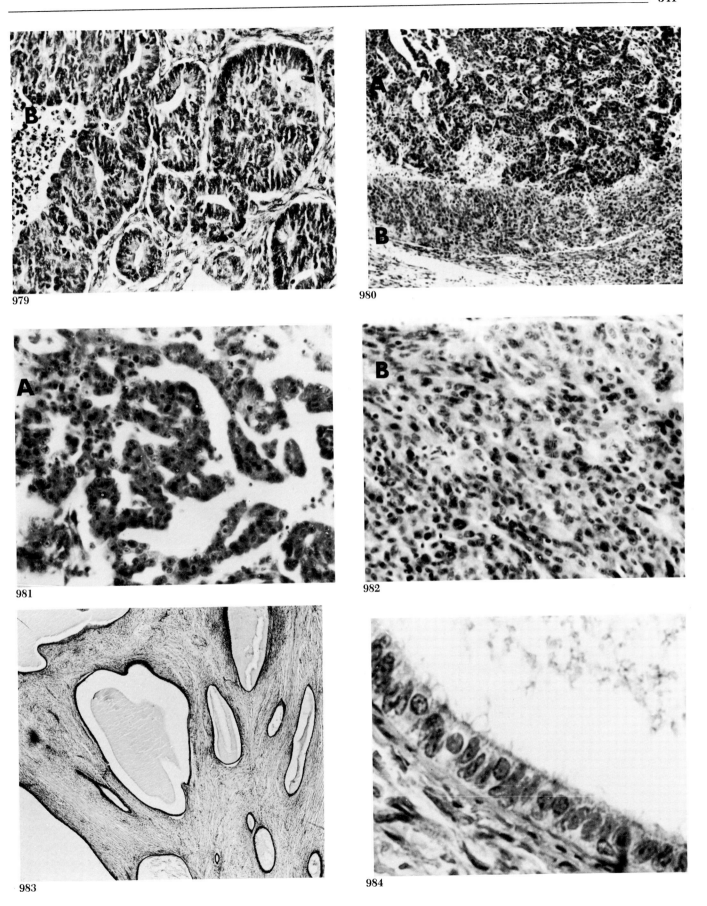

979

980

981

982

983

984

985 Cystadenofibroma of the ovary
Papillary structures are formed by dense fibrous connective tissue stroma and covered by a serous type of epithelium. Occasional cysts are seen. (H&E. ×25)

986 Cystadenofibroma developing from rete ovarii
Note the transition from well-preserved tubular structures of rete ovarii to cystadenofibroma. The rectangle is magnified in Fig. 987. (H&E. ×25)

987 Cystadenofibroma developing from rete ovarii
High magnification of Fig. 986. Area of rectangle. (H&E. ×50)

988 Carcinoma developing in a cystadenofibroma of the ovary
(H&E. ×25)

989 Carcinoma of the breast metastatic to a cystadenofibroma of the ovary
The arrow indicates metastatic cells. (H&E. ×25)

990 Carcinoma of the breast metastatic to a cystadenofibroma of the ovary
High magnification of Fig. 989. The area indicated with an arrow in Fig. 989 shows an accumulation of metastatic cuboidal cells with large hyperchromatic nuclei. (H&E. ×120)

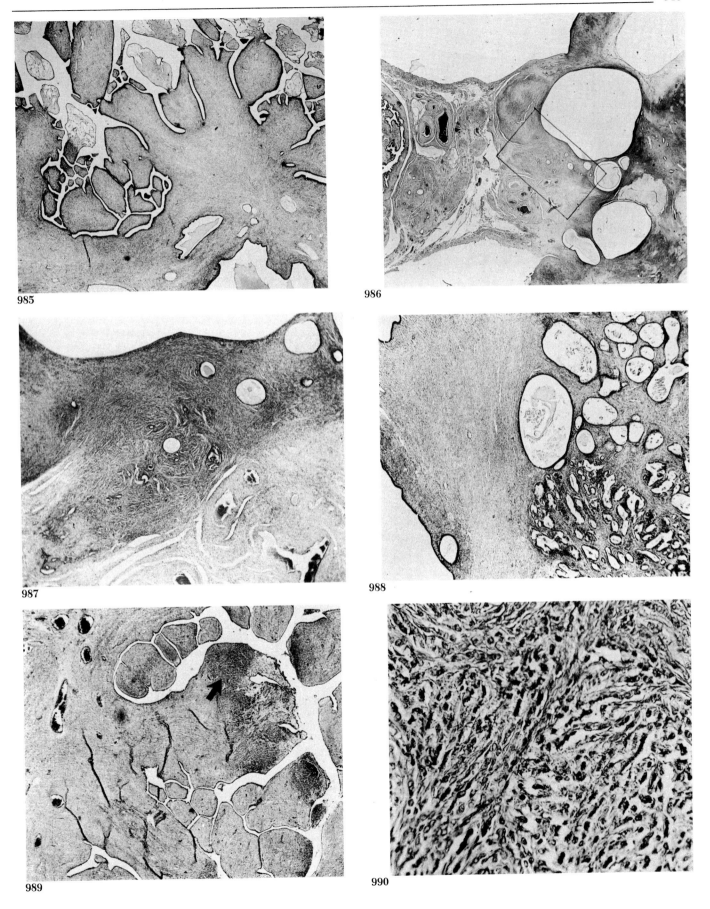

985

986

987

988

989

990

991 Surface papilloma of the ovary
The surface of an ovary shows numerous small and large papillary projections formed by cortical fibrous connective tissue and covered by hyperplastic epithelium. (H&E. ×25)

992 Surface papilloma of the ovary
High magnification of Fig. 991. Note the marked hyperplasia of the surface epithelium covering papillary projections. Compare this with the relatively normal germinal epithelium at the bottom of the picture. (H&E. ×100)

993 Surface papillary carcinoma of the ovary
The tumor is seen developing from the surface of an atrophic ovary. An entire ovary or a portion of it could be covered by surface papillary carcinoma. Irrespective of its small size, surface papilloma is notorious in producing extensive abdominal carcinomatosis by direct extension over the peritoneum and massive infiltration of the omentum and mesentery. (H&E. ×150)

994 Undifferentiated carcinoma of the ovary
The tumor is formed by masses of undifferentiated cells which do not have a morphologic or histochemical relationship to serous or mucinous carcinomas. (H&E. ×125)

995 Undifferentiated carcinoma of the ovary
This highly anaplastic tumor shows pronounced cellular and nuclear pleomorphism. Atypical mitotic figures are frequent. (H&E. ×125)

996 Miniature Brenner tumor of the ovary with hyalinized stroma
The two nests of epithelial cells are surrounded by hyalinized stroma. (H&E. ×50)

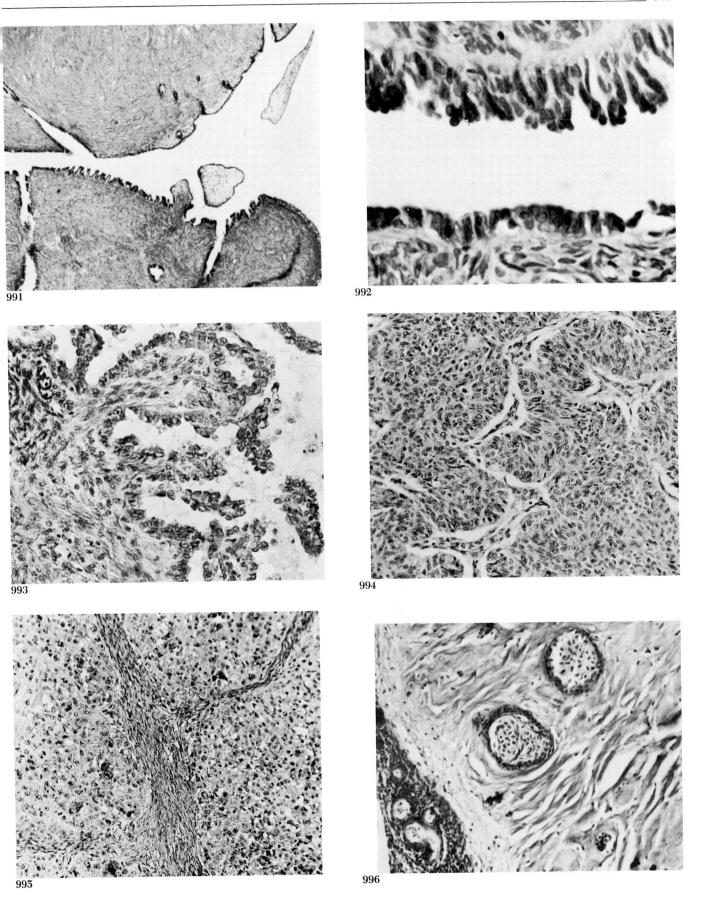

991

992

993

994

995

996

997   Miniature Brenner tumor of the ovary
Two nests of uniform ovoid epithelial cells are surrounded by circular fibers of connective tissue. This miniature Brenner tumor should be differentiated from Walthard cell rests resulting from invagination at the celomic epithelium. (H&E. ×50)

998   Solid Brenner tumor of the ovary
The fibroepithelial tumor is formed by islands of uniform ovoid cells resembling squamous or transitional epithelium and surrounded by neoplastic dense fibrous connective tissue stroma. Connective tissue stroma may show luteinization, in which case Brenner's tumor may be hormonally active. (H&E. ×50)

999   Epithelium of Brenner tumor island of the ovary
High magnification of Fig. 998. The detail of epithelial cells shows poorly demarcated cell borders. The nuclei are prominent with occasional distinct nucleoli. Some of the nuclei show longitudinal grooves, an observation not necessarily specific for Brenner epithelial cells. (H&E. ×350)

1000   Brenner tumor of the ovary with predominance of epithelial islands
The tumor is formed predominantly by numerous solid epithelial islands and scant fibrous connective tissue stroma. (H&E. ×62)

1001   Cystic Brenner tumor of the ovary
The tumor is composed of solid and cystic epithelial islands. Some of the cysts may reach considerable size. (H&E. ×15)

1002   Cystic Brenner tumor of the ovary
The cyst is lined by typical Brenner epithelial cells. Solid islands are seen adjacent to a cyst. (H&E. ×35)

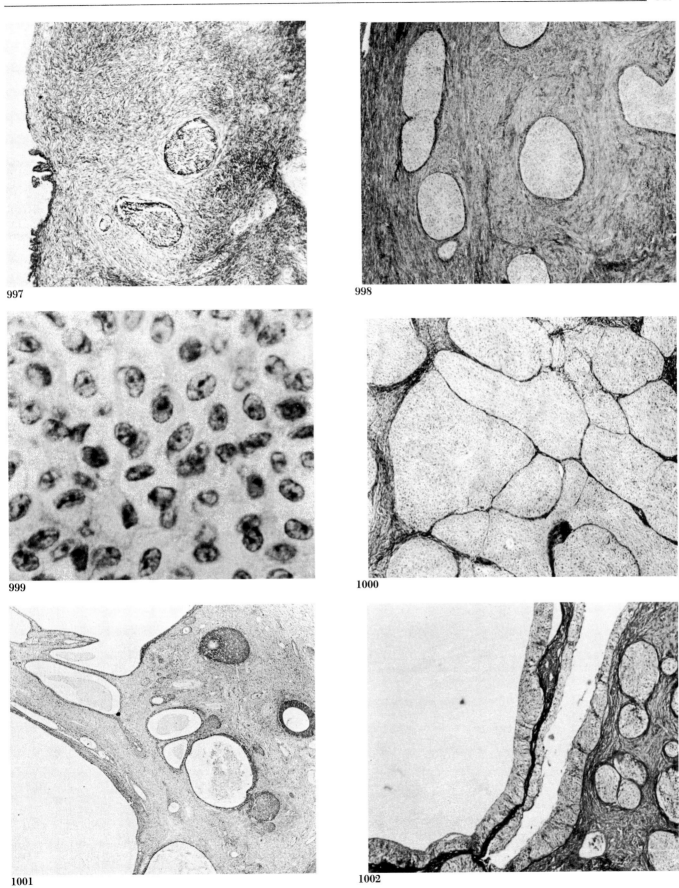

997

998

999

1000

1001

1002

1003   Cystic Brenner tumor of the ovary with mucinous epithelium

The epithelial island in Brenner's tumor shows the central cyst lined by tall columnar mucus-secreting epithelium. (H&E. ×150)

1004   Cystic Brenner tumor of the ovary with mucinous epithelium

Note the variation of epithelial cells in the cystic Brenner island. The cells close to the connective tissue stroma are cuboidal and those cells lining the cystic cavity are tall, columnar, and mucus-producing. (H&E. ×180)

1005   Brenner tumor of the ovary with mucinous epithelial metaplasia

There is variation of cells in the epithelial island. Some of the cuboidal cells become vacuolated and distended. Others undergo mucoid degeneration with the formation of microcysts. (H&E. ×220)

1006   Brenner tumor of the ovary with mucinous changes

Formation of microcysts is seen within epithelial islands. They contained PAS and Alcian blue positive material, identified as neutral and acid mucopolysaccharides. (PAS stain. ×50)

1007   Brenner tumor of the ovary with stromal calcifications

The connective tissue stroma of the tumor corresponds to a fibroma. Focal areas of calcification are occasionally seen, particularly adjacent to epithelial islands. (H&E. ×50)

1008   Brenner tumor of the ovary with extensive stromal edema

Two epithelial islands are surrounded by somewhat condensed fibrous connective tissue. The remaining stromal tissue shows marked edema. (H&E. ×50)

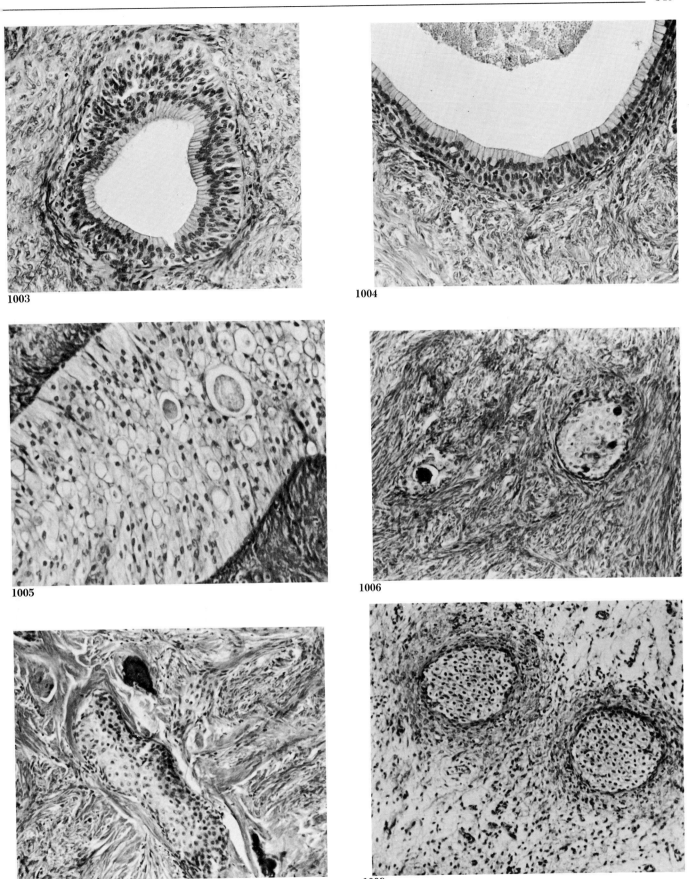

1003

1004

1005

1006

1007

1008

1009 Brenner cyst of the ovary
The large, unilocular cyst with a seromucinous content is lined by Brenner type epithelium showing foci of mucinous epithelial metaplasia. (H&E. ×45)

1010 Brenner cyst of the ovary with focal epithelial papillomatosis
The cyst is lined by typical Brenner type epithelium forming papillary projections. (H&E. ×25)

1011 Proliferating Brenner tumor of the ovary, possibly malignant
Epithelial islands are formed by proliferating epithelial cells. The nuclei show considerable hyperchromatism. Mitotic figures are inconspicuous. (H&E. ×150)

1012 Proliferating Brenner tumor of the ovary, possibly malignant
There is marked dysplasia of epithelium in a Brenner island. Note also the epithelial tendency for ramification and stromal invasion. (H&E. ×150)

1013 Malignant Brenner tumor of the ovary
To the right is seen a characteristic epithelial island. To the left, the epithelium of Brenner's island shows marked cellular pleomorphism and nuclear hyperchromatism. (H&E. ×125)

1014 Malignant Brenner tumor of the ovary
The epithelial island shows the characteristic picture of squamous cell carcinoma. Note the infiltration of the stroma by inflammatory cells. (H&E. ×100)

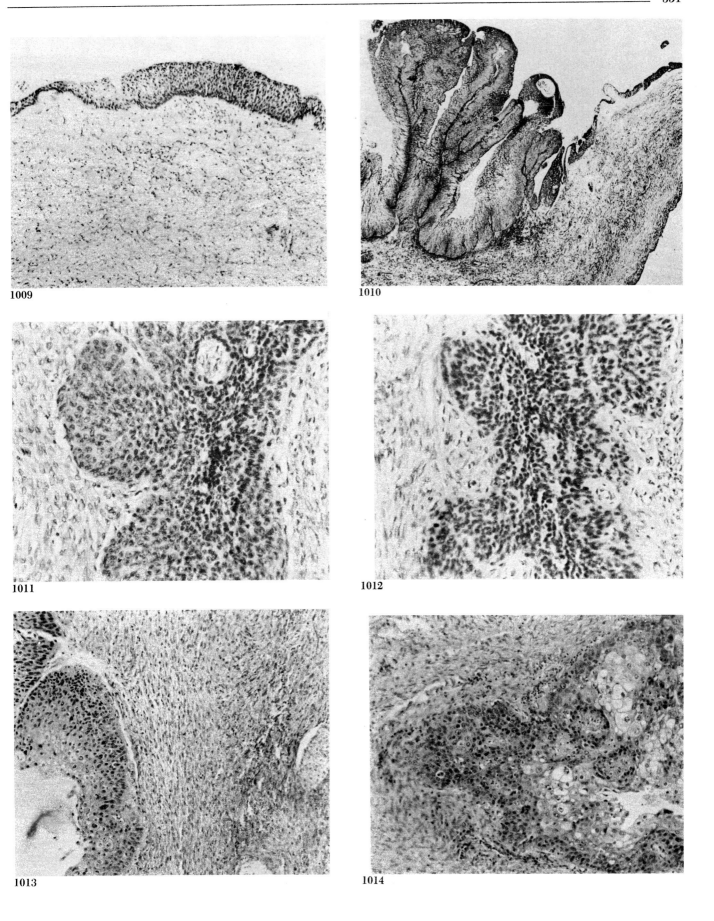

1009

1010

1011

1012

1013

1014

1015   Malignant Brenner tumor of the ovary
Brenner's epithelial islands are formed by highly atypical neoplastic cells showing cellular pleomorphism and the presence of bizarre nuclei. (H&E. ×280)

1016   Malignant Brenner tumor of the ovary with invasion of lymphatic channels
There is invasion of lymphatic channels of the stroma by plugs of malignant neoplastic epithelial cells. Note the marked nuclear hyperchromatism. (H&E. ×150)

1017   Adenomatoid tumor of the ovary
The cystic tumor is formed by irregular projections and islands. The neoplastic cells are forming cystlike or glandlike spaces. A considerable degree of stromal hyalinization is present. (H&E. ×24)

1018   Adenomatoid tumor of the ovary
High magnification of Fig. 1017. The tumor is formed of glandlike structures lined by flattened cells with prominent hyperchromatic nuclei. In adenomatoid tumor of the ovary, fibromuscular stroma is absent. Hyaline deposition is prominent. Lymphocytes are scattered throughout. (H&E. ×125)

1019   Adenomatoid tumor of the ovary
The cystic tumor shows numerous glandlike spaces. It is notoriously misdiagnosed as lymphangioma or some kind of vascular tumor. The tumor spaces are not lined by endothelial cells. Two hypotheses of derivation of this tumor are (1) from Müllerian epithelial vestiges, (2) from peritoneal (mesothelial) origin. Histochemical investigation favors Müllerian epithelial origin. (H&E. ×24)

1020   Adenomatoid tumor of the ovary
High magnification of Fig. 1019. Compare this tumor with adenomatoid tumors of the uterus and oviduct. Benign tumors in the ovary are known to reach considerable size. (H&E. ×150)

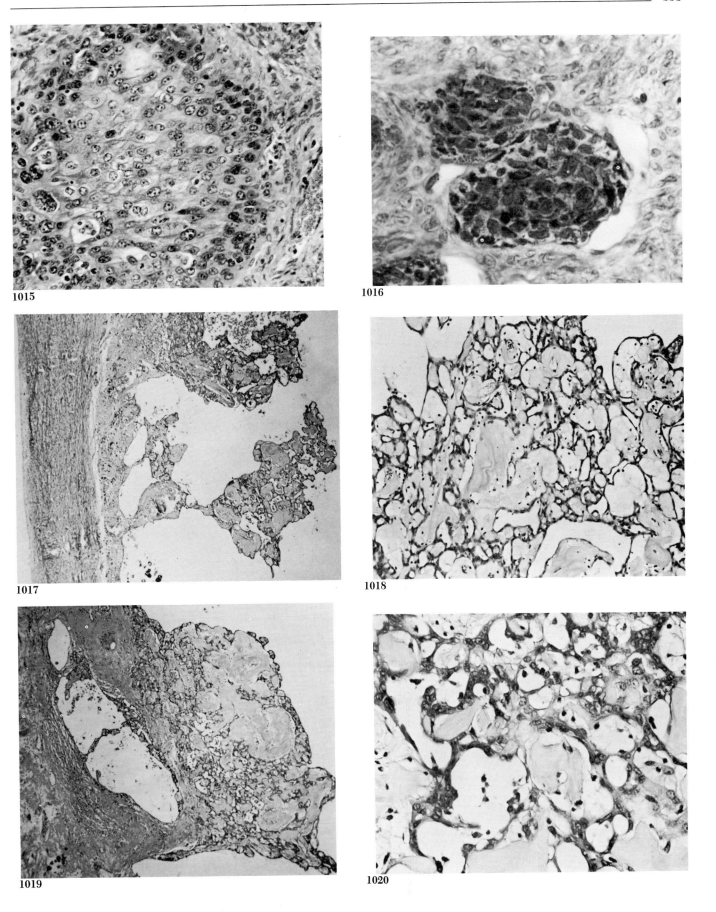

1015

1016

1017

1018

1019

1020

1021 Luteoma gravidarum of the ovary
This is an incidental finding at cesarean section. The ovary is replaced by a solid orange-yellow tumor. The origin of the tumor is most probably corpus luteum of pregnancy, although luteinized granulosa cells or theca cells should be taken into consideration. In some cases, it is difficult to make a precise distinction between a neoplasm and hyperplasia of luteal origin. (H&E. ×50)

1022 Luteoma gravidarum of the ovary
High magnification of Fig. 1021. The tumor is composed of polyhedral cells with numerous lipid droplets in the cytoplasm. Nuclei are prominent. Numerous intervening capillaries are present. (H&E. ×200)

1023 Luteoma gravidarum of the ovary
High magnification of Fig. 1021. The neoplastic cells vary in size. Cytoplasmic, round hyaline inclusion bodies are present as seen in corpus luteum of pregnancy. The cytoplasm is finely granular and contains brown pigment. (H&E. ×300)

1024 Luteoma gravidarum of the ovary
High magnification of Fig. 1021. Between the luteinized polyhedral cells are scattered dark cells with pyknotic nuclei. Calcium deposition may occur as seen in this case. (H&E. ×125)

1025 Undifferentiated lipid tumor of ovary in pregnancy
This rapidly growing ovarian tumor was detected in the second trimester of pregnancy. The unilateral, solid, orange-yellow soft tumor is seen replacing the ovary and invading neighboring structures. The tumor is formed by large irregular lipid-containing cells and small dark-staining cells. It is highly vascular. (H&E. ×50)

1026 Undifferentiated lipid tumor of ovary in pregnancy
High magnification of Fig. 1025. The large neoplastic cells show extensive vacuolization of cytoplasm. Variation in the size and chromatin content of the nuclei is evident. Atypical mitotic figures are present. The frozen section revealed a high lipid content. (H&E. ×125)

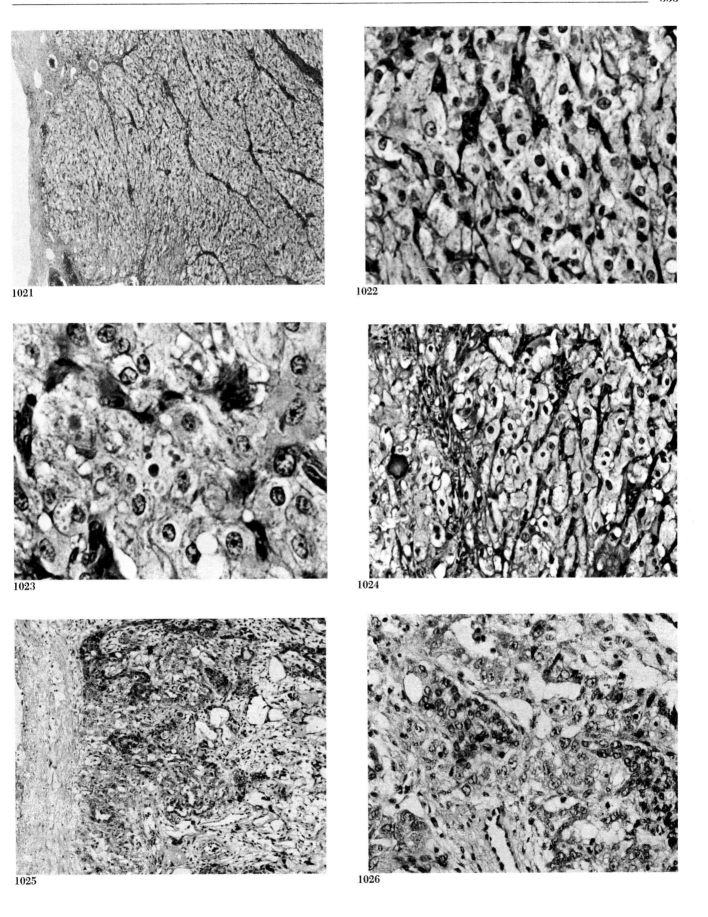

1021

1022

1023

1024

1025

1026

1027 Undifferentiated lipid tumor of ovary in pregnancy
High magnification of Fig. 1025. There is intra-cytoplasmic deposition of numerous round hyaline granules or bodies. Focal calcific deposition is present. Frequent bizarre hyperchromatic nuclei are seen. (H&E. ×180)

1028 Undifferentiated lipid tumor of ovary in pregnancy
High magnification of Fig. 1025. The highly luteinized tumor cells show hyperchromatic irregular nuclei and the presence of numerous round hyaline bodies. (H&E. ×180)

1029 Adrenal cortical rest tumor (heterotopic adrenal cell rest adenoma) of the ovary
The tumor is formed by cells closely resembling those of the adrenal cortex. The cytoplasm of the cells appears clear because of its content of lipid and glycogen. (H&E. ×30)

1030 Adrenal cortical rest tumor (heterotopic adrenal cell rest adenoma) of the ovary
High magnification of Fig. 1029. The histologic pattern of neoplastic ovarian tumor cells is indistinguishable from cells of zona glomerulosa and fascicularis of the adrenal cortex. (H&E. ×160)

1031 Adrenal cortical rest tumor (heterotopic adrenal cell rest adenoma) of the ovary
High magnification of Fig. 1029. The patient, 35 years of age, had a history of secondary amenorrhea and increasing hirsutism, deepening voice, and enlargement of the clitoris. Elevated urinary 17-keto-steroid, abnormal carbohydrate metabolism, and mild hypertension were present. (H&E. ×160)

1032 Malignant adrenal cortical rest tumor (heterotopic adrenal cell rest carcinoma) of the ovary
The tumor is formed by clear cells varying in size and in lipid content. Note the loss of organoid appearance and the presence of hyperchromatic nuclei. (H&E. ×50)

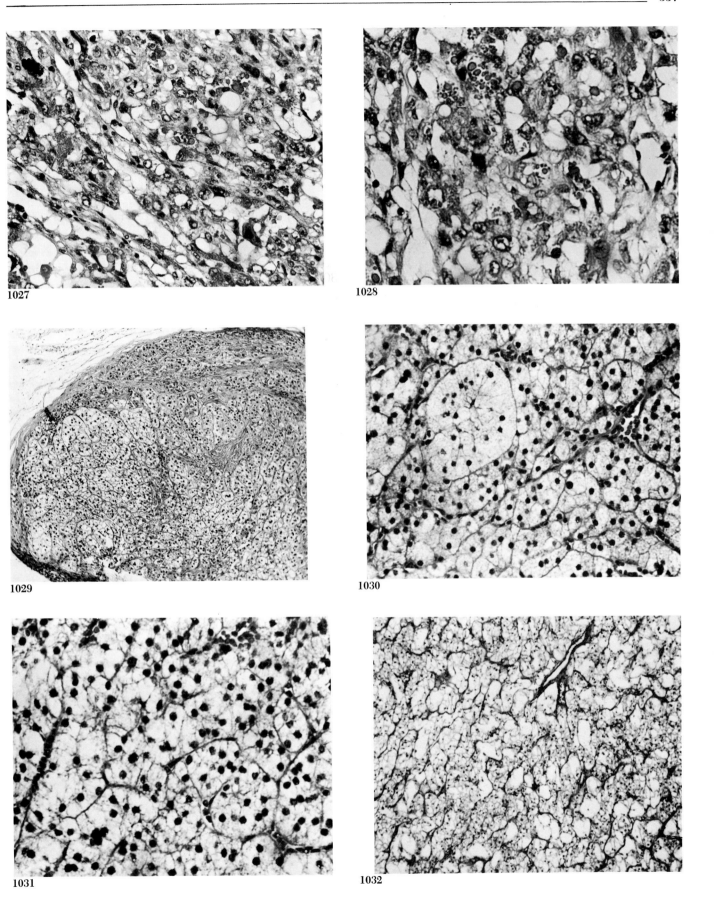

1027

1028

1029

1030

1031

1032

1033 Malignant adrenal cortical rest tumor (heterotopic adrenal cell rest carcinoma) of the ovary

High magnification of Fig. 1032. Nuclear atypism of tumor cells is seen. Neoplastic cells rich in lipid with atypical mitotic figures are present. The patient, a 14-year-old girl, had hirsutism and an enlarged clitoris. Androgen hyperactivity was confirmed by a high excretion of 17-ketosteroid. A poorly encapsulated tumor of the ovary was removed. (H&E. ×280)

1034 Malignant adrenal cortical rest tumor (heterotopic adrenal cell rest carcinoma) of the ovary

The ovarian tumor is formed by polyhedral neoplastic cells with large bizarre nuclei. Lipid vacuoles are prominent. The cytoplasm is finely granular and contains brown pigment. Administration of 2,000 units of chorionic gonadotropin, given intramuscularly on arising, will help in differentiating between adrenal cortical rest tumor of the ovary and hilus cell tumor and/or androblastoma. There will be no increase in androgen excretion in the urine specimen obtained during the next 24 hr in cases of adrenal cortical rest tumor. In cases of hilus cell tumor (Fig. 1042) or androblastoma, androgen excretion may be increased three to six times. (H&E. ×220)

1035 Malignant adrenal cortical rest tumor (heterotopic adrenal cell rest carcinoma) of the ovary

Different area of the tumor shown in Fig. 1034. Note the striking resemblance to the adrenal cortical carcinoma, suggesting an adrenal origin of the tumor. The patient, a 41-year-old woman, showed rapid defeminization followed by virilization. At laparatomy, a large ovarian tumor with metastasis to the liver was seen. (H&E. ×220)

1036 Hilus cell hyperplasia of the ovary

There is diffuse proliferation of cords of polyhedral cells scattered in and among nerves and blood vessels of the ovarian hilar area. The hilar cells measure 30 to 40 μ in diameter, have round, relatively hyperchromatic nuclei and marked eosinophilic cytoplasm. It is difficult to draw a precise distinction between hilus cell tumor and diffuse hyperplasia. (H&E. ×50)

1037 Hilus cell hyperplasia of the ovary

Crystalloids of Reinke are seen clearly in a section overstained with eosin. Heidenhain's iron-hematoxylin stain and Masson's trichrome stain are useful in the demonstration of these intracytoplasmic crystalloid inclusions. Note the presence of yellow-brown lipochrome pigment granules in the cytoplasm of occasional hilus (interstitial) cells. (H&E. ×150)

1038 Hilus cell tumor of the ovary

The tumor is formed by cords and islands of polyhedral cells, with the intervening stroma composed of elongated cells. The hilus cells show prominent round nuclei and contain lipid. The tumor originated from gonadal hilus cells. Hilus cell tumors of the ovary may be hormonally inactive or may give rise to postmenopausal bleeding (feminizing, rather than masculinizing behavior). Finally they may produce virilization with a normal or slight increase of total 17-ketosteroid output. (H&E. ×100)

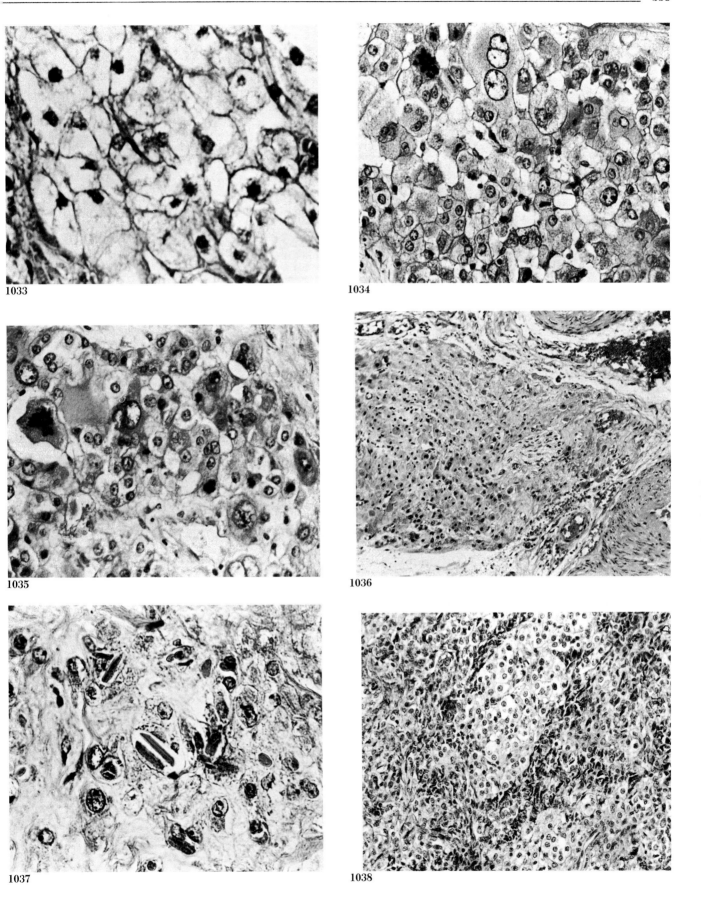

1033

1034

1035

1036

1037

1038

1039 Hilus cell tumor of the ovary
Vacuolization and granularity of the cytoplasm
are well recognized. The nuclei are somewhat
eccentric. Although clearly demarcated, no capsule is present around these tumors. The majority
of hilus cell tumors are benign. (H&E. ×125)

1040 Hilus cell tumor of the ovary
High magnification of Fig. 1039. The hilus cells
are arranged in an adenomatous pattern. Intervening connective tissue stroma is almost absent.
Uniform nuclei show prominent nucleoli.
Eosinophilic cytoplasm is finely granular and
shows the presence of lipochrome pigment.
Identification of crystalloid of Reinke is helpful
in diagnosing hilus cell tumor. Absence of
crystalloid, however, should not rule out hilus
cell tumor. (H&E. ×180)

1041 Hilus cell tumor of the ovary
The tumor is formed by trabeculae composed of
hilus cells. Hilus cells are identical with testicular interstitial (Leydig) cells. (H&E. ×50)

1042 Hilus cell tumor of the ovary
High magnification of Fig. 1041. The patient, 40
years old, showed hirsutism and had a history of
amenorrhea of 4 years duration. Hypertrophy of
the clitoris was present. The 17-ketosteroids
were slightly elevated. After administration of
chorionic gonadotropin, elimination of 17-keto-
steroid increased from 9.3 to 40 mg. The tumor
involved one ovary. The tumor is composed of
cords and islands of large, markedly eosinophilic hilus cells. (H&E. ×125)

**1043 Mesenchymal hilus cell tumor of the
ovary**
This virilizing ovarian tumor is formed by typical
lipid-containing epithelioid cells with round
nuclei and prominent nucleoli. Intervening are
elongated spindle cells with hyperchromatic
nuclei. The morphologic picture suggests, in this
case, development of hilus cells from mesenchymal connective tissue cells. (H&E. ×125)

**1044 Mesenchymal hilus cell tumor of the
ovary**
Elongated, closely packed spindle cells of
mesenchymal tissue origin are seen differentiating into hilus cells. The tumor produced marked
virilization, with an increase of 17-ketosteroids.
Hilus cell tumor should be differentiated from
a heterotopic adrenal cell rest adenoma of the
ovary. (H&E. ×125)

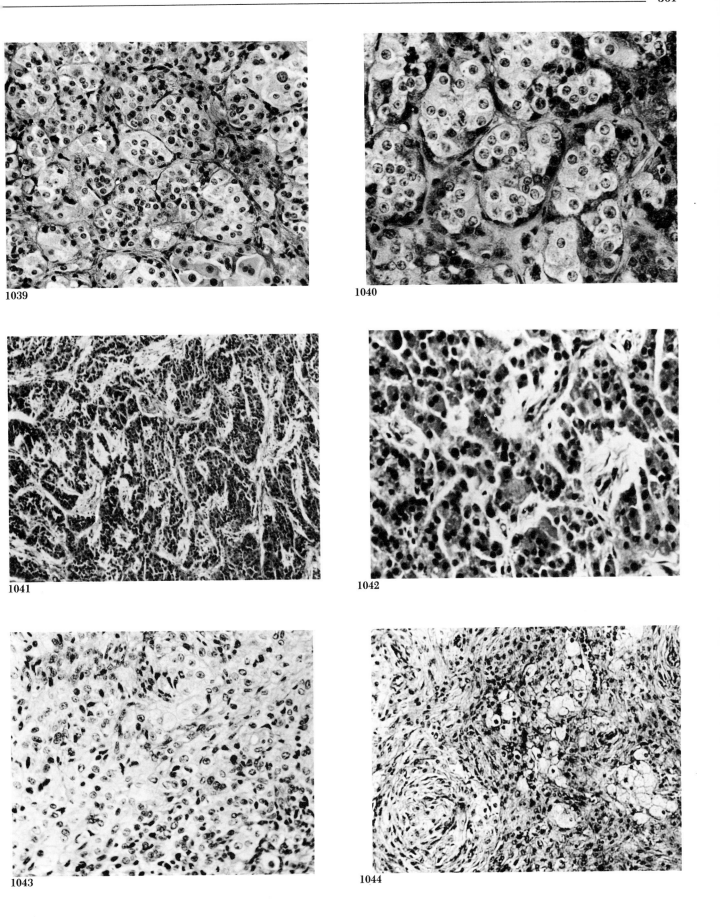

1039

1040

1041

1042

1043

1044

1045 Malignant hilus cell tumor of the ovary
The patient, 52 years old, had hirsutism, enlargement of the clitoris, and an ovarian mass. The 17-ketosteroids were consistently elevated. At laparotomy, a large ovarian tumor adherent to neighboring structures was found. The tumor shows cellular pleomorphism and marked nuclear atypism and hyperchromatism. Neoplastic cells are seen diffusely infiltrating the stroma. Lipid and lipochrome pigment is present within the cytoplasm of neoplastic cells. (H&E. ×125)

1046 Malignant hilus cell tumor of the ovary
Abortive alveolar arrangement of neoplastic hilus cells is seen. Note the presence of giant hilus cells and the perivascular deposition of hemosiderin. There is increased vascularity as compared with its benign counterpart. (H&E. ×125)

1047 Malignant hilus cell tumor of the ovary
The patient, 33 years old, had oligomenorrhea and mild virilization. An oophorectomy was performed for unilateral ovarian tumor 12 cm in diameter. The capsule was seemingly intact. The patient died of extensive metastases 4 years later. The tumor is composed of large irregular neoplastic hilus cells diffusely infiltrating the ovarian stroma. Irregular and hyperchromatic nuclei are present. (H&E. ×125)

1048 Malignant hilus cell tumor of the ovary
High magnification of Fig. 1047. There is a high degree of cellular and nuclear atypism and pleomorphism. Eosinophilic granular cytoplasm shows a decrease of lipid material. Anaplasia of hilus cells is correlated with the malignant course of the tumor. (H&E. ×220)

1050 Tubular type, well-differentiated feminizing androblastoma of the ovary, with lipid storage (Sertoli cell tumor)
The tubular structures are lined by Sertoli cells. The cytoplasm of these cells contains a large amount of lipid. There is close approximation of tubular structures with little intervening connective tissue stroma. The presence of lipid in Sertoli cells points to an endocrine function, predominantly estrogenic, of these cells. The patient, 58 years old, had a history of postmenopausal bleeding. A unilateral ovarian tumor was present. Curettings showed glandular cystic hyperplasia. The final diagnosis was feminizing androblastoma. (H&E. ×150)

1049 Tubular androblastoma (Pick's adenoma) of the ovary
The tumor is formed by tubular structures lined by tall columnar epithelial cells identical with Sertoli cells. Interstitial connective tissue contains scattered interstitial (Leydig) cells. This highly differentiated tumor is identical with the tubular adenomas encountered in undescended testes and in feminizing testes. Of all androblastomas, this one is least hormonally active, if not hormonally indifferent, and is the most well differentiated. (H&E. ×150)

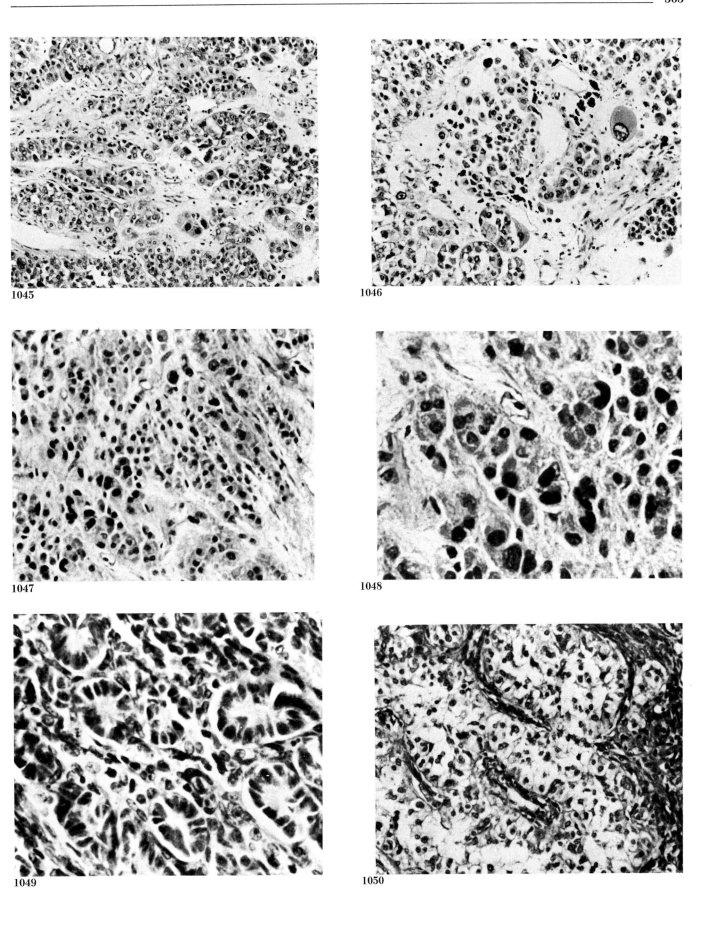

1045

1046

1047

1048

1049

1050

1051 Tubular type, well-differentiated andro-blastoma of the ovary, with lipoid storage

The tumor may be composed of Sertoli cells arranged in cords or tubules with various degrees of lipoid storage, interstitial (Leydig) cells, and mesenchymal cells in different stages of differentiation. Depending upon the predominance of the above-mentioned components, androblastoma may be feminizing, virilizing, or hormonally inert. (H&E. ×125)

1052 Tubular type androblastoma of the ovary with lipoid storage (androblastoma tubulare lipoides ovarii)

The tumor shows marked lipoid storage in the Sertoli cells lining the tubules. This was formerly misinterpreted as "folliculome lipidique." It is not to be confused with the virilizing "heterotopic adrenal cell rest adenoma" or mesonephric carcinoma. (H&E. ×125)

1053 Tubular type androblastoma of the ovary with lipoid storage (androblastoma tubulare lipoides ovarii)

The tumor is formed by well-differentiated tubular structures lined by overdistended Sertoli cells due to marked lipoid storage. Well-differentiated androblastomas, as a rule, are benign. With the loss of structural and cellular differentiation, the malignant potentiality of the tumor increases. (H&E. ×180)

1054 Tubular type androblastoma of the ovary with hilus cells

The tumor is composed of tubular structures lined by Sertoli cells. Intervening connective tissue contains cords formed by interstitial (Leydig) cells. They are identical with hilus cells. The patient, 30 years old, had secondary amenorrhea, progressive hirsutism, enlargement of the clitoris, and acne. The ovarian tumor was unilateral. Excretion of 17-ketosteroids was normal. After excision of the tumor, defeminization regressed. (H&E. ×125)

1055 Tubular type, moderately well-differentiated androblastoma of the ovary

The tumor is formed by ducts, glandlike and cystic structures lined by epithelial cells. The connective tissue stroma shows the presence of interstitial (Leydig) cells. There is differentiation of trabecular structures into tubules. This is a virilizing tumor. (H&E. ×80)

1056 Trabecular type androblastoma of the ovary

Trabecular arrangement of relatively poorly differentiated Sertoli cells is seen. The trabeculae are reminiscent of germ cords of the developing gonad. The connective tissue stroma is loose. This is a virilizing tumor. An intermediate stage of tumor development is shown. (H&E. ×80)

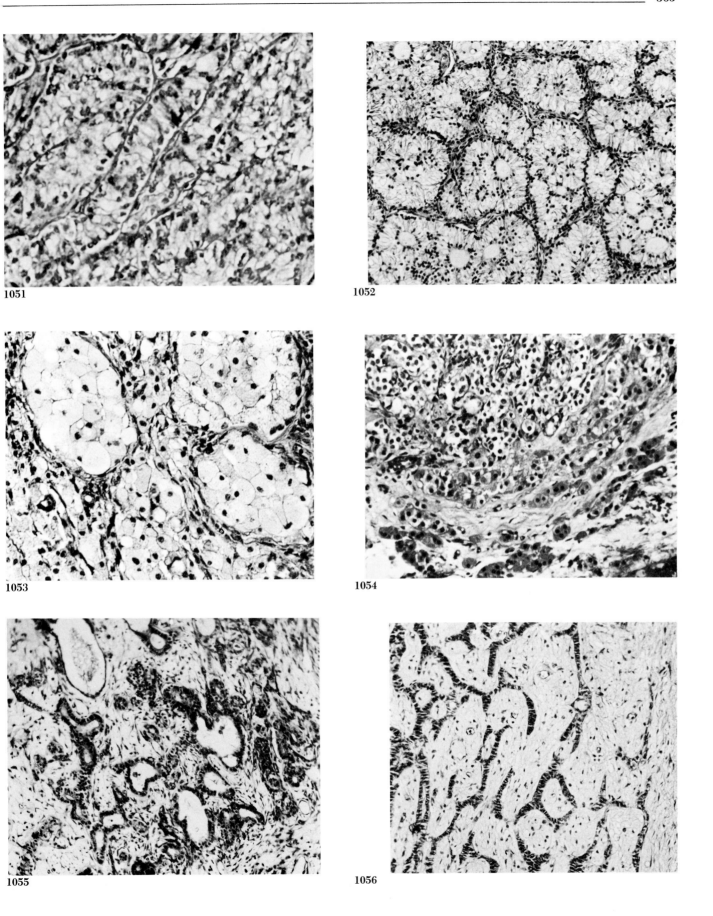

1051

1052

1053

1054

1055

1056

1057 Mesenchymal type androblastoma of the ovary

Diffuse arrangement of spindle-shaped mesenchymal cells is seen. There are scattered small groups of interstitial (Leydig) cells. This is a virilizing tumor. (H&E. ×125)

1058 Mesenchymal type androblastoma of the ovary

Note the attempted differentiation of cell cords amid undifferentiated mesenchymal cells. The patient, 50 years old, had a history of virilization and balding. (H&E. ×125)

1059 Mesenchymal type androblastoma of the ovary

This highly undifferentiated tumor is formed by pleomorphic cells of mesenchymal origin. The patient, 35 years old, had a history of amenorrhea, hirsutism, and enlargement of the clitoris in the past year. A unilateral, poorly encapsulated ovarian tumor is seen. The patient died of metastases 2 years later. (H&E. ×150)

1060 Mesenchymal type androblastoma of the ovary

This poorly differentiated tumor is formed by diffusely distributed ovoid and spindle-shaped cells. Note the presence of round, relatively large hyaline bodies. (H&E. ×120)

1061 Mixed type (tubular and mesenchymal) androblastoma of the ovary

The tumor is formed by tubular structures lined by Sertoli cells and large areas of diffusely distributed poorly differentiated pleomorphic mesenchymal cells. (H&E. ×50)

1062 Mixed type (tubular and mesenchymal) androblastoma of the ovary

The tumor is composed of diffuse stromal areas and tubular structures lined by Sertoli cells. This is a virilizing tumor. (H&E. ×125)

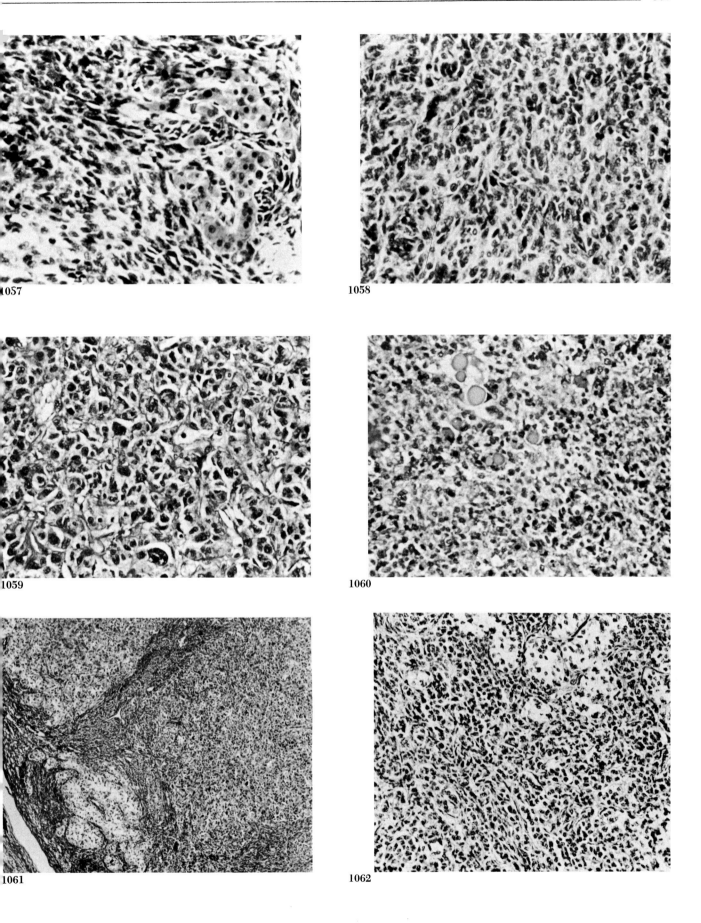

1057

1058

1059

1060

1061

1062

1063 Tubular feminizing androblastoma (so-called Sertoli cell tumor) of the ovary
The patient, 58 years old, had marked feminization. Curettings showed glandular cystic hyperplasia. A large amount of estrogen was detected chemically and biologically in ovarian tumor tissue and in the patient's urine. Such tumors have been reported as Sertoli cell tumors on the assumption that Sertoli cells lining tubular structures produce estrogen. However, histochemical investigation revealed that hormonal activity was limited to interstitial (Leydig) cells in this case. (H&E. ×80)

1064 Tubular, feminizing androblastoma (so-called Sertoli cell tumor) of the ovary
Sudan black stain of the specimen shown in Fig. 1063. Interstitial (Leydig) cells contain dark-staining lipid granules and most probably produce estrogens. Note the complete absence of lipid granules in the Sertoli cells. (×80)

1065 Tubular feminizing androblastoma (so-called Sertoli cell tumor) of the ovary
The patient, 54 years old, had marked feminization and irregular postmenopausal bleeding. In urine and ovarian tumor tissue, estrogens and androgens were isolated showing the following values: 4.69 μg and 5.34 μg estrogens per gram of tissue and/or urine, and 1.6 μg androgens per gram of tissue only. The tumor was formed by well-differentiated tubular structures lined by Sertoli cells. The arrow indicates the presence of numerous interstitial (Leydig) cells in intervening connective tissue stroma. (H&E. ×80)

1066 Tubular feminizing androblastoma (so-called Sertoli cell tumor) of the ovary
Sudan black stain of the specimen shown in Fig. 1065. Note the lipid granules in the interstitial (Leydig) cells. They are considered to produce estrogens and androgens. The feminizing properties of androblastomas are explained by the secretion of estrogen in these tumors by cells that are analogous to Sertoli cells and potentially capable of estrogen production. This is probably so in some cases. The ambivalent character of interstitial (Leydig) cells is most probably the correct explanation of the feminizing characteristic in the majority of such tumors. (×150)

1067 Granulosa cell rest of the ovarian cortex in a 2-year-old child
Following degeneration of an ovum, the surrounding follicular cells clump and form a pseudotubular structure. (H&E. ×320)

1068 Granulosa cell rest of the cortex of the ovary
Granulosa cells are seen forming several Call-Exner bodies. A mild theca cell reaction is present. Granulosa cells may proliferate in an atretic follicle. (H&E. ×180)

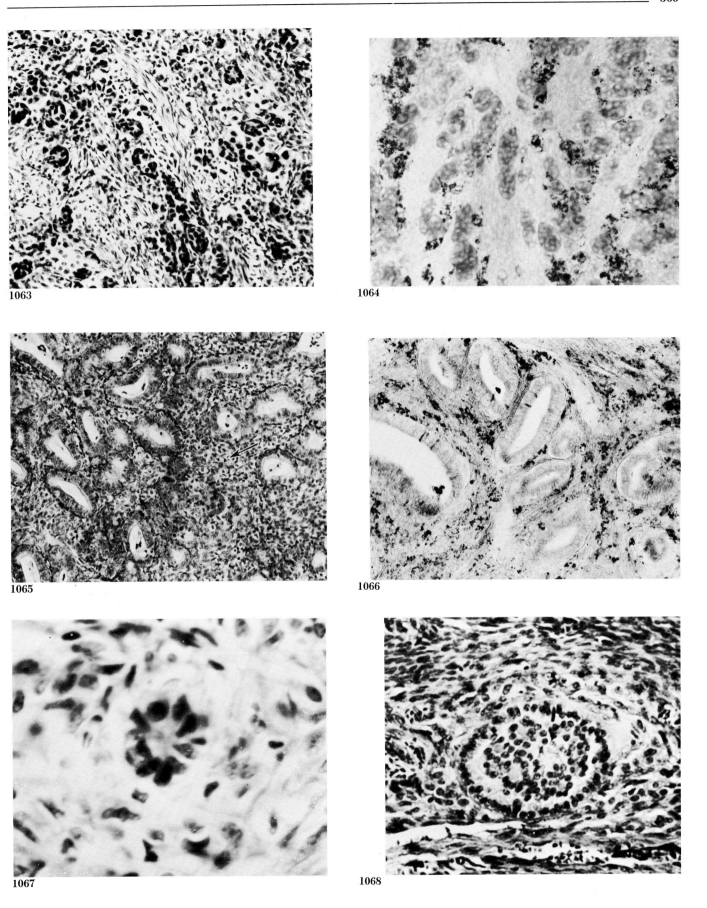

1063

1064

1065

1066

1067

1068

1069 Granulosa cell rests of the ovary
Multiple granulosa cell rests are seen in the ovarian cortex. Differentiation between multiple granulosa cell rests, granulosa cell hyperplasia, and an early granulosa cell tumor is difficult. They may likewise represent embryonic nests of granulosa cells, so-called granulosa-ballen. (H&E. ×150)

1070 Miniature granulosa cell tumor of the ovary
Several foci of proliferating granulosa cells form miniature granulosa cell tumors. (H&E. ×60)

1071 Miniature granulosa cell tumor of the ovary
Note the presence of miniature granulosa cell tumor in the ovarian cortex of an otherwise atrophic ovary. This was an incidental finding. The patient, 60 years old, had an adenocarcinoma of the endometrium. (H&E. ×90)

1072 Cystic granulosa cell tumor of the ovary
These large cysts remind one of graafian follicles. They are lined with granulosa cells showing numerous Call-Exner bodies. By attempting to reproduce mature follicles, cystic tumors show the highest degree of tumor differentiation. (H&E. ×25)

1073 Cystic granulosa cell tumor of the ovary with Call-Exner bodies
High magnification of Fig. 1072. Granulosa cell layer of a cyst is seen. Note the Call-Exner bodies. Several mitotic figures are seen. The presence of mitotic figures is important in assessing the malignant potentiality of a tumor. (H&E. ×300)

1074 Follicular type granulosa cell tumor of the ovary
The tumor is formed by islands of fairly uniform granulosa cells. They are separated by strands of connective tissue. Granulosa cells are arranged in a follicular pattern. The patient, 52 years old, had postmenopausal bleeding and an ovarian tumor. (H&E. ×125)

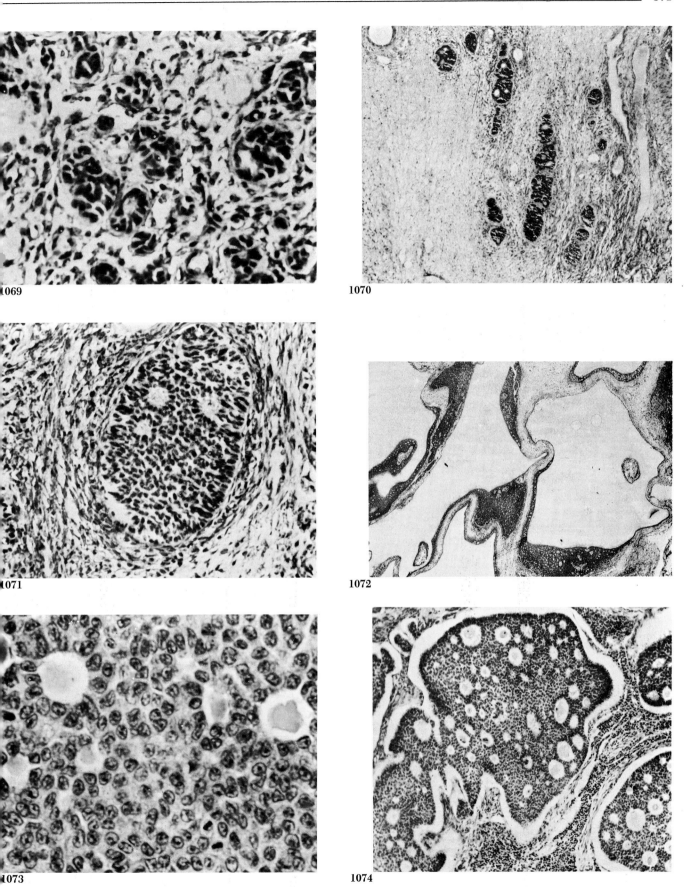

1069

1070

1071

1072

1073

1074

1075   Alveolar type granulosa cell tumor of the ovary

Granulosa cells are arranged in an alveolar pattern. The connective tissue strands show early hyalinization. The majority of granulosa cell tumors produce excessive estrogen; some are endocrinologically indifferent. An occasional granulosa cell tumor has been androgenically active. The reason for this aberration is not clear. (H&E. ×125)

1076   Alveolar type granulosa cell tumor of the ovary with stromal hyalinization

Note the alveolar arrangement of granulosa cells with extensive hyalinization of connective tissue stroma. (H&E. ×50)

1077   Alveolar type granulosa cell tumor of the ovary

Alveolar arrangement of granulosa cells is seen. Note the luteinization of connective tissue stroma similar to theca interna in graafian follicle. (H&E. ×135)

1078   Trabecular type granulosa cell tumor of the ovary

Granulosa cells are arranged in a trabecular pattern. Connective tissue stroma is loose and edematous. This represents an intermediate stage of differentiation of the granulosa cell tumor. (H&E. ×135)

1080   Mesenchymal type granulosa cell tumor of the ovary

The tumor is formed by poorly differentiated cells with diffuse distribution. This anaplastic form of granulosa cell tumor is also referred to as the "sarcomatous pattern." Note the masses of dark and light nuclei. The histologic diagnosis should be correlated with the clinical picture. The frozen section reveals fine lipid granules in the cytoplasm of these cells. (H&E. ×160)

1079   Trabecular type granulosa cell tumor of the ovary

Trabecular arrangement of granulosa cells is seen with sparse connective tissue stroma. (H&E. ×135)

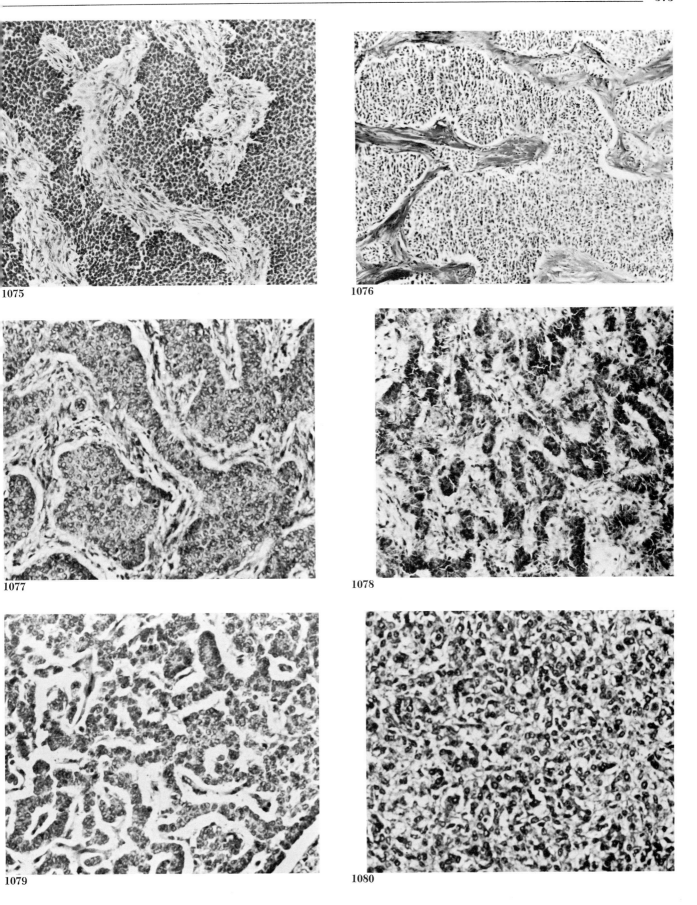

1075

1076

1077

1078

1079

1080

1081 Mesenchymal type granulosa cell tumor of the ovary
This highly undifferentiated tumor is formed by poorly outlined cells with ovoid hyperchromatic nuclei. Mitotic figures are very frequent. Approximately 30 per cent of all granulosa cell tumors show malignant behavior. (H&E. ×180)

1082 Atypical granulosa cell tumor of the ovary
Granulosa cells form broad bands with microcyst formation. (H&E. ×125)

1083 Atypical granulosa cell tumor of the ovary
Elongated granulosa cells, with plump hyperchromatic nuclei, are arranged in rosettes. (H&E. ×150)

1084 Granulosa cell tumor of the ovary with luteinization (folliculome lipidique of Lecène)
A partly alveolar, partly trabecular type of granulosa cell tumor with pronounced luteinization of granulosa cells. This form of granulosa cell tumor is known as "folliculome lipidique of Lecène." Curettings revealed glandular cystic hyperplasia of the endometrium with pronounced predecidual stromal reaction. This is sometimes misinterpreted as tubular type androblastoma with lipoid storage (androblastoma tubulare lipoides ovarii). (H&E. ×100)

1085 Mixed theca–granulosa cell tumor of the ovary
The tumor is formed by equal participation of granulosa cells and theca cells. Theca externa stroma is prominent. (H&E. ×220)

1086 Mixed theca–granulosa cell tumor of the ovary
Islands of granulosa cells are separated by broad strands of theca cells. (H&E. ×150)

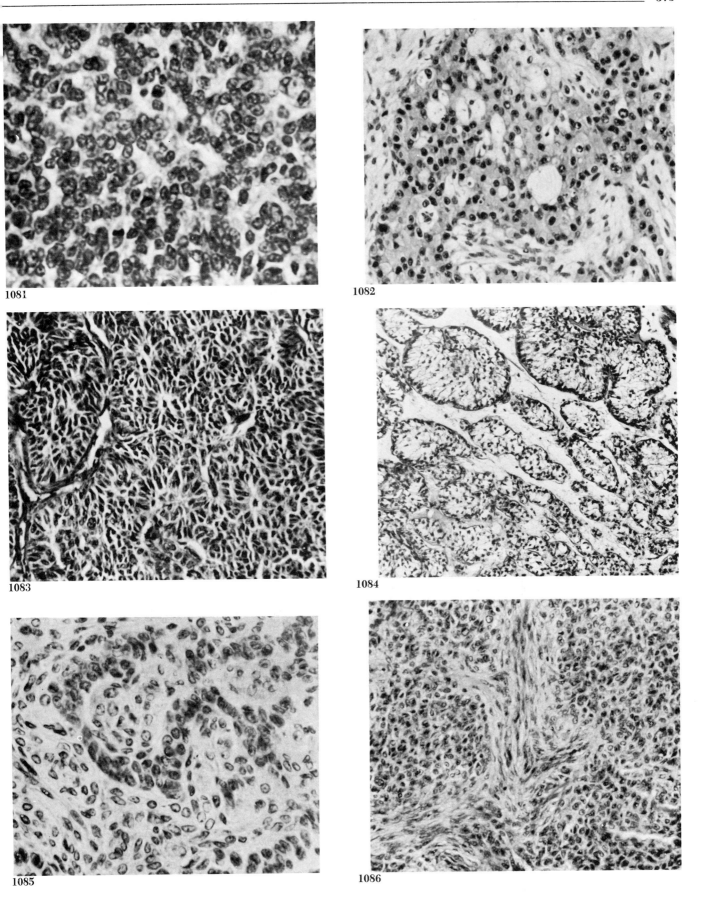

1081

1082

1083

1084

1085

1086

1087   Mixed theca–granulosa cell tumor of the ovary
There is predominance of plump elongated theca cells surrounding trabecular structures and alveolar groups of granulosa cells. (H&E. ×100)

1088   Mixed theca–granulosa cell tumor of the ovary
The follicular island of granulosa cells is surrounded by a solid mass of theca cells. (H&E. ×100)

1089   Thecoma of the ovary
The tumor is composed of spindle-shaped and plump cells forming whorls. Lipid is demonstrated in the cytoplasm of the cells and in the connective tissue stroma. This benign feminizing tumor occurs most frequently after the menopause. (H&E. ×150)

1090   Thecoma of the ovary with luteinization
Cross section of a theca cell tumor. The nuclei appear round. Cytoplasm is markedly vacuolated and contains lipoid material. Occasionally stromal hyalinization may occur. The frozen section reveals abundant lipid material. (H&E. ×200)

1091   Thecoma of the ovary with edema
Marked interstitial edema is seen in a thecoma. Difficulties arise in differentiating theca cell tumors from an ovarian fibroma. The presence of lipid material in the tumor suggests a diagnosis of theca cell tumor. Willis stated that many fibromas of the ovary are variants of theca cell tumors. (H&E. ×150)

1092   Malignant theca cell tumor of the ovary
The tumor is formed by spindle-shaped cells with marked nuclear pleomorphism. Lipid material is present in the frozen section. (H&E. ×62)

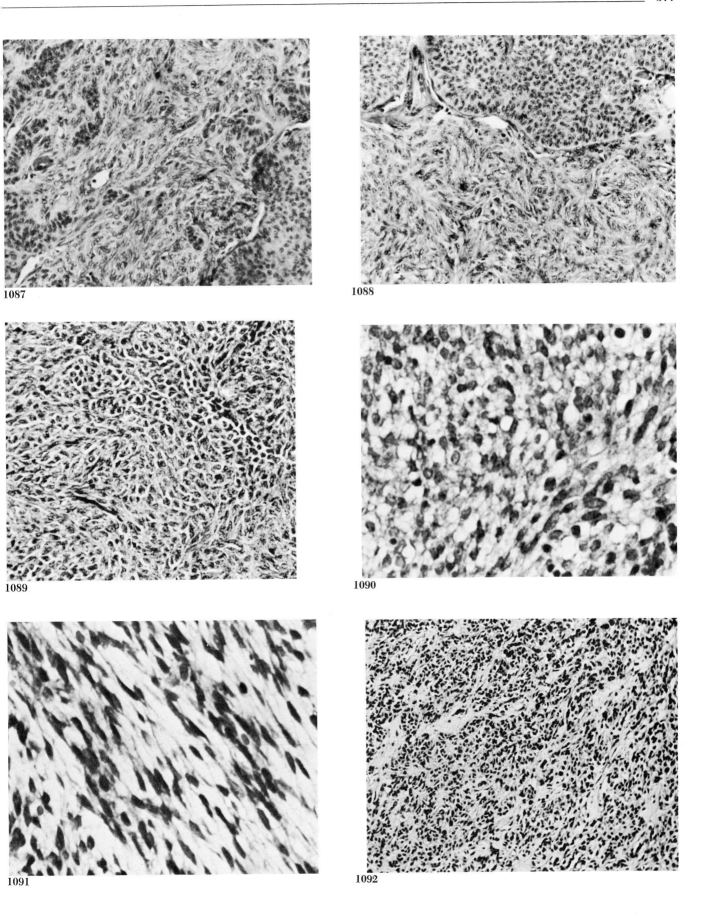

1087

1088

1089

1090

1091

1092

1093   Malignant theca cell tumor of the ovary
High magnification of Fig. 1092. There is marked cellular and nuclear pleomorphism. Atypical mitotic figures are present. Note the vacuolization of cytoplasm and the presence of lipoid material. (H&E. ×380)

1094   Gynandroblastoma of the ovary
The tumor is formed by two distinct components. To the right are the tubular structures of an androblastoma. To the left is the typical granulosa cell tumor. Hormonally, such a tumor may be virilizing, feminizing, or silent. (H&E. ×125)

1095   Gynandroblastoma of the ovary
The tumor is formed by androblastoma and granulosa cell constituents. Both tumor parts must be demonstrated in order to make the diagnosis. At the top of the picture, tubular structures are lined by Sertoli cells. The bottom of the picture shows the follicular pattern of the granulosa cell tumor with Call-Exner bodies. The tumor arises from undifferentiated gonadal mesenchyme which has bisexual potentialities. (H&E. ×125)

1096   Gonadoblastoma of the ovary
The tumor is formed by large round germ cells, occasional dark oval cells, and infiltrating lymphocytes. This area of the tumor shows a similarity to a dysgerminoma. A gonadoblastoma may be virilizing, feminizing, or hormonally indifferent. (H&E. ×62)

1097   Gonadoblastoma of the ovary
The tumor is formed by neoplastic germ cells with large round nuclei. Interspersed are mesenchymal small cells with pycnotic nuclei. Note the presence of large hyaline structures. Gonadoblastomas occur in dysgenetic gonads. Absence of connective tissue stroma and lack of lymphocytic infiltration are important differential diagnostic clues favoring gonadoblastoma. (H&E. ×125)

1098   Gonadoblastoma of the ovary
The tumor is formed by large germ cells, small cells, or cell cords which are prototypes of Sertoli cells and/or granulosa cells. In addition, the connective tissue stroma contains interstitial (Leydig) cells. Teter uses the term gonocytoma III for this type of tumor and states that gonadoblastoma usually occurs in patients with (1) a female phenotype, (2) signs of masculinization, and (3) a negative sex chromatin pattern. Feminizing mixed germ cell tumor is called gonocytoma II by the same investigator. (H&E. ×50)

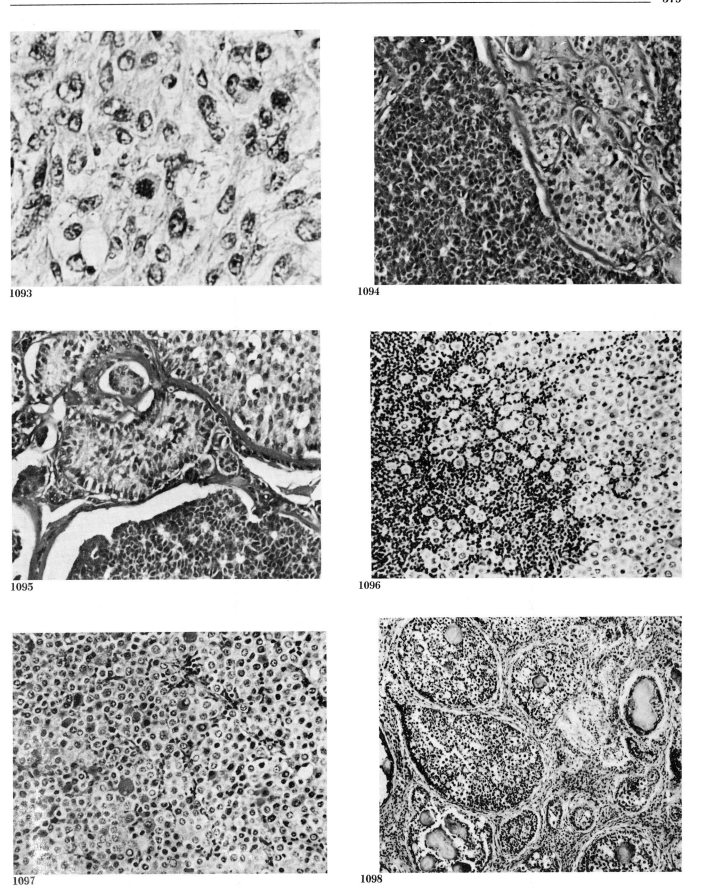

1093

1094

1095

1096

1097

1098

1099   Gonadoblastoma of the ovary
High magnification of Fig. 1098. Germ cells are surrounded by small dark cells. The presence of psammoma bodies or irregular calcified masses in neoplastic islands is pathognomonic for this neoplasm. A gonadoblastoma represents a mixed germ cell tumor, whereas a dysgerminoma is a pure germ cell tumor. (H&E. ×125)

1100   Gonadoblastoma of the ovary
This is a masculinizing tumor. The large neoplastic nests are composed of Sertoli granulosa cells and large round germ cells. Typical foci of calcification and hyalinization are present. (H&E. ×260)

1101   Gonadoblastoma of the ovary
This is a masculinizing tumor. Small cells are arranged in a "coronal" fashion around germ cells. The arrow indicates a collection of interstitial (Leydig) cells. (H&E. ×180)

1102   Dysgerminoma of the ovary
The germ cell tumor is composed of large vesicular cells with prominent round nuclei arranged in islands, alveolar structures, or strands separated by a variable amount of connective tissue and infiltrated by lymphocytes. (H&E. ×90)

1103   Dysgerminoma of the ovary
Round tumor cells are diffusely distributed. The sparse connective tissue stroma is infiltrated by lymphocytes. The cytoplasm of dysgerminoma cells contains varying amounts of glycogen. (H&E. ×50)

1104   Dysgerminoma of the ovary
The tumor shows alveolar distribution of large germ cells. Diffuse infiltration with lymphocytes and the formation of lymphoid follicles are pathognomonic for dysgerminoma. (H&E. ×62)

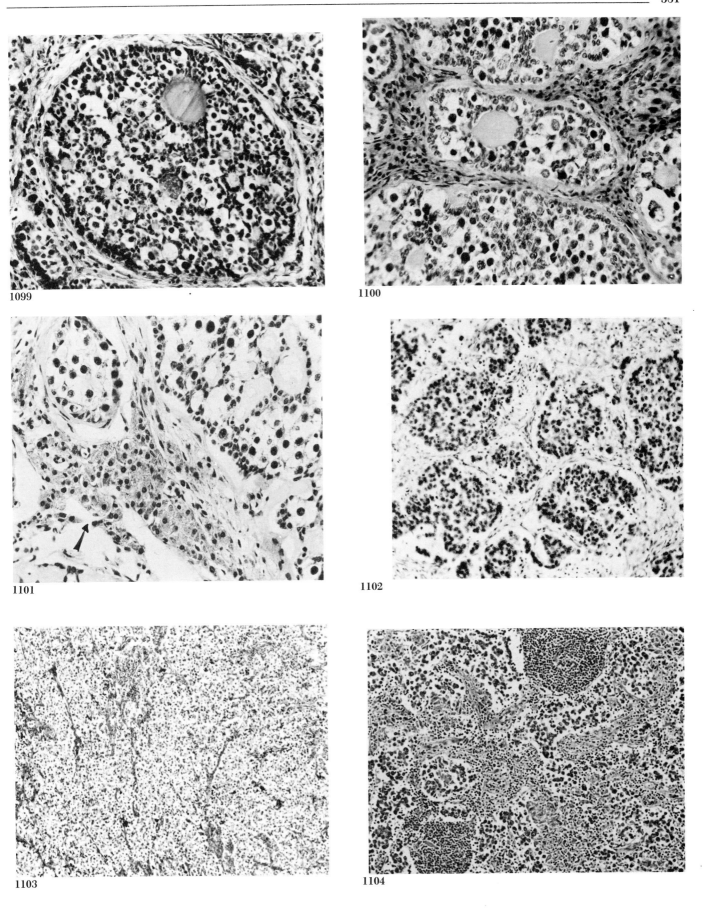

1099

1100

1101

1102

1103

1104

1105 Dysgerminoma of the ovary
High magnification of Fig. 1104. Large vesicular cells, 16 to 24 μ in diameter, show prominent centrally placed nuclei with several nucleoli. Mitotic figures are frequent. The glycogen content of cytoplasm is high. (H&E. ×150)

1106 Dysgerminoma of the ovary
Several multinucleated giant cells occur in areas of tumor necrosis. They originate from stromal cells. Tumor giant cells originating from germ cells may occasionally be seen. (H&E. ×180)

1107 Mesonephric tumor of the ovary
The tumor is formed by small cysts with intracystic projections and very cellular intervening stroma. Tumors may develop from vestiges of mesonephrons, mesonephric tubules, or rete ovarii. This malignant tumor with extensive abdominal spread occurred in a 21-year-old patient. (H&E. ×62)

1108 Mesonephric tumor of the ovary
This tumor forming numerous cysts is lined by cuboidal epithelium with round hyperchromatic nuclei. Tumorous papillary projections seen within the cystic space simulate glomerular tufts. These may contain abundant capillaries. Mitotic activity is always present. (H&E. ×125)

1109 Mesonephric tumor of the ovary
The tumor is composed of cysts and tubules lined by "hobnail" cells. Mayer's mucicarmine stain is particularly useful for demonstration of mitotic activity. (H&E. ×50)

1110 Mesonephric tumor of the ovary
The tumor is formed by numerous papillary projections lined by cuboidal cells with prominent round hyperchromatic nuclei. The connective tissue stroma is relatively sparse. Mesonephric tumors of the ovary are invariably malignant. (H&E. ×150)

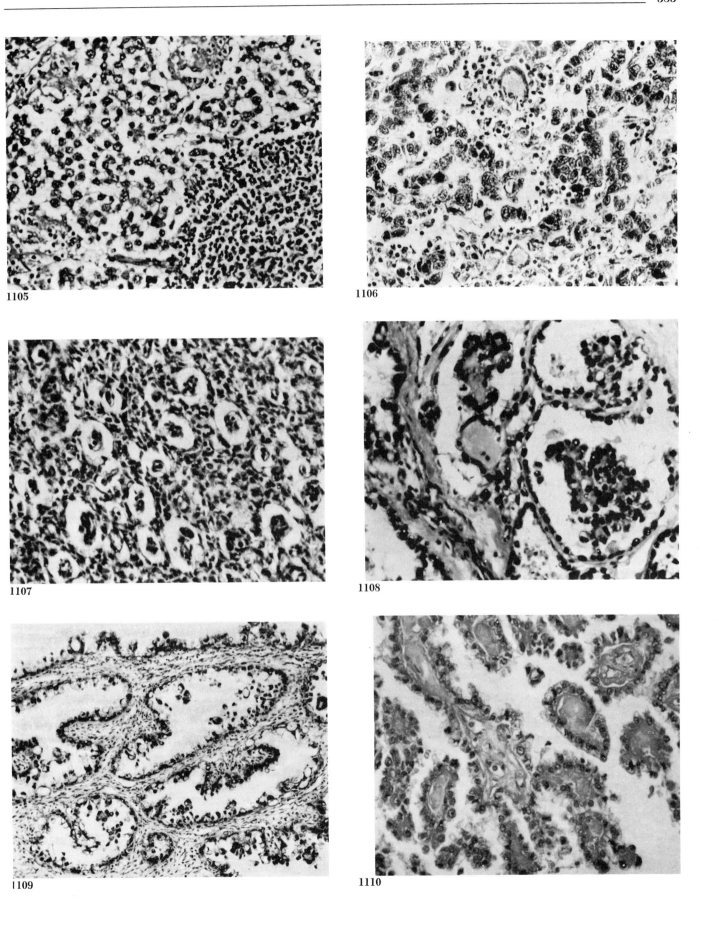

1105

1106

1107

1108

1109

1110

1111   Mesonephric tumor of the ovary
Numerous papillary projections are covered by proliferating clear cells with prominent hyperchromatic nuclei. The cytoplasm may contain glucoprotein. Alcian blue and Mayer's mucicarmine stains are negative. Fatty material may be detected in areas of necrosis and degeneration. Intervening connective tissue is sparse. (H&E. ×125)

1112   Mesonephric tumor of the ovary
The tumor shows alveolar arrangement of clear cells. Atypical mitotic figures are frequent. Intervening connective tissue is sparse. The Best carmine-positive granules may be detected in the cytoplasm of clear cells. (H&E. ×125)

1113   Mesonephric tumor of the ovary
There is an alveolar arrangement of clear cells with extensive hyaline degeneration of the intervening stroma. Mesonephric tumors of the ovary are initially extremely responsive to chemotherapy and irradiation. The dramatic response will not prevent future recurrence which is then nonresponsive to both means of therapy. (H&E. ×75)

1114   Mesonephric tumor of the ovary
Pseudorosette formation by clear cells is seen surrounding hyaline bodies. (H&E. ×200)

1116   Fibroma of the ovary
The tumor is formed by interlacing bundles of fibrous connective tissue cells. Spindle-shaped fibroblasts are seen producing collagen. Difficulties may be encountered in differentiating this tumor from thecoma. Fibromas, as a rule, do not contain lipoid material. (H&E. ×85)

1115   Mesonephric tumor of the ovary
The cystic tumor is lined by clear mesonephric cells showing degeneration with ballooning. (H&E. ×180)

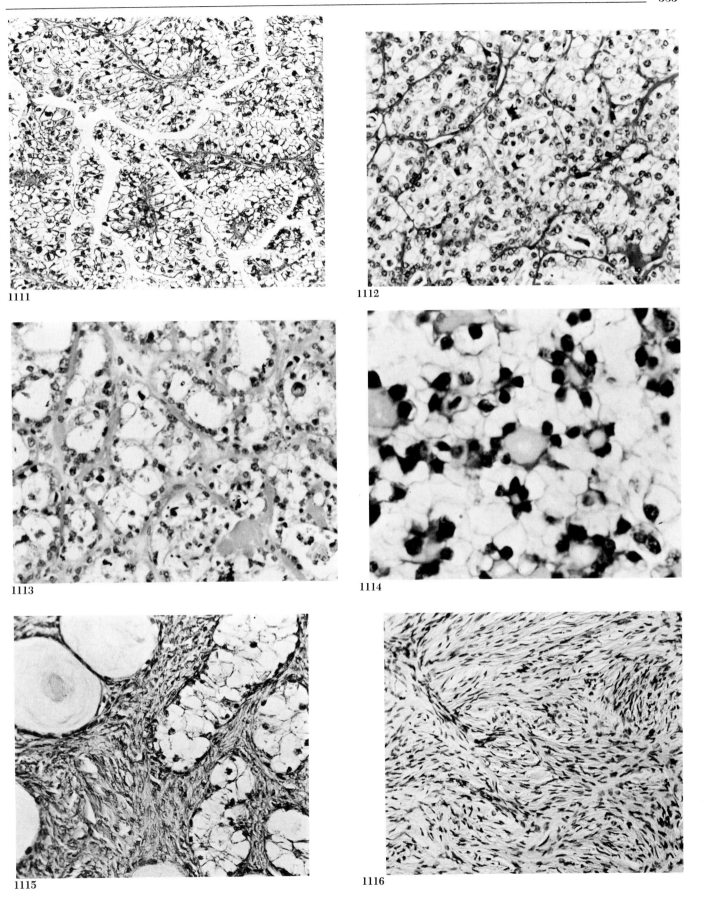

1111

1112

1113

1114

1115

1116

1117 Fibrosarcoma of the ovary
This well-differentiated fibrosarcoma is composed of fibroblasts and shows occasional mitotic figures. (H&E. ×90)

1118 Myxofibrosarcoma of the ovary
This tumor is formed by elongated cells and stellate cells with a myxomatous matrix. Nuclear pleomorphism, hyperchromatism, and atypical mitotic figures are present. (H&E. ×85)

1119 Cavernous hemangioma of the ovary
This tumor is composed of large vascular spaces replacing ovarian cortex. The vascular spaces are lined by endothelial cells containing blood. Intervening connective tissue stroma is sparse. (H&E. ×50)

1120 Hemangioendothelioma of the ovary
The tumor is composed of vascular spaces lined by proliferating neoplastic endothelial cells. (H&E. ×55)

1121 Hemangioendothelioma of the ovary
High magnification of Fig. 1120. Proliferating atypical endothelial cells with marked nuclear pleomorphism line the vascular spaces. (H&E. ×220)

1122 Hemangiopericytoma of the ovary
The tumor is composed of a central capillary with concentrically arranged elongated pericytes. Silver impregnation demonstrates capillary sheath and extravascular proliferation of tumor cells. (H&E. ×180)

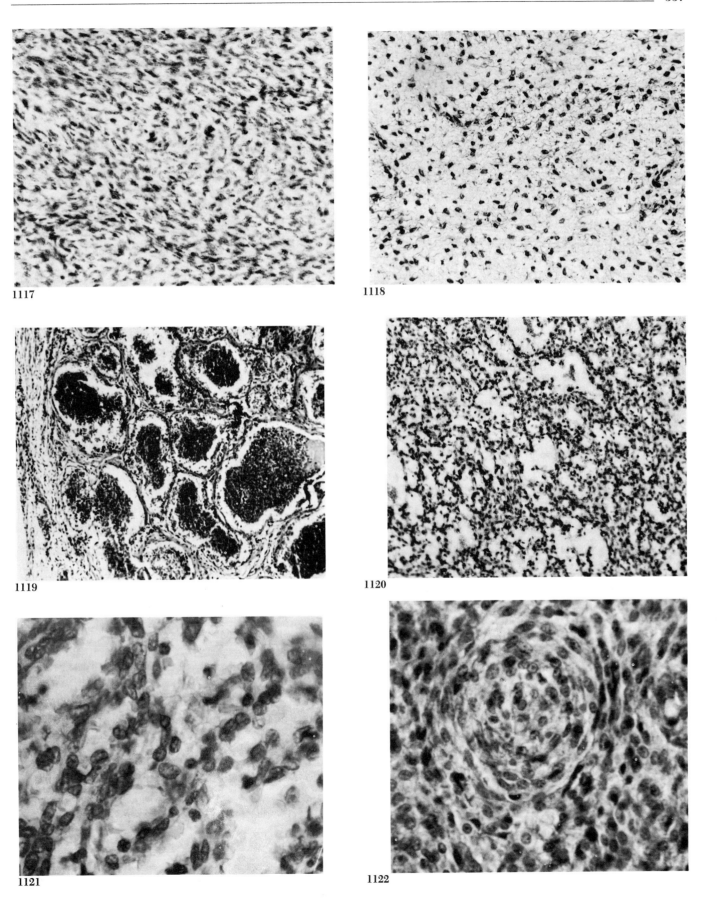

1117

1118

1119

1120

1121

1122

1123 Lymphangioma of the ovary
The cortical portion of an ovary contains a poorly defined tumor composed of vascular channels identified as lymphatic vessels. There is no malignant potential in this tumor. (H&E. ×50)

1124 Pleomorphic undifferentiated sarcoma of the ovary
Sarcomas of pelvic tissues or organs other than the ovary should be excluded prior to establishing a diagnosis of ovarian sarcoma. The tumor is formed by highly anaplastic pleomorphic cells. (H&E. ×220)

1125 Chondrosarcoma of the ovary
The tumor consists of large areas of neoplastic cartilaginous tissue. The cartilage cells are pleomorphic and show bizarre and hyperchromatic nuclei and atypical mitotic figures. The surrounding tissue shows hemorrhage and necrosis. (H&E. ×50)

1126 Mixed mesodermal tumor of the ovary
The tumor is formed by proliferating connective tissue stroma and numerous cystlike structures lined by neoplastic epithelium. This is a slow growing, repeatedly recurring ovarian tumor. It is frequently misdiagnosed as a benign ovarian tumor. (H&E. ×24)

1127 Mixed mesodermal tumor of the ovary
High magnification of Fig. 1126. Proliferating relatively well-differentiated stromal cells surround abortive glandular structures. They are lined by cuboidal epithelial cells, some of which are mucin-producing. (H&E. ×150)

1128 Mixed mesodermal tumor of the ovary
High magnification of Fig. 1126. Clusters of poorly differentiated mesenchymal cells are located in myxomatous matrix around vascular spaces and glandlike structures. (H&E. ×110)

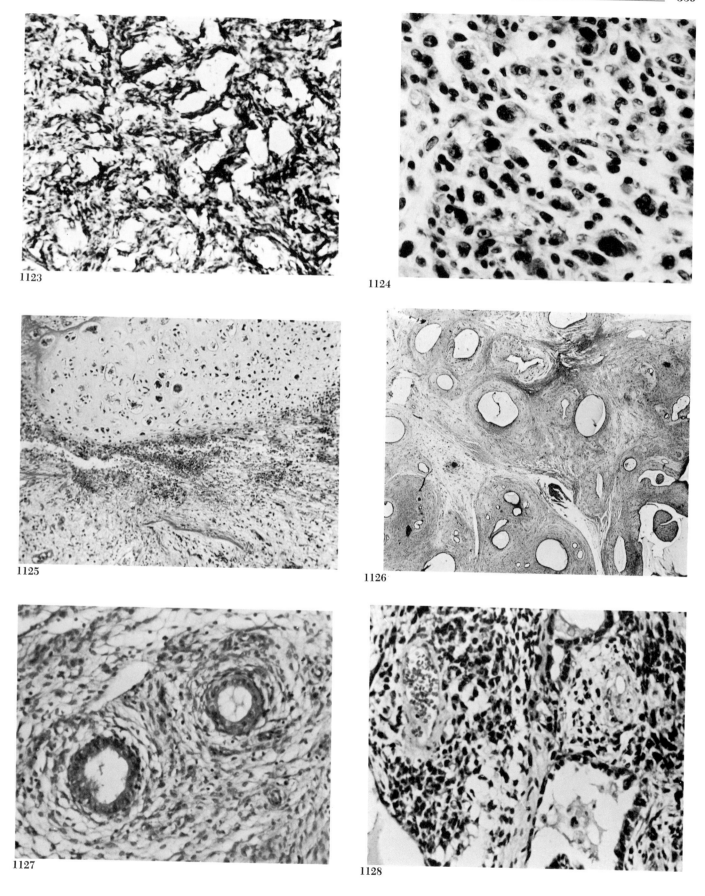

1123

1124

1125

1126

1127

1128

1129   Carcinosarcoma of the ovary
The tumor is formed by islands of neoplastic epithelial cells showing all the characteristics of a carcinoma and a distinctly sarcomatous connective tissue stroma. This is a highly malignant mixed mesodermal tumor of the ovary. (H&E. ×125)

1130   Benign cystic teratoma of the ovary
The cyst wall shows a variety of tissues: epidermis, numerous sebaceous glands, sweat glands, cartilage, muscle tissue, and adipose tissue. (H&E. ×45)

1131   Benign cystic teratoma of the ovary
This cystic teratoma is lined by cuboidal cells showing differentiation toward squamous epithelium. The connective tissue stroma shows hyalinization. No other structures are present. (H&E. ×155)

1132   Foreign bodies reaction in the wall of a benign cystic teratoma of the ovary
Foreign-body giant cells surround hair shafts in the cyst wall. (H&E. ×62)

1134   Choroid plexus in a cystic teratoma of the ovary
Choroid plexus is formed by papillary projections which are lined by cuboidal cells with uniform round nuclei. Like many other well-differentiated tissue in a cystic teratoma, the choroid plexus serves a functional role. The fluid produced by this organ whether by dialysis, secretion, or transudation, in many respects, resembles cerebrospinal fluid. The protein electrophoretic pattern bespeaks its origin from blood serum, the source of cerebrospinal fluid. (H&E. ×125)

1133   Benign cystic teratoma of the ovary
The cyst wall contains mature cerebral and cerebellar tissue with formation of an abortive ventricle. (H&E. ×12)

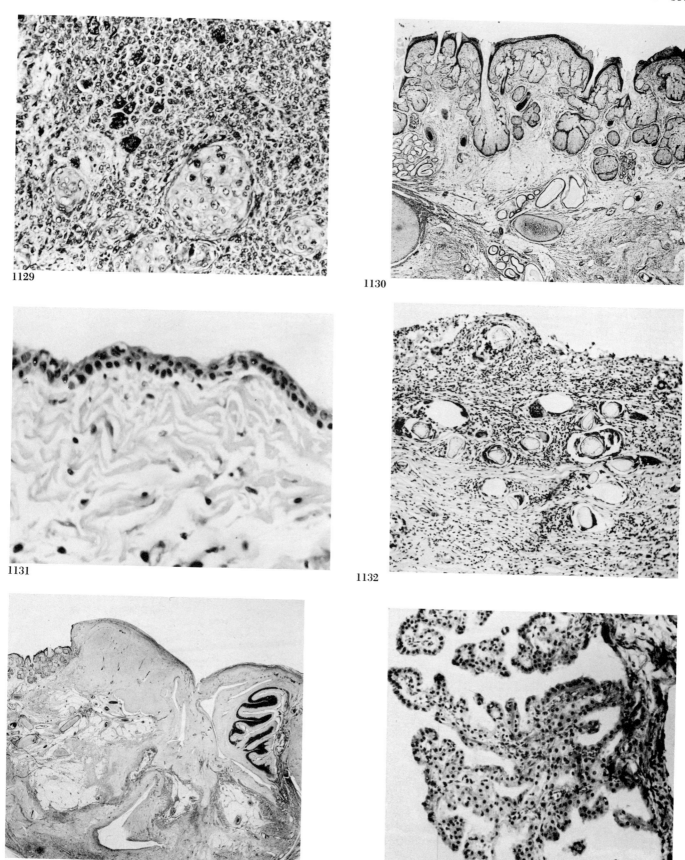

1129

1130

1131

1132

1133

1134

1135 Solid, mature benign teratoma of the ovary

This is much rarer than a cystic teratoma. The tumor is formed by solid strands of adipose tissue, sebaceous glands, and a few cysts lined by squamous epithelium. It is surrounded by dense fibrous connective tissue. Solid teratomas occur most frequently in children and young adults. (H&E. ×81)

1136 Struma ovarii

This benign cystic teratoma of the ovary consists exclusively or predominantly of thyroid tissue. The latter may resemble the normal thyroid, or it may manifest all the pathologic changes seen in the thyroid gland, including adenomatous goiter, hyperplasia, benign and malignant thyroid neoplasms. Occasionally it may be associated with ovarian cystadenoma. The tumor is formed by acini, some of which are small and others large and distended with colloid. (H&E. ×50)

1137 Adenoma developing in struma ovarii

This solid tumor is formed by relatively large cells with clear cytoplasm and uniform nuclei. The thyroid tissue is devoid of follicles and suggestive of embryonal adenoma. Such an adenoma arising in struma ovarii represents a biologic problem inasmuch as the behavior and malignant potentiality of adenomas developing in teratomas are not known. (H&E. ×200)

1138 Malignant struma ovarii (adenocarcinoma of the thyroid arising in struma ovarii)

Note the thyroid tissue with acini and cords of thyroid carcinoma. (H&E. ×40)

1139 Carcinoid occurring in cystic teratoma of the ovary

This tumor is occasionally associated with a solid teratoma or mucinous cystadenoma of the ovary. Adjacent to the cartilage in the cystic teratoma are numerous islands formed by round cells with uniform nuclei. These cells show chromaffinity and argentaffinity. Mitotic figures are rare. This is a malignant neoplasm with a slow growth rate. (H&E. ×24)

1140 Carcinoid occurring in cystic teratoma of the ovary

High magnification of Fig. 1139. The uniform cells contain round nuclei and prominent nucleoli. They are derived from enterochromaffin. Kultschitzky cells of the intestine are present. The tumor cells elaborate serotonin, a vasoconstrictive agent, giving rise to the so-called malignant carcinoid syndrome. (H&E. ×180)

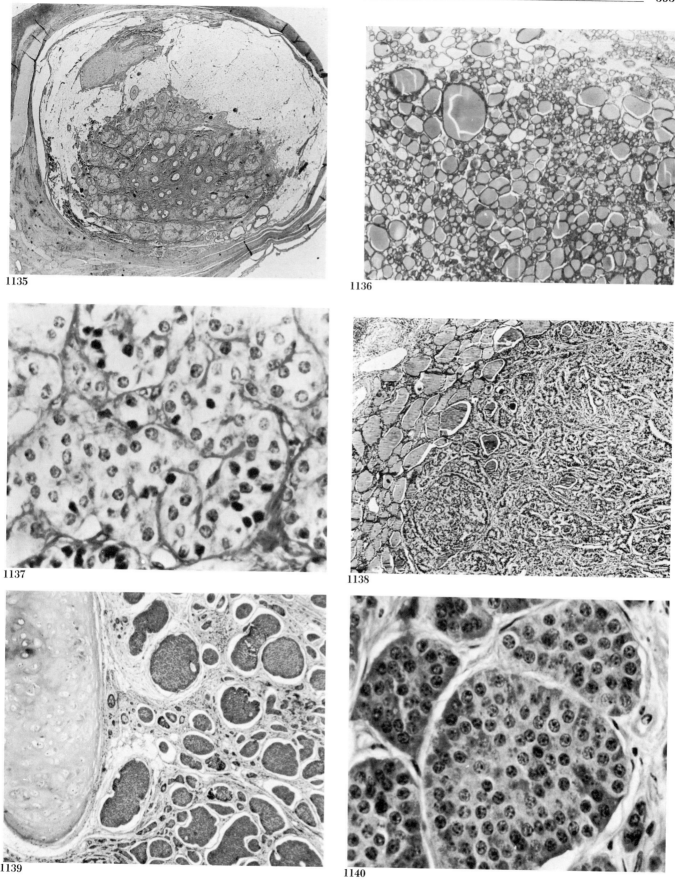

1135

1136

1137

1138

1139

1140

1141 Sebaceous adenoma developing in a teratoma of the ovary
This is a specialized form of cystic or solid teratoma. Marked hyperplasia and neoplasia of sebaceous glands form an adenoma. (H&E. ×50)

1142 Sebaceous adenoma developing in a teratoma of the ovary
High magnification of Fig. 1141. The tumor is formed by typical lipid-containing mature sebaceous cells and aggregates of young dark-staining small cells. Scattered microcysts with sebum are present. (H&E. ×150)

1143 Carcinoma developing in a benign cystic teratoma of the ovary
The arrow indicates an area of carcinoma developing in the wall of a benign cystic teratoma. (H&E. ×55)

1144 Carcinoma developing in a benign cystic teratoma of the ovary
High magnification of Fig. 1143. Proliferating atypical neoplastic epithelial cells are invading connective tissue stroma. (H&E. ×100)

1145 Teratocarcinoma of the ovary
The tumor is composed of various immature or embryonal structures derived from three blastodermic layers. (H&E. ×30)

1146 Teratocarcinoma of the ovary
Teratocarcinoma, as a rule, is a solid tumor. The masses of embryonic tissue of all varieties show bizarre histologic patterns. This tumor is highly malignant. (H&E. ×70)

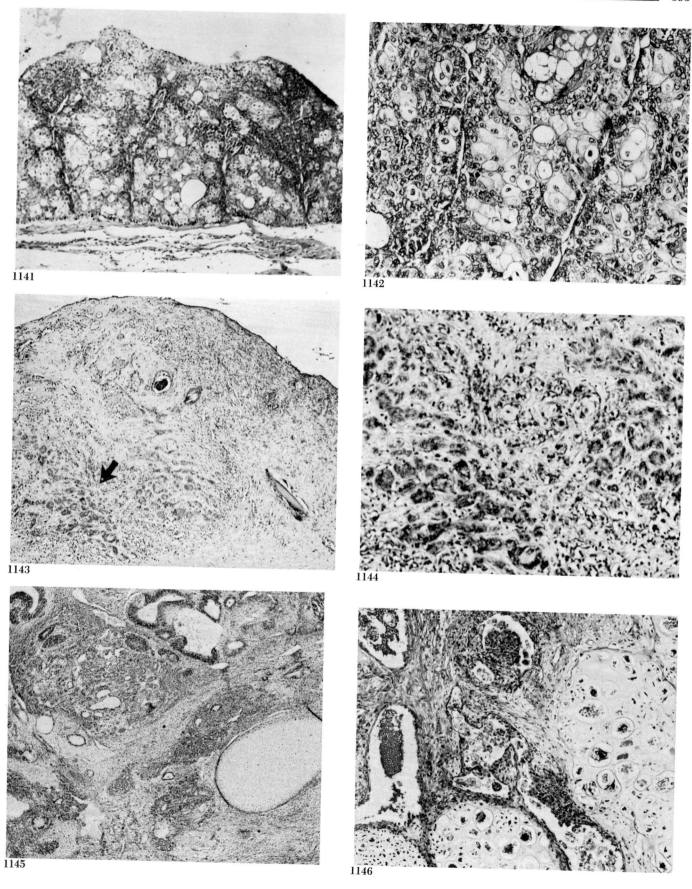

1141

1142

1143

1144

1145

1146

1147   Teratocarcinoma of the ovary
The highly immature neoplastic tissue shows poor cellular organization. (H&E. ×70)

1148   Rhabdomyosarcoma occurring in a primary teratocarcinoma of the ovary
Adjacent to a carcinomatous area there is a portion of very cellular tumor formed by elongated tumor cells and primitive muscle fibers. (H&E. ×50)

1149   Rhabdomyosarcoma occurring in a primary teratocarcinoma of the ovary
High magnification of Fig. 1148. There is cross striation of primitive muscle fiber. (H&E. ×350)

1150   Endodermal sinus tumor (embryonal carcinoma) of the ovary, Teilum
This highly malignant germ cell tumor occurs in young women. The extraembryonic membrane tumor contains yolk-sac endoderm and extra-embryonic mesoblast. It is frequently misdiagnosed as nongerminal carcinoma, mesonephroma, endothelioma, or angiosarcoma. The characteristic feature is the peculiar sinusoid formation. (H&E. ×72)

1151   Endodermal sinus tumor (embryonal carcinoma) of the ovary, Teilum
Note the typical glomeruluslike unit, to the left, the so-called endodermal sinus of Duval. (H&E. ×125)

1152   Endodermal sinus tumor (embryonal carcinoma) of the ovary, Teilum
The system of small cystic cavities and channels are lined by layers of irregular cells with large hyperchromatic nuclei. (H&E. ×300)

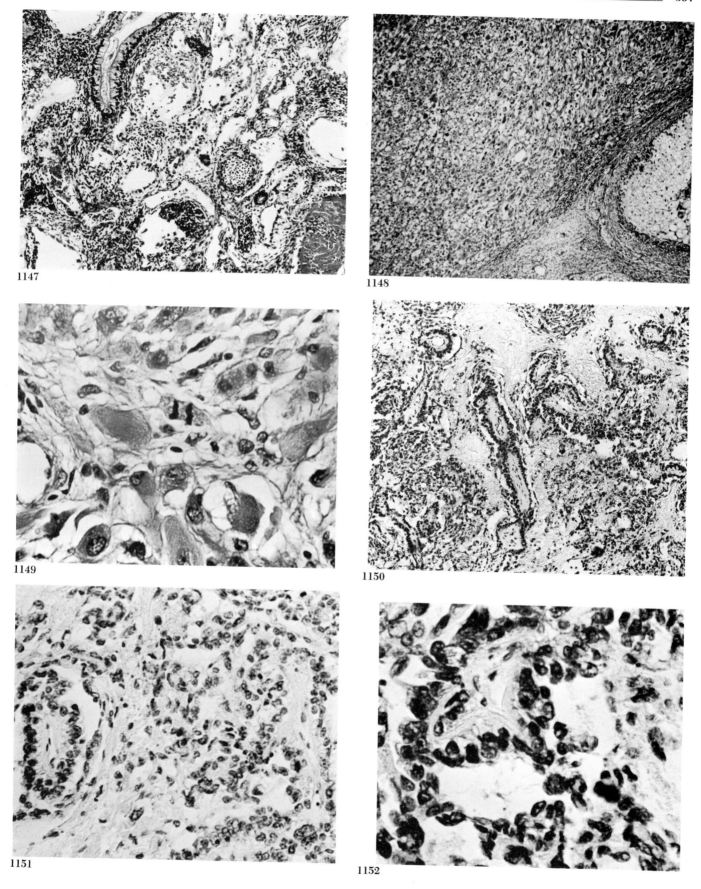

1147

1148

1149

1150

1151

1152

1153 Endodermal sinus tumor (embryonal carcinoma) of the ovary, Teilum
The mesoblastic component of an ovarian tumor shows stellated endothelial mesodermal cells forming a reticular network. (H&E. ×100)

1154 Primary choriocarcinoma of the ovary
Besides being primary, this tumor may arise in an ovarian pregnancy. It is formed by vacuolated cytotrophoblasts and multinuclear syncytiotrophoblasts. There is absence of villi. The tumor cells produce gonadotropin. (H&E. ×125)

1155 Primary choriocarcinoma of the ovary
There are extensive areas of hemorrhagic necrosis and a massive growth of destructive cytotrophoblasts. The tumor occurs in girls and young adults. Prior to establishing the diagnosis of a primary choriocarcinoma of the ovary, metastases from a choriocarcinoma elsewhere and an ovarian teratocarcinoma with trophoblastic elements should be excluded. (H&E. ×125)

1156 Malignant lymphoma (lymphoblastic lymphosarcoma) of the ovary
There is diffuse infiltration of ovarian cortex by uniform lymphoma cells. Note the obliteration of ovarian structure. The ovarian involvement is mostly secondary. In Burkitt's tumor (African lymphoma syndrome) there is very frequent bilateral ovarian involvement occurring in female children. (H&E. ×50)

1157 Malignant lymphoma (lymphoblastic lymphosarcoma) of the ovary, Burkitt's tumor
The round neoplastic cells are relatively large and resemble lymphoblasts. There is diffuse infiltration of ovary by tumor cells. (H&E. ×125)

1158 Malignant lymphoma (lymphocytic lymphosarcoma) of the ovary
The infiltration of the ovarian cortex by round cells forms neoplastic lymphatic aggregates. (H&E. ×50)

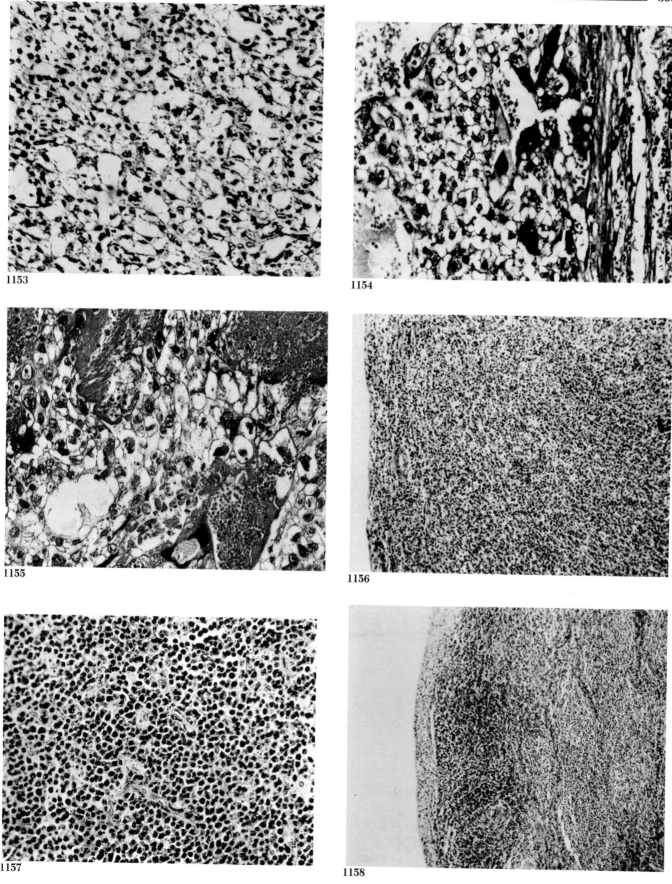

1153

1154

1155

1156

1157

1158

**1159   Malignant lymphoma (lymphocytic lym-
phosarcoma) of the ovary**
High magnification of Fig. 1158. The tissue is infiltrated with relatively small round cells resembling lymphocytes. (H&E. ×85)

1160   Reticulum cell sarcoma of the ovary
The ovarian cortex is infiltrated by pleomorphic
cells with prominent round nuclei. (H&E. ×50)

1162   Krukenberg tumor of the ovary
Krukenberg tumor usually represents metastatic gastric carcinoma to the ovary. Individual
epithelial cells, strands of epithelioid cells, and
glandlike structures are seen intermingled with
proliferating connective tissue stroma. Signet-
ring cells have a mucoid content and nuclei
placed at the periphery of the cells. (H&E. ×95)

1161   Reticulum cell sarcoma of the ovary
High magnification of Fig. 1160. Large reticulum
cells are seen with prominent nuclei and accentuated nucleoli. (H&E. ×150)

1163   Krukenberg tumor of the ovary
High magnification of Fig. 1162. Typical muci-
carminophilic signet-ring cells are present.
(H&E. ×80)

1164   Krukenberg tumor of the ovary
Note the prominent signet-ring cell pattern.
(H&E. ×125)

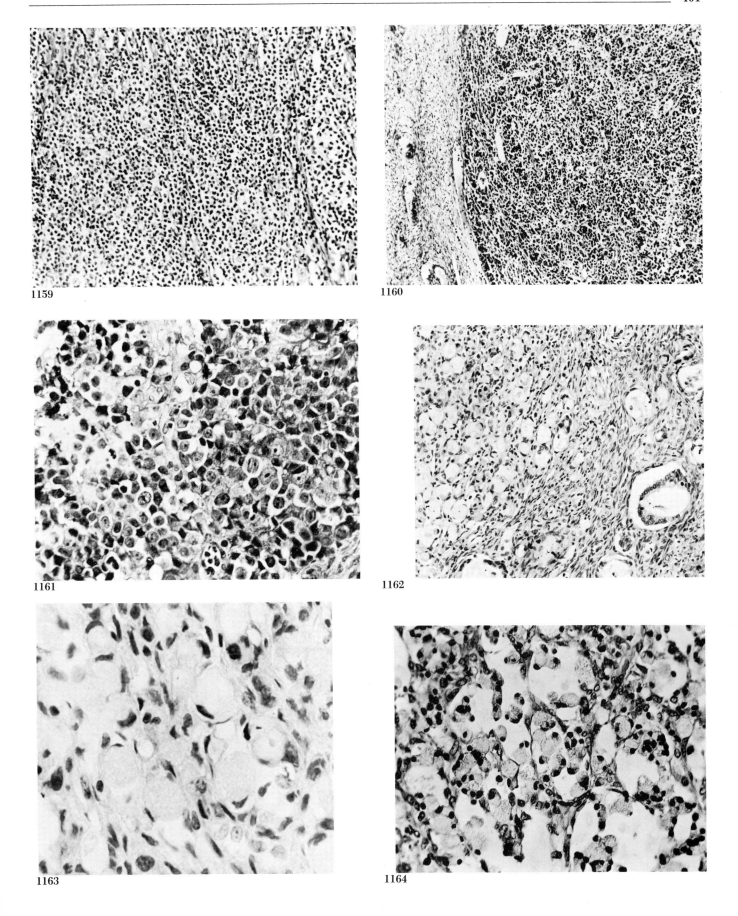

1159

1160

1161

1162

1163

1164

1165 Krukenberg tumor of the ovary
Clusters of epithelial cells and glands infiltrate the connective tissue stroma. (H&E. ×50)

1166 Carcinoma of the breast metastatic to the ovary
(H&E. ×50)

1167 Carcinoma of the breast metastatic to the ovary
(H&E. ×125)

1168 Carcinoma of the breast metastatic to the ovary
(H&E. ×62)

1169 Carcinoma of the breast metastatic to the ovary with theca cell reaction
(H&E. ×100)

1170 Adenocarcinoma of the pancreas metastatic to the ovary
(H&E. ×50)

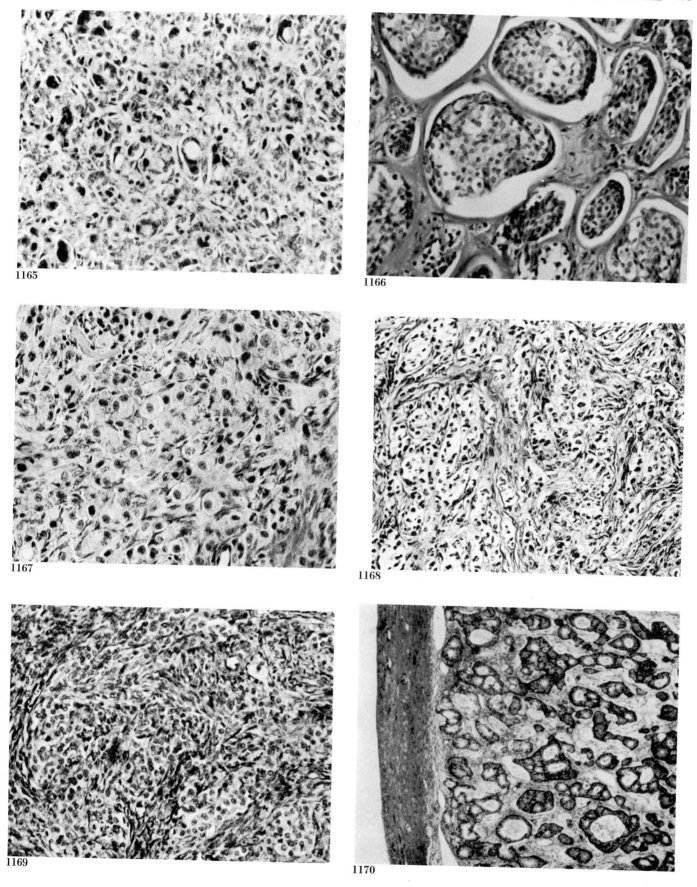

1165

1166

1167

1168

1169

1170

1171   Adenocarcinoma of the large intestine metastatic to the ovary
(H&E. ×24)

1172   Adenocarcinoma of the large intestine metastatic to the ovary
High magnification of Fig. 1171. (H&E. ×80)

1173   Adenocarcinoma of the sigmoid metastatic to the ovary
(H&E. ×160)

1174   Papillary adenocarcinoma of the oviduct metastatic to the ovary
(H&E. ×80)

1175   Adenocarcinoma of the endometrium metastatic to the ovary
(H&E. ×160)

1176   Malignant melanoma of the eye metastatic to the ovary
(H&E. ×50)

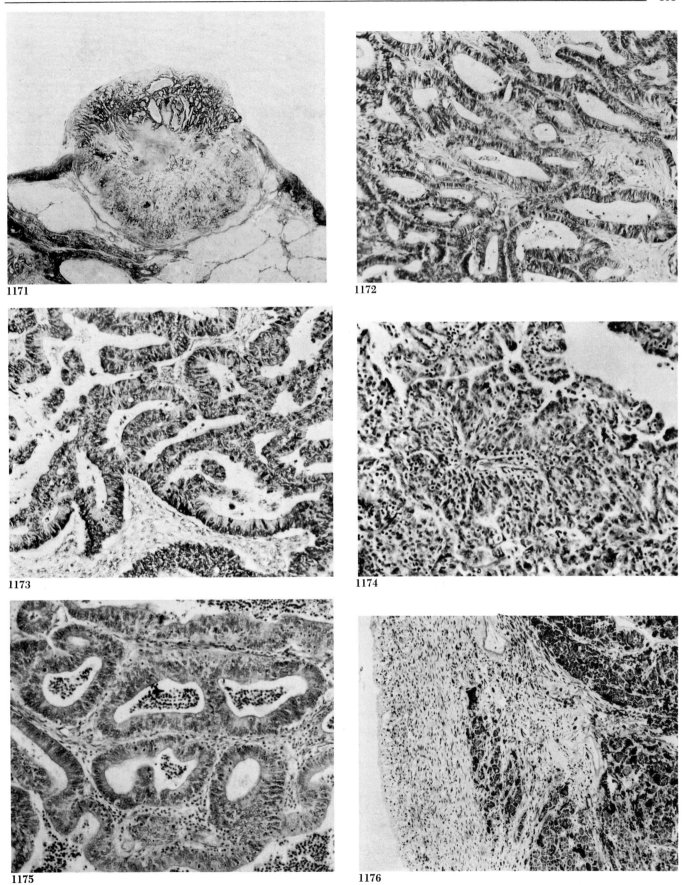

1171

1172

1173

1174

1175

1176

COLOR PLATES
Chapter 7
Diseases of the Ovary
Plates 13, 14, 15, and 16

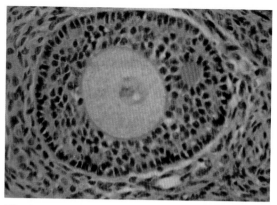

73 Growing follicle Note the formation of a Call-Exner's body by granulosa cells. There is a deeply staining cell membrane around the ovum (zona pellucida). (H&E. ×320)

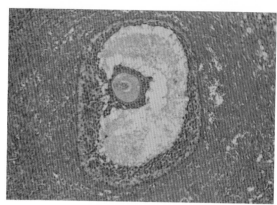

74 Perifollicular hemorrhage Perifollicular hemorrhage is present in theca cell layers of the graafian follicle. (H&E. ×110)

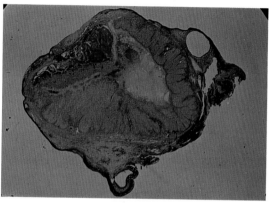

75 Hemorrhage into corpus luteum of menstruation At onset of menstruation, hemorrhage may occur into the corpus luteum. (H&E. ×5)

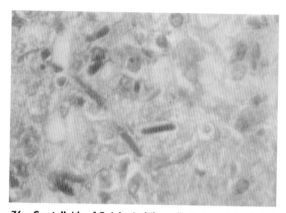

76 Crystalloids of Reinke in hilus cells (interstitial cells) of the ovary Crystalloids of Reinke are cellular inclusions of protein origin present in a very low percentage of hilus cells. In the hilus cells of the senile ovary, they may be present in greater number. Overstaining with eosin is helpful in demonstrating these crystalloids. (H&E. ×125)

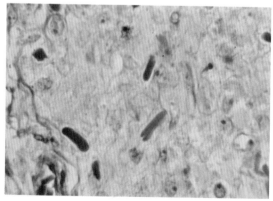

77 Crystalloids of Reinke in hilus cells (interstitial cells) of the ovary Crystalloids of Reinke are stained dark black with Heidenhain's iron hematoxylin. (×125)

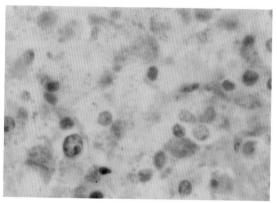

78 Lipochrome pigment in hilus cells (interstitial cells) of the ovary Note the presence of yellow-brown lipochrome pigment in the cytoplasm of hilus cells. (H&E. ×125)

Plate 13

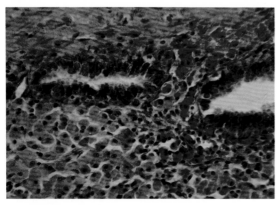

79 Endometriosis of the ovary with macrophages Numerous polyhedral macrophages surround endometrial glands and contain brown pigment granules. (H&E. ×275)

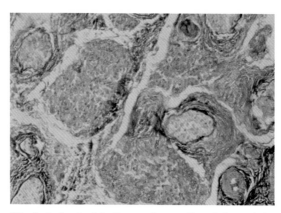

80 Testicular feminization syndrome There is hyperplasia of interstitial Leydig cells. They appear orange-red. The seminiferous tubules show extensive peritubular fibrosis. (Masson's trichrome stain. ×50)

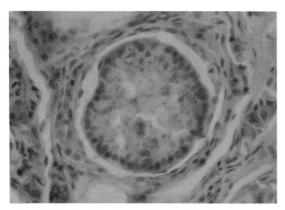

81 Testicular feminization syndrome Note the presence of lipid granules in the cytoplasm of Leydig and Sertoli cells. Both cells may be involved in estrogen production. (Oil red 0. ×70)

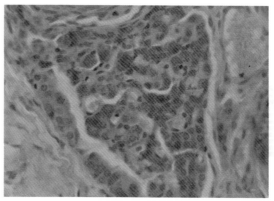

82 Testicular feminization syndrome The lipid content of interstitial Leydig cells is high. (Oil red 0. ×70)

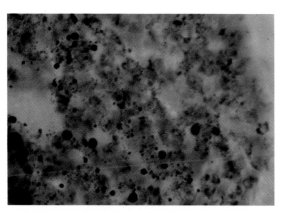

83 Testicular feminization syndrome Cholesterol and its esters are seen in interstitial Leydig cells. This is a Schultze modification of the Liebermann-Burchard reaction. (×100)

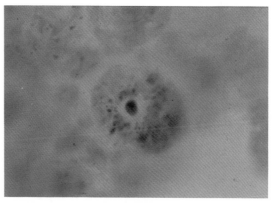

84 Testicular feminization syndrome Note the cholesterol within a lumen of a seminiferous tubule and the presence of brown pigment granules in Sertoli cells. This is a Schultze modification of the Liebermann-Burchard reaction. (×125)

Plate 14

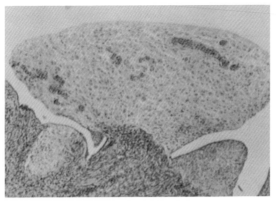

85 Cortical decidual reaction (deciduosis) of the ovary following nor-ethisterone administration (H&E. ×24)

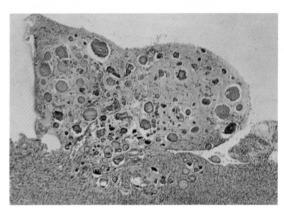

86 Psammoma bodies of the ovary Note the accumulation of psammoma bodies in the ovarian cortex and the periovarian adhesion. (H&E. ×75)

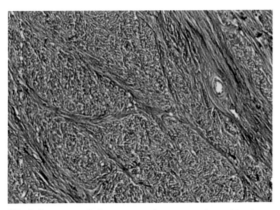

87 Leiomyoma of the ovary The tumor is formed by bundles of smooth muscle fibers replacing ovarian stroma. (Masson's trichrome stain. ×62)

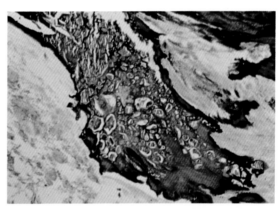

88 Leiomyoma of the ovary with ossification and calcification Very frequently leiomyoma of the ovary shows regressive changes with areas of calcification and/or ossification. (Von Kóssa's stain. ×62)

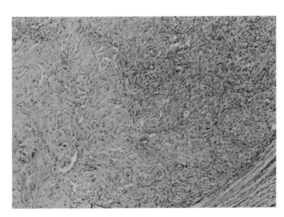

89 Sclerosing thecoma of the ovary The tumor shows extensive hyalinization. (H&E. ×55)

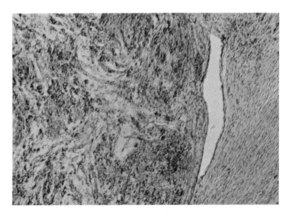

90 Sclerosing thecoma of the ovary Note the lipid granules in preserved theca cells amid extensive areas of hyalinization. (Sudan III. ×55)

Plate 15

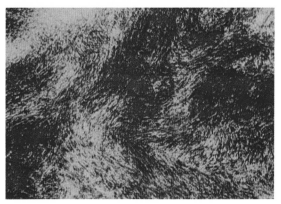

91 Thecoma of the ovary Note the lipid within the tumor cells and connective tissue stroma. (Oil red 0. ×50)

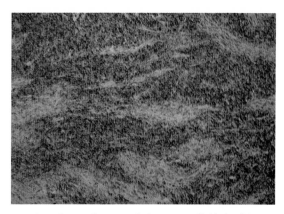

92 Granulosa cell tumor of the ovary Lipid droplets are present in the cytoplasm of granulosa cells and occasional theca cells. (Oil red 0. ×90)

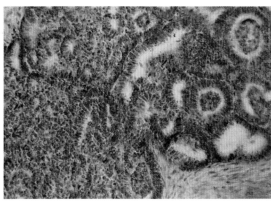

93 Tubular type androblastoma of the ovary Lipid is present in the cytoplasm of cells lining tubular structures of the tumor. (Oil red 0. ×50)

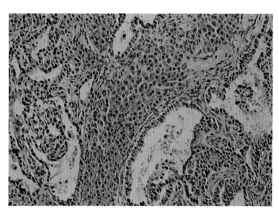

94 Carcinoma of the ovary with luteinization of stromal cells (thecomatosis) Such a thecomatous response of ovarian stroma has been observed in primary ovarian neoplasms as well as with different types of metastatic tumors to the ovary. Endocrine manifestations particularly of androgenic nature have been associated with stromal thecomatosis. (H&E. ×70)

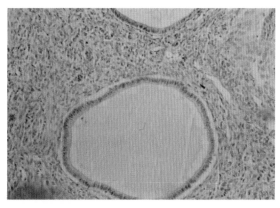

95 Krukenberg tumor associated with mucinous cystadenoma of the ovary Metastatic gastric carcinoma is seen in a preexisting mucinous cystadenoma of the ovary. A mucinous cyst and stroma containing tumor cells are seen. (H&E. ×50)

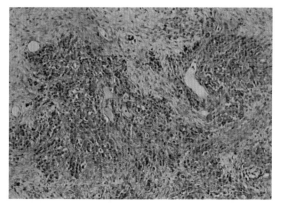

96 Krukenberg tumor of the ovary Numerous mucicarminophilic signet-ring cells are present. (Mayer's mucicarmine stain. ×70)

Plate 16

8

Diseases of the Uterine Ligaments and Parametrium

1177 Mesonephric rest of the mesosalpinx in a 3-year-old girl
The tubule is lined by columnar cells with elongated nuclei and is surrounded by a smooth muscle coat. (H&E. ×180)

1178 Mesonephric rest of the mesosalpinx in a woman of reproductive age
The mesonephric tubule is lined by cuboidal cells with round nuclei and distinct nucleoli. Smooth muscle fibers surround the tubule. A small amount of diastase-resistant, weakly PAS-positive material is present within epithelial cells of mesonephric origin. (H&E. ×150)

1179 Mesonephric cyst of the mesosalpinx (cyst of Kobelt's tubule)
The cyst located in the mesosalpinx contains smooth muscle fibers in its wall and is lined by mesonephric epithelium. Usually a small cyst is difficult to enucleate. (H&E. ×50)

1180 Mesonephric cyst of the mesosalpinx
High magnification of Fig. 1179. The lining of the mesonephric cyst is formed by cuboidal cells with prominent ovoid hyperchromatic nuclei. (H&E. ×250)

1181 Hyperplasia of mesonephric rests of the mesosalpinx
Numerous small glandular structures are lined by cuboidal epithelial cells. Differentiation from adenoma is difficult. Collagen and reticulum stain establish the presence of basement membrane in the mesonephric rests and mesonephric adenoma. (H&E. ×50)

1182 Anlage of a parovarian cyst of the mesosalpinx in a 22-cm fetus
The arrow indicates anlage of a parovarian cyst in the mesosalpinx. (H&E. ×8)

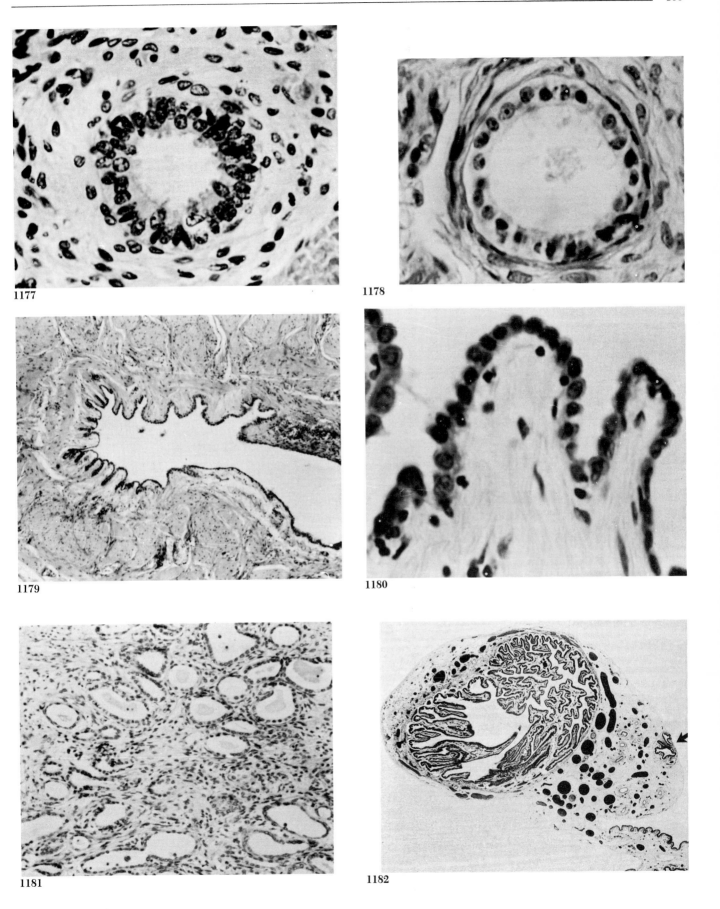

1177

1178

1179

1180

1181

1182

1183   Paramesonephric (Müllerian) rests of the mesosalpinx in a 4-year-old child
The cluster of glandular structures is lined by columnar to cuboidal epithelial cells. There is differentiation into three types of cells: ciliated, nonciliated, or secretory and intercalated (peg) cells. The smooth muscle coat is absent. (H&E. ×125)

1184   Lining of an early paramesonephric cyst of the mesosalpinx
The paramesonephric (Müllerian) cyst in the mesosalpinx is lined by epithelium identical with oviductal epithelium. (H&E. ×150)

1185   Paramesonephric cyst of the mesosalpinx in a 17-year-old girl
A paramesonephric (Müllerian) cyst is seen within connective tissue stroma of the mesosalpinx. The lumen of the oviduct is to the right. The loose surrounding connective tissue permits ready enucleation. This is characteristic of a paramesonephric cyst. (H&E. ×6)

1186   Paramesonephric cyst of the mesosalpinx
High magnification of Fig. 1185. Tubal epithelium with small epithelial projections line the thin connective tissue wall. Loose connective tissue stroma surrounds the cyst wall. (H&E. ×50)

1187   Wall of a large paramesonephric cyst
Nondistinct flattened epithelium lines the fibrous and hyalinized cyst wall. The arrow indicates the plane of cleavage between the cyst and mesosalpingeal connective tissue. The presence of a plane of cleavage is pathognomonic of a paramesonephric cyst. (H&E. ×50)

1188   Paramesonephric cyst with stalk (so-called hydatid of Morgagni or paramesonephric appendix)
The paramesonephric cyst is attached by a relatively long stalk to the infundibular portion of the oviduct. (H&E. ×10)

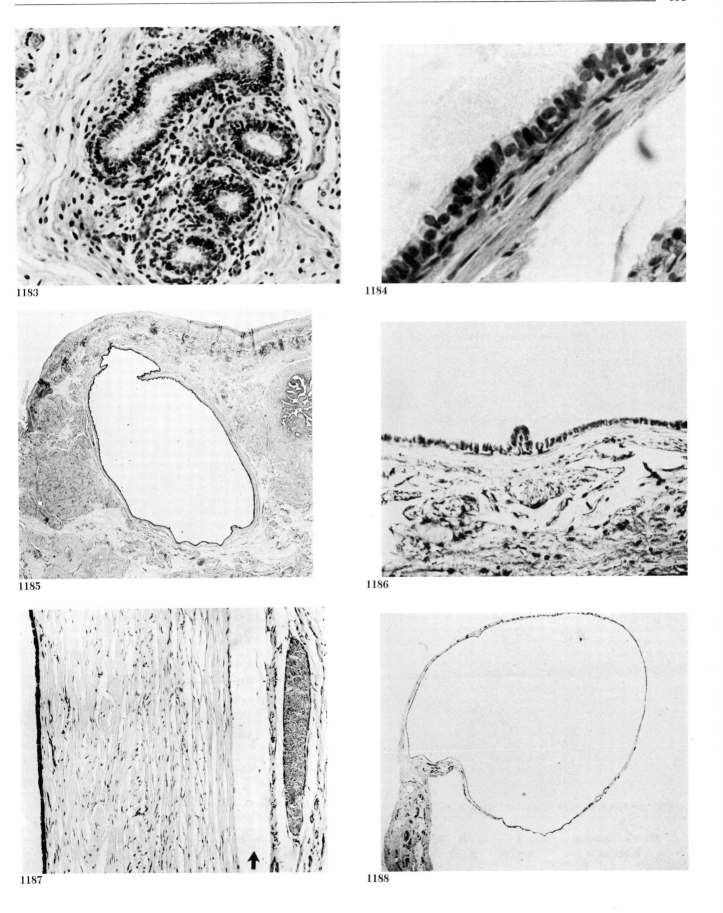

1183

1184

1185

1186

1187

1188

1189 Papillary serous cystadenoma developing in a paramesonephric cyst of the mesosalpinx
The paramesonephric cyst shows a fibrous wall and a distinct plane of cleavage. Multiple coarse papillary projections arise from the cyst wall. Some appear detached. This tumor is strikingly similar to an ovarian serous cystadenoma. The oviduct is normal. (H&E. ×8)

1190 Papillary serous cystadenoma developing in a paramesonephric cyst of the mesosalpinx
This papillary tumor is composed of dense collagen fiber cores which are covered by a single layer of tubal epithelial cells. Malignant transformation may occur. (H&E. ×25)

1191 Papillary serous cystadenoma developing in a paramesonephric cyst of the mesosalpinx
High magnification of Fig. 1190. The papillary projections are lined by oviductal epithelium. PAS, Alcian blue, and Mayer's mucicarmine stains are positive, indicating the presence of neutral and acid mucopolysaccharides. Such tumors give credence to the theory of paramesonephric rest origin of some ovarian tumors. (H&E. ×62)

1192 Paramesonephric cyst of the mesosalpinx with inspissated secretions
(H&E. ×12)

1193 Adrenal rest in the mesovarium of a newborn
The ovoid structure to the left represents accessory adrenal tissue in the mesovarium. The ovary is to the right. (H&E. ×25)

1194 Adrenal rest in the mesovarium of a newborn
High magnification of Fig. 1193. The well-encapsulated adrenal cortical tissue shows a peripheral "adult" zone and central "fetal" zone. (H&E. ×62)

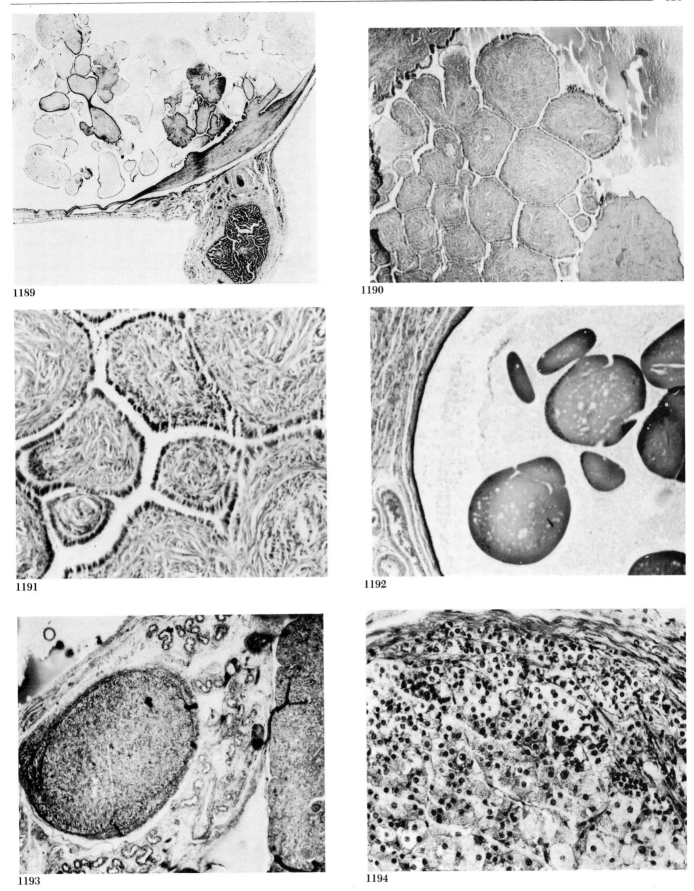

1189

1190

1191

1192

1193

1194

1195 Adrenal rest of the mesosalpinx
Accessory adrenal cortical tissue is composed of a central area with dense cells and a peripheral zone with large lipid-containing cells. (H&E. ×10)

1196 Peripheral zone of adrenal rest of the mesosalpinx
High magnification of Fig. 1195. The large pale cells contain abundant lipid. (H&E. ×150)

1197 Central zone of adrenal rest of the meso-salpinx
High magnification of Fig. 1195. "Compact cells" contain finely granular eosinophilic cytoplasm and decreased lipid content. Note the marked vascularity of this zone. Compact cells resemble Leydig's cells. (H&E. ×150)

1198 Nodular fasciitis of the round ligament
Proliferation of fibroblasts and capillaries, minute foci of fat necrosis, and inflammatory cell infiltration are present. This benign lesion is occasionally misdiagnosed as a sarcoma. (H&E. ×30)

1199 Nodular fasciitis of the round ligament
High magnification of Fig. 1198. Note the proliferation of fibroblasts, the presence of lipid-containing histiocytes, and infiltration with lymphocytes and plasma cells. The tumor originates from round ligament fascia. This inflammatory granuloma has bizarre cellular proliferation. Recurrence is frequent if it is inadequately excised. (H&E. ×90)

1200 Unclassified cyst of the round ligament
(H&E. ×7)

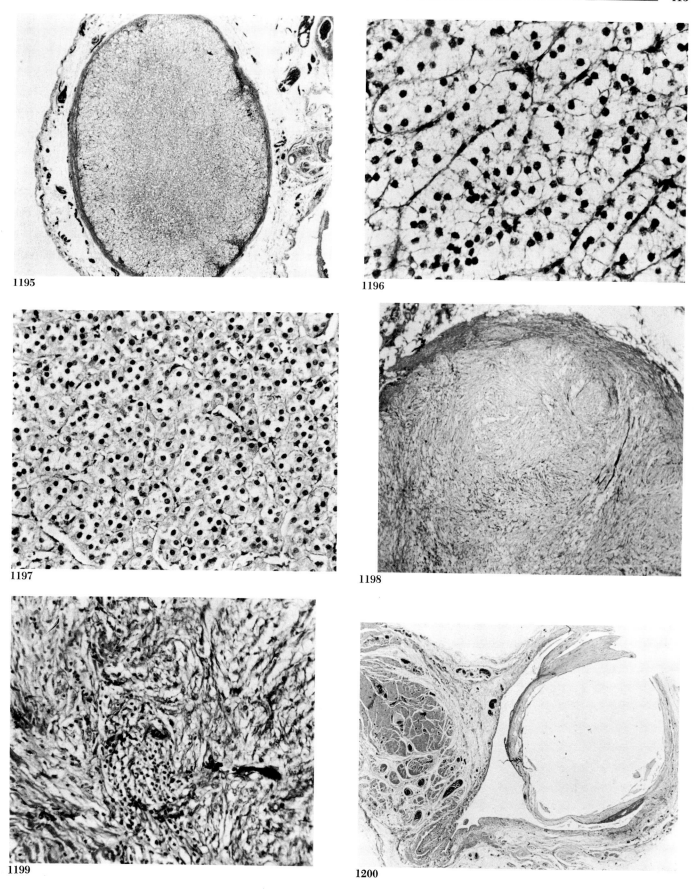

1195

1196

1197

1198

1199

1200

1201 Round ligament cyst, not otherwise specified
High magnification of Fig. 1200. The cyst lining is not discernible. (H&E. ×40)

1202 Endometriosis of the round ligament
The fibromuscular tissue of the round ligament contains numerous glandular structures surrounded in places by endometrial stromal cells. Some heterotopic endometrial glands are filled with blood. (H&E. ×10)

1203 Endometriosis of the round ligament
High magnification of Fig. 1202. Heterotopic endometrial glands and stromal cells are seen in the round ligament. (H&E. ×18)

1204 Neurilemmoma of the round ligament
The tumor is formed by fibriles and clusters of nuclei in a palisading arrangement. This form of neurilemmoma is known as Antoni type A. A neurilemmoma with myxomatoid changes and cystic spaces is known as Antoni type B. This benign tumor has the capacity for local recurrence. It should be differentiated from neurofibroma, which may become malignant. (H&E. ×55)

1205 Leiomyoma of the round ligament
There is pronounced hyaline degeneration in this leiomyoma. A residual of compressed dark nuclei of smooth muscle fibers is seen. (H&E. ×55)

1206 Leiomyoma of the round ligament
High magnification of Fig. 1205. (H&E. ×110)

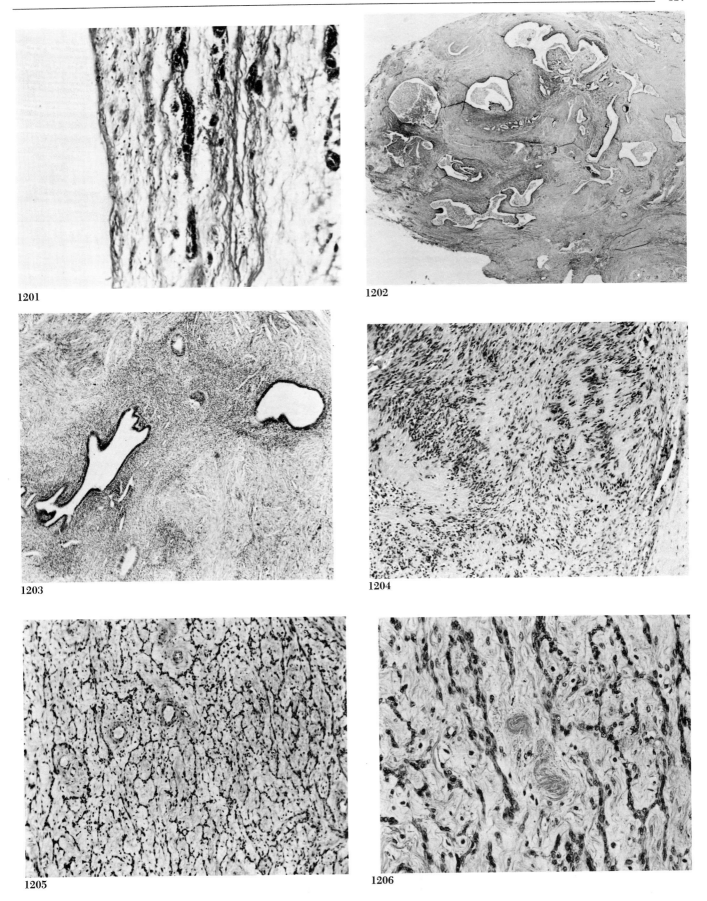

1201

1202

1203

1204

1205

1206

1207 Talc powder granuloma of the broad ligament
This foreign-body granuloma contains crystals. Such a granuloma may develop from talc used in surgical gloves or following the application of sulfonamide powder. Microchemical examination of the crystals is desirable. Tuberculous granuloma and sarcoidosis with secondary crystal formation must be considered in the differential diagnosis. (H&E. ×125)

1208 Lipoma of the broad ligament
This poorly encapsulated tumor is composed of lobules of mature fat cells. (H&E. ×45)

1209 Leiomyoma of the broad ligament
The tumor is formed by smooth muscle fibers showing extensive areas of hyaline degeneration with liquefaction and pseudocyst formations. (H&E. ×8)

1210 Leiomyoma of the broad ligament
High magnification of Fig. 1209. Islands of hyaline degeneration and areas of disintegrating tumorous smooth muscle fibers can be seen. (H&E. ×85)

1211 Primary adenocarcinoma of the mesosalpinx, probably dysontogenetic of paramesonephric (Müllerian) origin
This primary, moderately well-differentiated carcinoma occurring in the mesosalpinx has some resemblance to endometrial adenocarcinoma. (H&E. ×90)

1212 Mesonephroma of the mesosalpinx
This tumor developed from mesonephric rests in the mesosalpinx. The tumor is composed of irregular cells with clear cytoplasm and large hyperchromatic nuclei. (H&E. ×90)

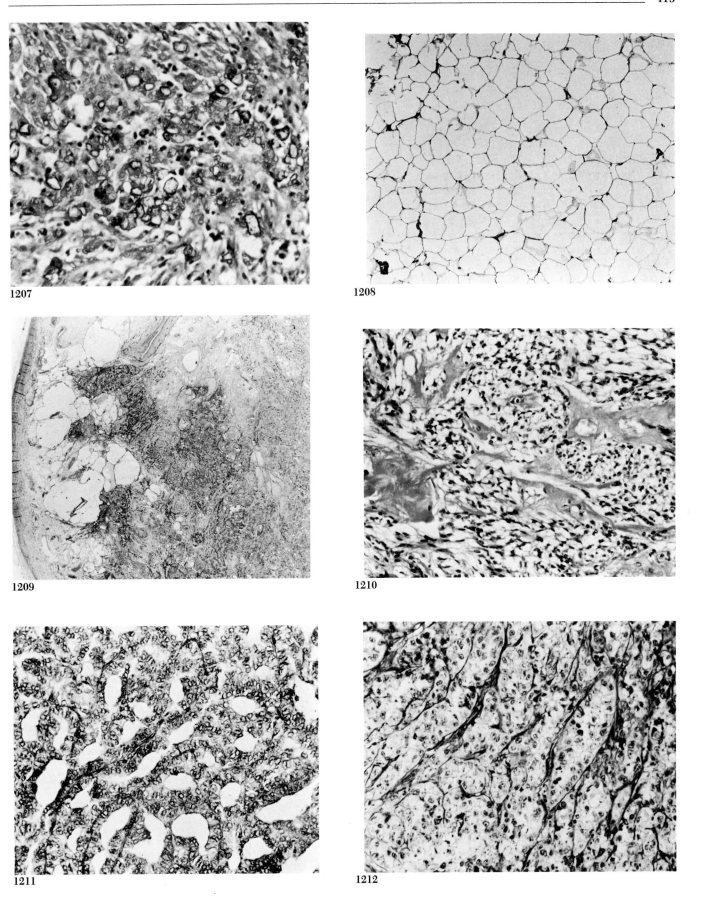

1207

1208

1209

1210

1211

1212

1213 Mesonephroma of the mesosalpinx
Papillary and alveolar arrangements of tumor cells are seen. Such morphologic appearance of the tumor may lead to an unfounded assumption of its origin as a variant of an ovarian serous cystadenocarcinoma. Histochemical examination as outlined previously will help in reaching a definite diagnosis. (H&E. ×75)

1214 Mesonephroma of the mesosalpinx
High magnification of Fig. 1213. Alveolar spaces and tuftlike projections are lined by cuboidal mesonephric epithelium. The round nuclei show prominent nucleoli. Atypical mitoses are frequent. (H&E. ×180)

1215 Leiomyosarcoma of the broad ligament
This leiomyosarcoma has developed from a pre-existing leiomyoma. Fasciculation of muscle fibers is preserved. Atypical mitoses are frequent, an important diagnostic criterion. Intervening connective tissue stroma is absent. (H&E. ×180)

1216 Leiomyosarcoma of the broad ligament
This leiomyosarcoma developed from a pre-existing leiomyoma. Fasciculation is in part preserved. Pleomorphic cells with bizarre hyperchromatic nuclei are present. The tumor cells exhibit degenerative changes. (H&E. ×180)

1217 Hemangioendotheliosarcoma of the broad ligament
The tumor is composed of vascular spaces lined by neoplastic, proliferating endothelial cells (endothelioblasts). The neoplastic endothelial cells vary in appearance and contain large hyperchromatic nuclei. Mitotic figures are frequent. (H&E. ×90)

1218 Reticulum cell sarcoma of the broad ligament
The base of the broad ligament is infiltrated by a tumor composed of pleomorphic round cells. (H&E. ×3)

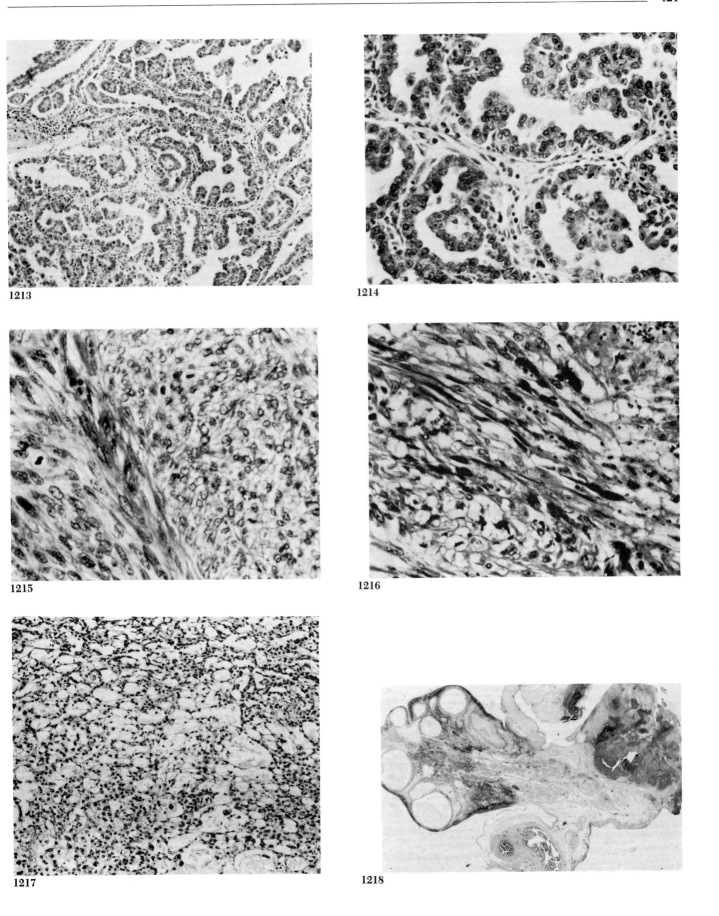

1213

1214

1215

1216

1217

1218

1219 Reticulum cell sarcoma of the broad ligament

High magnification of Fig. 1218. The reticulum cells present a pleomorphic appearance. Nuclei show prominent nucleoli. Mitoses are frequent. Reticulum stain is useful in differentiating this tumor from other malignant lymphomas. (H&E. ×140)

1220 Squamous cell carcinoma of the cervix, in the lymphatic channels of parametrium

Islands of squamous cell carcinoma are seen in dilated lymphatics of the parametrium. (H&E. ×45)

1221 Adenocarcinoma of the large intestine metastatic to parametrium

Parametric connective tissue and the mesosalpinx are invaded by adenocarcinoma. (H&E. ×10)

1222 Pelvic ganglion cells in a normal parametrium

These normal non-irradiated pelvic ganglion cells were removed at a hysterectomy in a patient 49 years old. (H&E. ×111)

1223 Effect of betatron irradiation on pelvic ganglion cells of the parametrium

Pelvic ganglion as seen in a patient receiving betatron external radiation, approximately 5,000 r, 9 weeks after irradiation. Note the marked proliferation of connective tissue cells with cicatrization and fragmentation of pelvic ganglion. There is infiltration with chronic inflammatory cells. (H&E. ×100)

1224 Effects of betatron irradiation on pelvic ganglion cells of the parametrium

Note the variation in size of the ganglionic cells. Nuclear pyknosis and cellular margination are striking. (Wilder's reticulum stain. ×400)

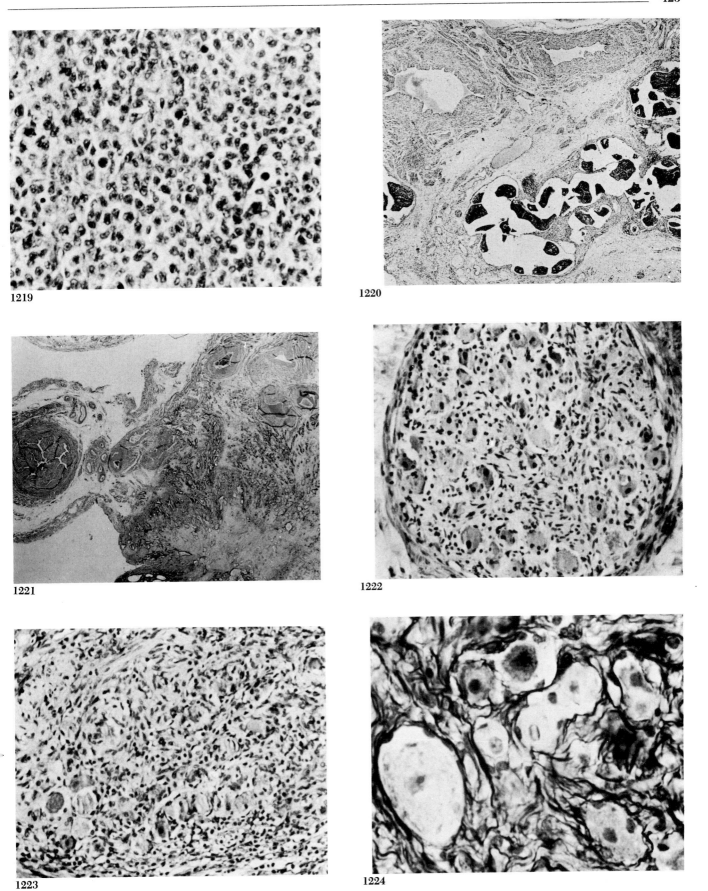

1219

1220

1221

1222

1223

1224

COLOR PLATES

Chapter 8

Diseases of the Uterine Ligaments and Parametrium

Plate 17

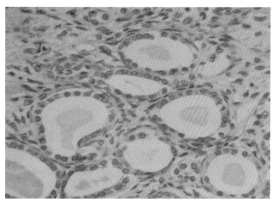

97 Mesonephric rest of the mesosalpinx The tubular structures are lined by cuboidal epithelium and contain glucoprotein within their lumens. (H&E. ×50)

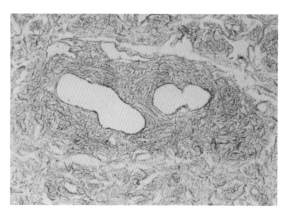

98 Mesonephric rest of the mesosalpinx There is concentric arrangement of reticulum fibers. (Wilder's reticulum stain. ×62)

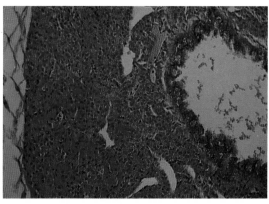

99 Adrenal rest of the mesosalpinx with central calcification Central calcification is seen in the accessory adrenal tissue in the mesosalpinx. (H&E. ×125)

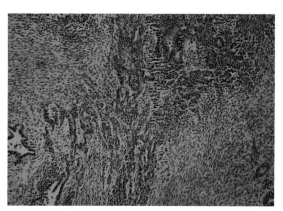

100 Carcinosarcoma of the broad ligament The tumor is formed by carcinomatous epithelial elements and sarcomatous stromal elements. It represents a form of mixed mesodermal tumor. (H&E. ×75)

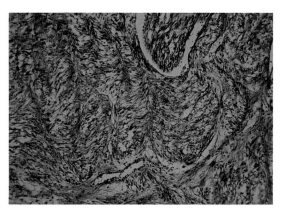

101 Poorly differentiated sarcoma of the broad ligament Elongated neoplastic cells form whorls. Mitoses are frequent. (PTAH. ×75)

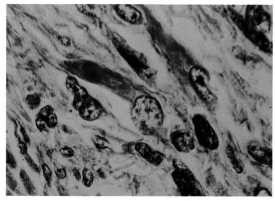

102 Rhabdomyosarcoma of the broad ligament The tumor is formed by elongated rhabdomyoblasts with distinct striation. This malignant mesenchymal tumor shows predominance of rhabdomyoblasts. (Masson's trichrome stain. ×600)

Plate 17

9

Diseases of the Pelvic Peritoneum, Omentum, Retroperitoneum, and Pelvic Lymph Nodes

1225 Mesothelial lining of normal pelvic peritoneum
A single layer of cuboidal cells rests is seen on a fibrous base. (H&E. ×160)

1226 Early acute pelvic peritonitis
The vessels underneath the mesothelium are dilated, lined by swollen endothelium, and contain leukocytes, some of which are marginated. Leukocytes have migrated into the fibrous tissue. The mesothelial cells themselves show some edema. (H&E. ×120)

1227 Organizing pelvic peritonitis
The membrane is denuded of mesothelium. Flakes of fibrin lie on the free surface, but there has been proliferation of fibroblasts in the connective tissue base, and the exudate is predominantly lymphocytic. (H&E. ×62)

1228 Peritoneal inclusion cyst
A simple cyst lined by a layer of flattened cells. (H&E. ×95)

1229 Tuberculous peritonitis
A noncaseating granuloma composed of epithelioid cells and Langhans' giant cells with lymphocytic reaction lies under the mesothelial surface, the mesothelial cells themselves being denuded. (H&E. ×50)

1230 Pseudomyxoma peritonei
Note the absence of mesothelial cell lining. Lakes of mucoid material dilate the lymphatic channels. A modest perivascular lymphocytic infiltrate is seen deep in the lesion. The lesion followed rupture of an ovarian mucinous cystadenoma. (H&E. ×25)

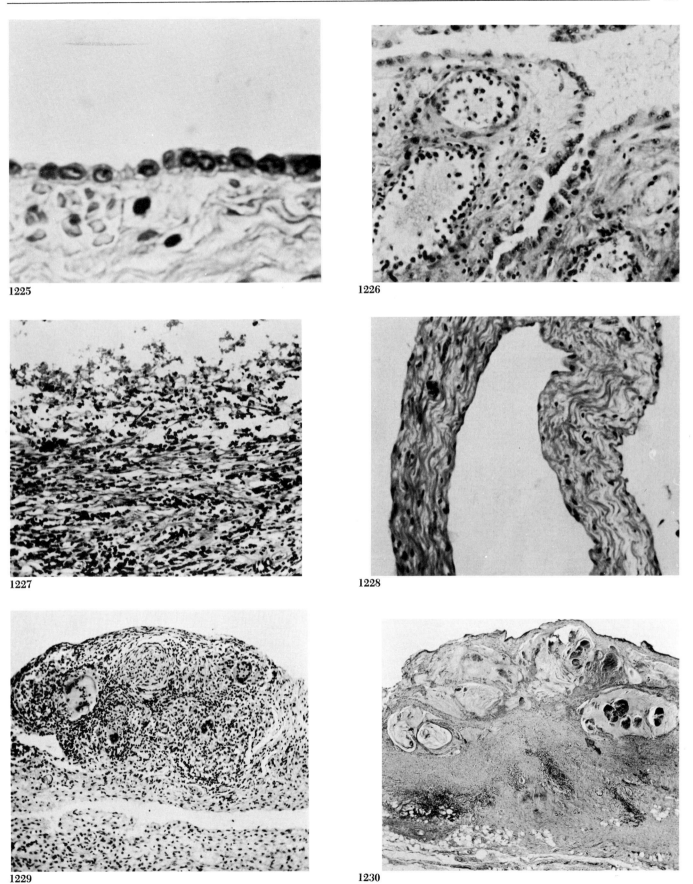

1225

1226

1227

1228

1229

1230

1231   Mesothelioma in situ of the pelvic peritoneum
A somewhat atypical proliferation of the mesothelial cell layer is shown. (H&E. ×125)

1232   Mesothelioma of the pelvic peritoneum
Bland papillary projections composed of a fibrous core with variable lymphocytic component project into the peritoneal cavity. The mesothelial cells themselves are taller than average and show a mild degree of pleomorphism. (H&E. ×110)

1233   Mesothelioma of the pelvic peritoneum
The papillary architecture is less well preserved than in Fig. 1232. Proliferation of mesothelial cells is evident, and the cells show loss of cohesion as well as pseudorosette formation. (H&E. ×125)

1234   Mesothelioma of the pelvic peritoneum
The papillary pattern is retained, but the noncohesive mesothelial cells form broad sheets, and there is marked cellular pleomorphism, nuclear hyperchromasia, and other stigmas of neoplasia. (H&E. ×135)

1235   Mesothelioma of the pelvic peritoneum
An even less well-differentiated area is seen. (H&E. ×180)

1236   Carcinomatosis of the peritoneum, secondary to papillary serous cystadenocarcinoma of the ovary
A well-preserved papillary pattern is seen in the implant. (H&E. ×50)

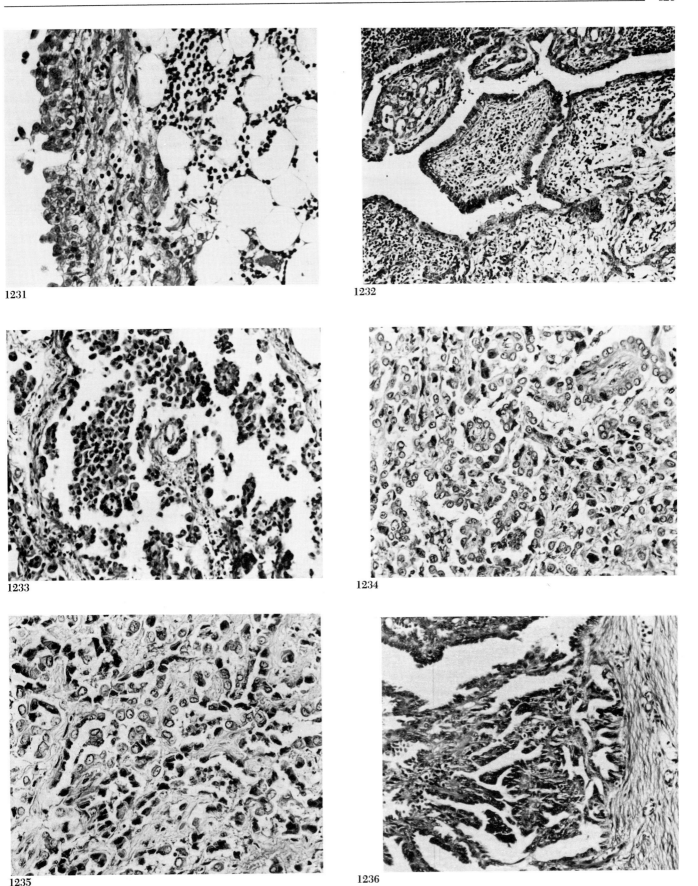

1231

1232

1233

1234

1235

1236

1237   Fat necrosis of the omentum
The completely necrotic adipose tissue in the center is surrounded by a sharply demarcating zone of mixed lymphocytes and foam cells. (H&E. ×90)

1238   Necrotizing arteritis of the omentum, with surrounding granulomatous reaction
Fibrinoid necrosis of the entire wall of the artery is shown. An intense surrounding reaction containing epithelioid cells and a few giant cells is present. (H&E. ×65)

1239   Granulomatous omentitis of undetermined cause
Epithelioid cells, giant cells, and a lymphocytic component are present. No foreign body, parasite, or fungus was identified; there was no intestinal perforation, history of trauma or previous surgical procedure. (H&E. ×150)

1240   Endometriosis of the omentum
A central space mimicking the cavum uteri is lined by a mucosa containing endometrial glands and stroma. A zone of fibrosis and organizing hemorrhage surround it. (H&E. ×8)

1241   Endosalpingiosis of the omentum
Multicystic structures are seen within the fibrofatty stroma of omentum. The lining of cysts shows striking resemblance to tubal epithelium. (H&E. ×50, ×200)

1242   Papillary serous cystadenocarcinoma of the ovary invading omentum
Contrast with Fig. 1236 in which the implanted carcinoma has not invaded. (H&E. ×62)

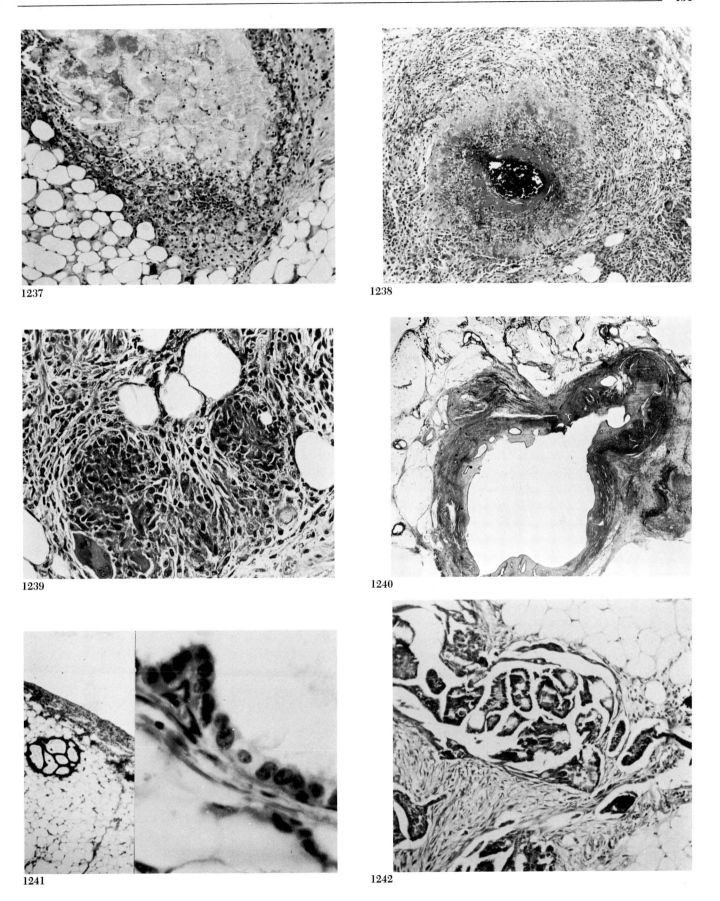

1237

1238

1239

1240

1241

1242

1243 Solid adenocarcinoma of the ovary metastatic to the omentum
Neoplastic glands infiltrate the fibroadipose omentum. (H&E. ×90)

1244 Mesonephroma of the ovary metastatic to the omentum
The metastatic tumor is forming papillary structures. (H&E. ×24)

1245 Mesonephroma of the ovary metastatic to the omentum
According to the criteria in Fig. 1213, the tumor should be differentiated from ovarian papillary serous cystadenocarcinoma. (H&E. ×50)

1246 Reticulum cell sarcoma of the omentum
Although the lesion is usually more diffuse, the isolated perivascular accumulation of large dark cells is a pattern often seen, often as a satellite of larger aggregates. (H&E. ×50)

1248 Carcinomatosis of the omentum and peritoneum after yttrium (Y⁹⁰) therapy
Most of the tumor cells have disappeared, leaving only degenerated nuclei and scattered granules of elementary yttrium behind. A colloidal suspension of 30 mc of yttrium chloride (Y^{90}) was administered intraabdominally. Y^{90} is a pure beta emitter with a half-life of 61 hr, a maximum energy of 3.2 mev, and a maximum beta-particle range in tissue of 1.1 cm. (H&E. ×50)

1247 Reticulum cell sarcoma of the omentum
High magnification of Fig. 1246. There is infiltration of omental fat by a patternless sheet of medium to large cells without epithelial architecture. (H&E. ×150)

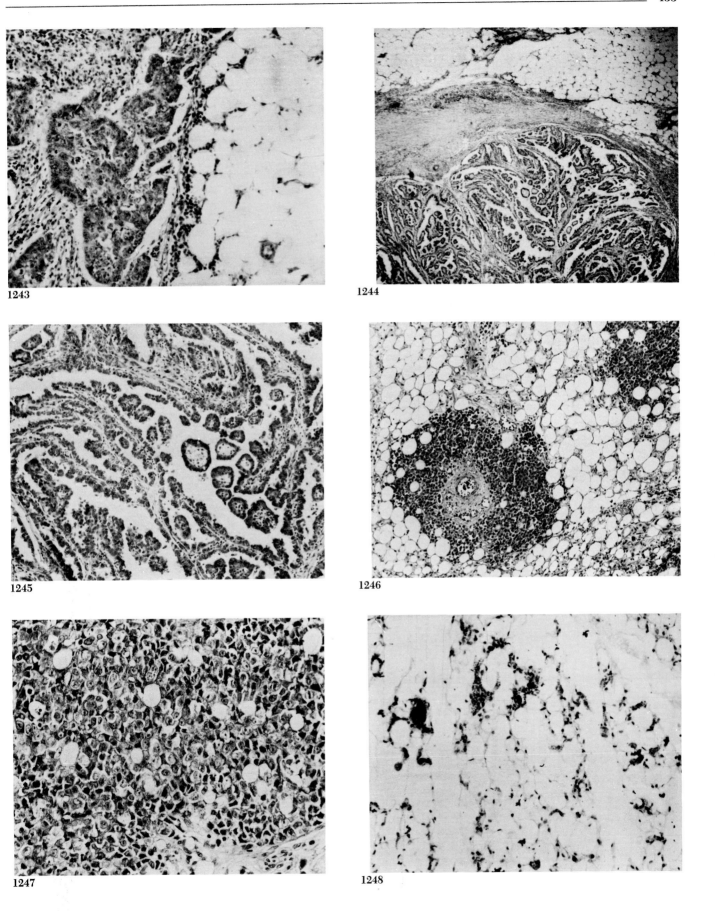

1243

1244

1245

1246

1247

1248

1249 Peritoneal carcinomatosis after yttrium (Y⁹⁰) therapy

High magnification of Fig. 1248. Isolated damaged tumor cells lie free amid necrotic debris and leukocytes. The arrow points to granules of elementary yttrium. (H&E. ×150)

1250 Actinomycosis of the pelvic connective tissue

A large conglomeration of the microorganism forming granules with clubs is surrounded by chronic inflammatory exudate including foam cells. (H&E. ×30)

1251 Actinomycosis of pelvic connective tissue

High magnification of Fig. 1250. The foam cells show an admixture of lymphocytes and a few neutrophiles. This picture is typical of pseudo-xanthomatous inflammation. (H&E. ×140)

1252 Xanthogranuloma of the retroperitoneal tissue

The well-vascularized, heavily collagenized connective tissue contains foci of foam cells and a light sprinkling of inflammatory cells. The cause is undetermined. (H&E. ×50)

1253 Xanthogranuloma of the retroperitoneal tissue

High magnification of Fig. 1252. A cluster of foam cells and chronic inflammatory cells is surrounded by dense fibrous connective tissue. (H&E. ×125)

1254 Xanthogranuloma of the retroperitoneal tissue

An occasional giant cell of the Touton type is surrounded by numerous foam cells or xanthoma cells. The latter have small, dark nuclei and doubly refractile lipid droplets, predominantly cholesterol. Lipid can be demonstrated in a frozen section using Sudan stains. (H&E. ×125)

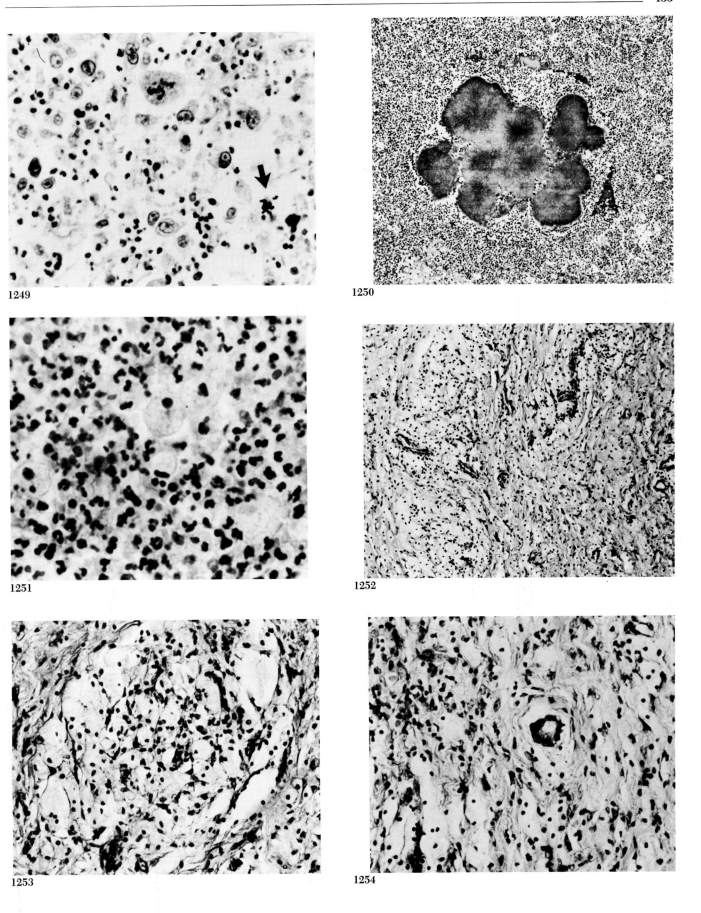

1249

1250

1251

1252

1253

1254

1255 Idiopathic retroperitoneal sclerosis (Ormon's disease)
The retroperitoneal fat is converted to a collagenized scar with accumulations of lymphoid tissue. (H&E. ×40)

1256 Idiopathic retroperitoneal sclerosis (Ormon's disease)
High magnification of Fig. 1255. Collagen fibers and aggregates of inflammatory cells are seen replacing retroperitoneal fatty tissue and producing sclerosis. (H&E. ×62)

1257 Idiopathic retroperitoneal sclerosis (Ormon's disease)
Collagen fibers are deposited between single fat cells and a more diffuse distribution of lymphocytes. (H&E. ×55)

1258 Myxosarcoma of the pelvic connective tissue
Note the neoplastic proliferation of stellate cells in a loose, mucicarmine-positive reticular myxoid network. (H&E. ×85)

1259 Myxosarcoma of the pelvic connective tissue
High magnification of Fig. 1258. Stellate cells and the delicate matrix of myxoid ground substance are seen. The nuclei are irregular and hyperchromatic. (H&E. ×350)

1260 Myxoid type liposarcoma of the retroperitoneum
The tumor is composed of lipoblasts, a network of capillaries, and myxoid ground substance. (H&E. ×62)

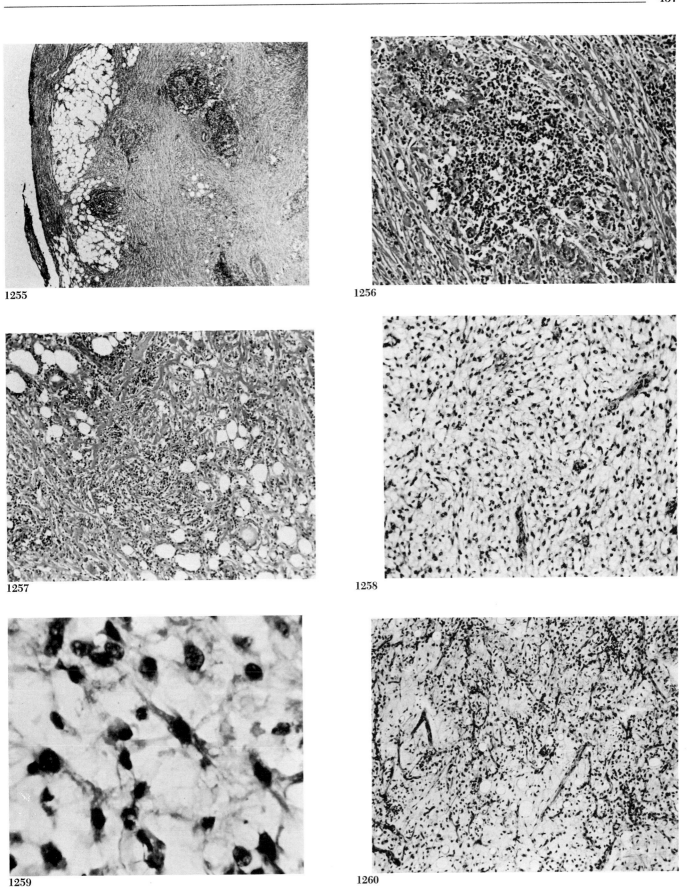

1255

1256

1257

1258

1259

1260

**1261 Myxoid type liposarcoma of the retro-
peritoneum**
High magnification of Fig. 1260. Hyperchromatic
pleomorphic lipoblasts, some in bipolar form,
are seen in a myxoid matrix. (H&E. ×160)

**1262 Alveolar rhabdomyosarcoma of the recto-
vaginal septum**
A pseudoglandular pattern is present as poorly
cohesive tumor cells seem to line spaces and
exfoliate into a preformed lumen. (H&E. ×80)

**1263 Alveolar rhabdomyosarcoma of the recto-
vaginal septum**
High magnification of Fig. 1262. Neoplastic
cells do not line up as an epithelium and in
other places form multinucleated strap cells
typical of a tumor derived from skeletal muscle.
(H&E. ×180)

1264 Paraganglioma of the pelvis
Nests of fairly uniform polyhedral cells with
clear cytoplasm form this tumor. There is a rich
capillary network. (H&E. ×100)

1265 Paraganglioma of the pelvis
High magnification of Fig. 1264. There is relative uniformity of the nuclei. Occasional binu-
cleated tumor cells are seen. Small islands of
cells are enveloped in delicate connective tissue
stroma. (H&E. ×180)

1266 Ganglioneuroblastoma of the pelvis
This is a tumor of the sympathetic nervous system. Small and large ganglioneuroblasts are seen
diffusely infiltrating connective tissue stroma.
(H&E. ×50)

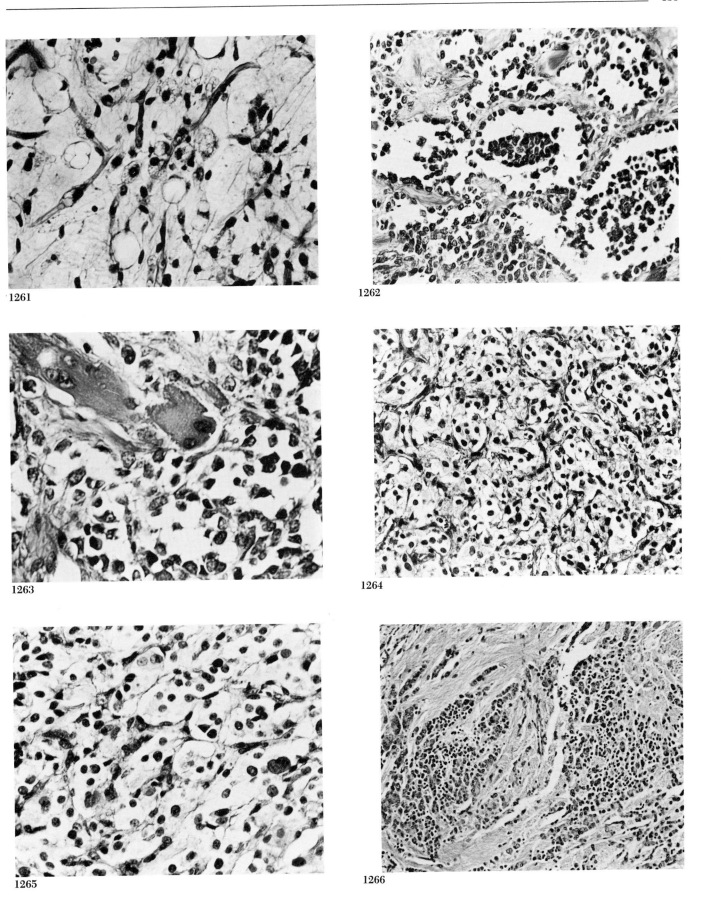

1261

1262

1263

1264

1265

1266

1267   Ganglioneuroblastoma of the pelvis
High magnification of Fig. 1266. This tumor shows considerable pleomorphism, differentiated and undifferentiated cells, and rosette formation. Intervening tissue shows a fine "fibrillary" network. (H&E. ×160)

1268   Ganglioneuroma of the pelvis
The tumor is composed of well-differentiated ganglionic cells and intervening neuroglial tissue. (H&E. ×75)

1269   Ganglioneuroma of the pelvis
High magnification of Fig. 1268. The ganglionic cells contain Nissl substance. Large round nuclei show prominent nucleoli. The intervening stroma consists of spindle cells and collagen fibers. (H&E. ×265)

1270   Neuroblastoma of the pelvis
The neoplasm is composed of large sheets of small dark tumor cells with almost no stroma. A suggestion of lobular pattern is present. (H&E. ×62)

1271   Neuroblastoma of the pelvis
High magnification of Fig. 1270. Uniform, nondescript tumor cells are composed of an immature nuclei and surrounded by almost invisible wisps of cytoplasm. An abortive attempt at rosette formation can be seen. (H&E. ×150)

1272   Myxoid type neurofibroma of the pelvis
The tumor is formed by coarse, wavy fibers and myxomatoid stroma. (H&E. ×50)

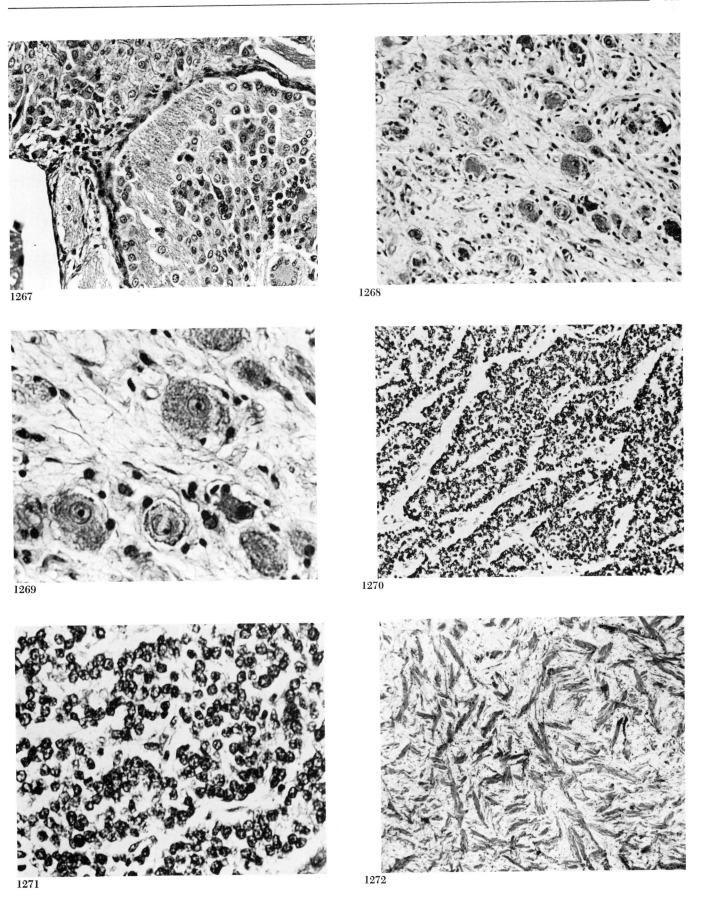

1267

1268

1269

1270

1271

1272

1273 Myxoid type neurofibroma of the pelvis
The tumor is formed by strands of wavy neuro-fibrils and myxomatous stroma infiltrated by occasional lymphocytes. (H&E. ×62)

1274 Myxoid type neurofibroma of the pelvis
Interlacing fiber bundles show prominent elongated nuclei. The intervening connective tissue stroma is myxoid and contains stellate cells. (H&E. ×150)

1275 Extramedullary ependymoma of the retro-peritoneum
The tumor is composed of sheets of small cells growing with a faint suggestion of a papillary pattern from delicate fibrovascular septums. (H&E. ×50)

1276 Extramedullary ependymoma of the retro-peritoneum
High magnification of Fig. 1275. Pleomorphic small dark cells are seen growing from a fibrovascular core. Fibrillary strands radiate from the stromal stalk into the nearby tumor cells while others lie free. (H&E. ×150)

1277 Extramedullary ependymoma of the retro-peritoneum
High magnification of Fig. 1275. A clearly defined papillary epithelial pattern with formation of pseudorosettes can be seen. (H&E. ×220)

1278 Extramedullary ependymoma of the ret-roperitoneum
The tumor is composed of papillary structures covered by epithelium-like cells. Connective tissue cores show the presence of mucicarmine-positive material. (H&E. ×220)

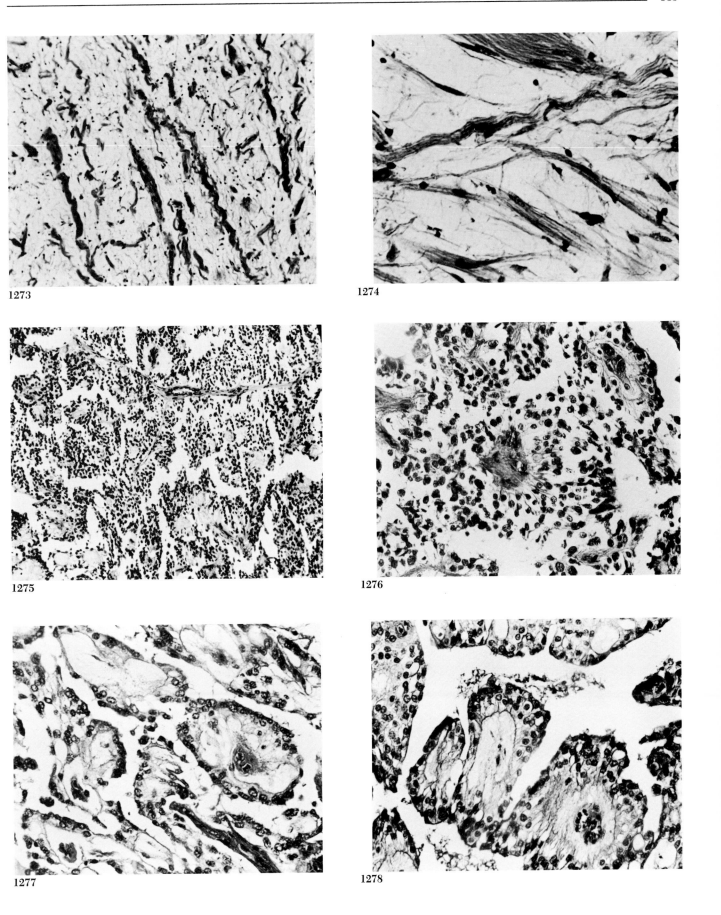

1273

1274

1275

1276

1277

1278

1279   Chordoma of the retroperitoneum
The tumor is composed of large cells growing
with a suggestion of nests in a quasi-chondroid
matrix resembling embryonic notochord. (H&E.
×62)

1280   Chordoma of the retroperitoneum
High magnification of Fig. 1279. The sheet of
large cells shows sharply defined cell walls and
clear cytoplasm. These are the so-called physaliferous cells, i.e., bubble-bearing cells. (H&E.
×150)

1281   Chordoma of the retroperitoneum
The tumor is formed by relatively small cells.
PAS stain may be positive in some cells. Mitoses
are absent. This tumor recurs and metastasizes.
(H&E. ×62)

1282   Chordoma of the retroperitoneum
The physaliferous cells grow in sheets with a
suggestion of epithelial cohesiveness. (H&E.
×120)

1284   Teratocarcinoma of the retroperitoneum
The tumor is formed by immature tubular structures and cartilage. The intervening cellular
mesenchymal matrix shows numerous mitotic
figures. This tumor is highly malignant. (H&E.
×50)

1283   Teratocarcinoma of the retroperitoneum
The tumor is composed of well-formed tubules
in a mesenchymal matrix. (H&E. ×24)

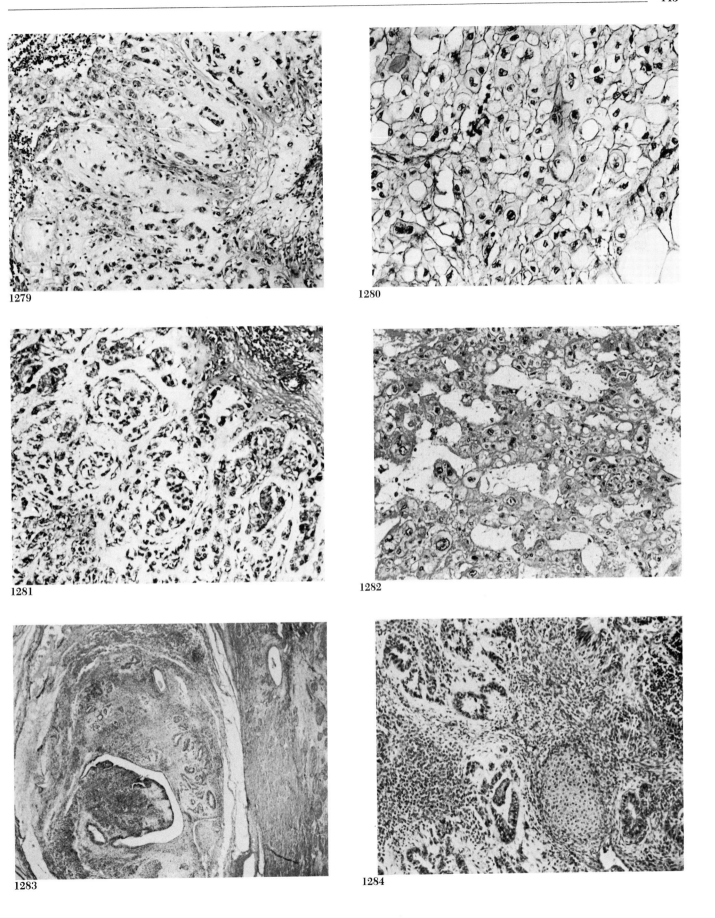

1279

1280

1281

1282

1283

1284

1285 Local sarcoid tissue reaction (pseudosarcoid reaction) in a pelvic lymph node
This discrete noncaseating granuloma is composed chiefly of epithelioid cells with an occasional giant cell. The patient had an invasive squamous cell carcinoma of the cervix. There was no clinical evidence of sarcoidosis. (H&E. ×50)

1286 Pseudosarcoid reaction in an irradiated pelvic lymph node
The numerous noncaseating granulomas show extensive hyalinization. The sarcoid tissue reaction occurring in an irradiated lymph node may be confused with sarcoidosis. (H&E. ×50)

1287 Endometriosis of a pelvic lymph node, showing secretory activity
An endometrial gland included in the pelvic lymph node shows secretory activity. Predecidual alteration of endometrial stromal cells is present. (H&E. ×50)

1288 Paramesonephric inclusion of a pelvic lymph node
A small epithelial-lined glandlike structure is present in the substance of a pelvic lymph node. It is lined with nondescript columnar cells which cannot be distinguished from any of the possible derivatives of the Müllerian duct. There is no evidence to support an embolic theory in such cases. These nests have been found in pelvic lymph nodes of stillborn female infants and presumably represent sequestration of buds of either coelom or coelom-derived paramesonephric duct epithelium during the course of lymph node formation in the embryo. (H&E. ×50)

1289 Paramesonephric inclusion in a pelvic lymph node
Such glandlike inclusions of paramesonephric origin may become cystically dilated, eventually producing obstructive uropathy. (H&E. ×24)

1290 Paramesonephric inclusion in a pelvic lymph node
High magnification of Fig. 1289. Epithelial lining of a cystic inclusion is seen. As a rule, there is an increase of pericystic connective tissue separating it from surrounding lymphoid tissue. (H&E. ×60)

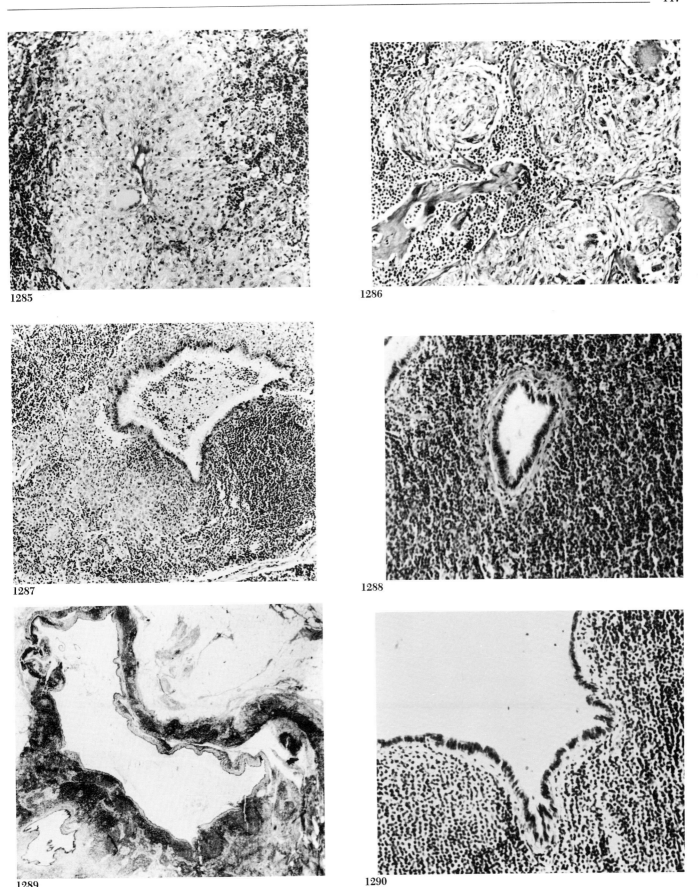

1285

1286

1287

1288

1289

1290

1291 Multiple paramesonephric inclusions in a pelvic lymph node
Paramesonephric inclusions may become cystically dilated reaching considerable size and occasionally, if they impinge on the ureters, may produce obstructive uropathy. (H&E. ×50)

1292 Lining epithelium of paramesonephric inclusions in a pelvic lymph node
High magnification of Fig. 1291. Note the tall columnar epithelial cyst lining. (H&E. ×180)

1293 Papillary carcinoma developing in a paramesonephric inclusion of a pelvic lymph node
This was an incidental finding in a lymph node removed during a Wertheim operation for squamous cell carcinoma of the cervix, stage I. The endometrium and ovaries were normal. Papillary projections within the cyst are lined by neoplastic cells. (H&E. ×50)

1294 Papillary carcinoma developing in a paramesonephric inclusion of a pelvic lymph node
High magnification of Fig. 1293. (H&E. ×150)

1295 Multiple paramesonephric inclusions of a pelvic lymph node with a coexisting unrelated metastatic squamous carcinoma of the cervix
(H&E. ×72)

1296 Partial fatty tissue replacement of a pelvic lymph node with a coexisting unrelated foci of metastatic squamous cell carcinoma of the cervix
(H&E. ×50)

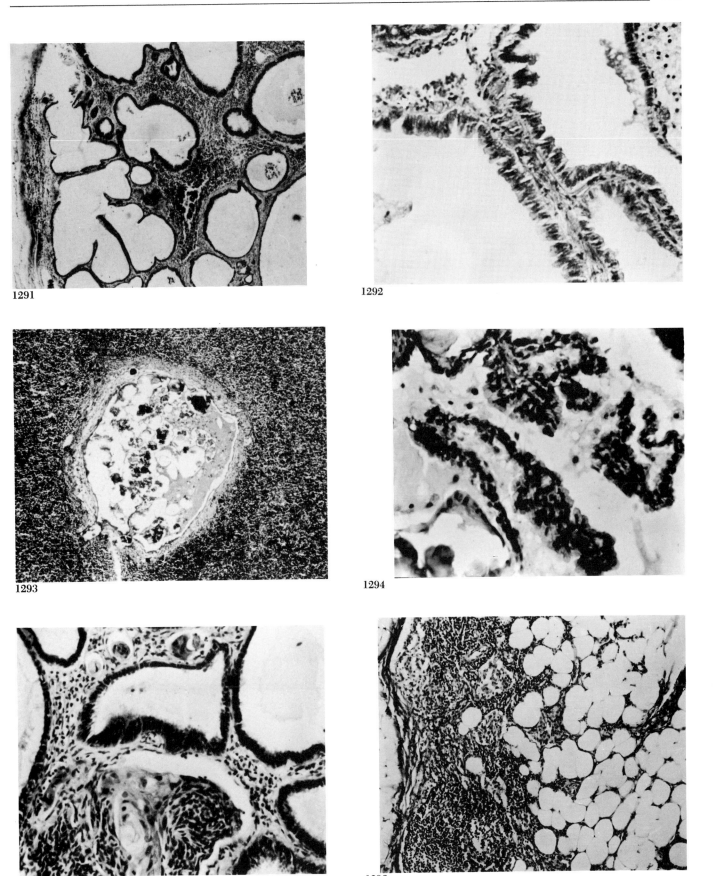

1291

1292

1293

1294

1295

1296

1297 Squamous cell carcinoma of the cervix metastatic to a pelvic lymph node
(H&E. ×50)

1298 Squamous cell carcinoma of the cervix metastatic to a pelvic lymph node
(H&E. ×70)

1299 Adenocarcinoma of the endometrium metastatic to a pelvic lymph node
(H&E. ×110)

1300 Papillary serous cystadenocarcinoma of the ovary metastatic to a pelvic lymph node
(H&E. ×60)

1301 Dysgerminoma of the ovary metastatic to a pelvic lymph node
(H&E. ×25)

1302 Malignant melanoma of the vulva metastatic to a pelvic lymph node
(H&E. ×70)

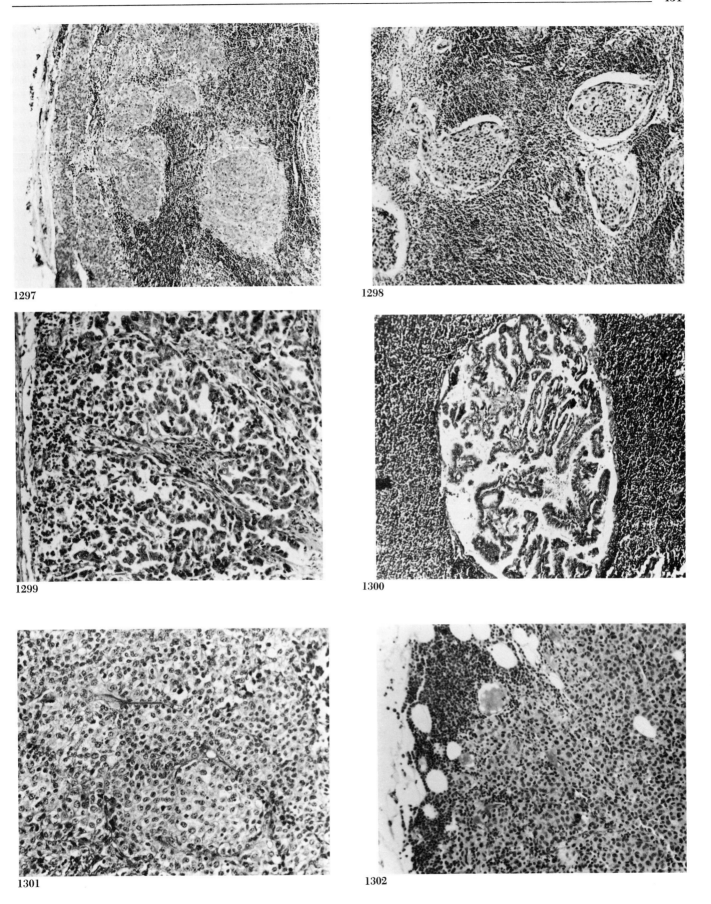

1297

1298

1299

1300

1301

1302

10

Diseases of the Adrenals of Gynecologic Interest

**1303 Congenital adrenal cortical hyperplasia
in adrenogenital syndrome**
This infant showed female pseudohermaphroditism. The syndrome was manifest at birth. The pathogenesis of the syndrome is excessive production of androgenic hormones by hyperplastic adrenals. Adrenal hyperplasia should be differentiated in female infants from masculinization of the external genitalia resulting from treatment of the mother with progestational agents or due to maternal androblastoma. The greatly enlarged adrenal gland shows encapsulated hyperplastic nodules. (H&E. ×20)

**1304 Congenital adrenal cortical hyperplasia
in adrenogenital syndrome**
High magnification of Fig. 1303. Hyperplasia of the zona reticularis can be seen. (H&E. ×50)

**1305 Congenital adrenal cortical hyperplasia
in adrenogenital syndrome**
High magnification of Fig. 1303. (H&E. ×100)

1306 Adrenal cortical carcinoma
The tumor is formed by large cells showing a marked variation in the size and shape of nuclei. Microscopic findings are not helpful in differentiating hormonal abnormalities. (H&E. ×62)

1307 Adrenal cortical carcinoma
High magnification of Fig. 1306. The large tumor cells show bizarre hyperchromatic nuclei. The cytoplasm is finely granular with prominent lipid vacuoles. Multinucleated tumor giant cells may be present. (H&E. ×120)

1308 Adrenal cortical carcinoma
High magnification of Fig. 1306. This adrenal tumor was developing in a 3-year-old girl with marked androgenic changes: clitoris hypertrophy, appearance of pubic hair, and advanced skeletal maturation. (H&E. ×200)

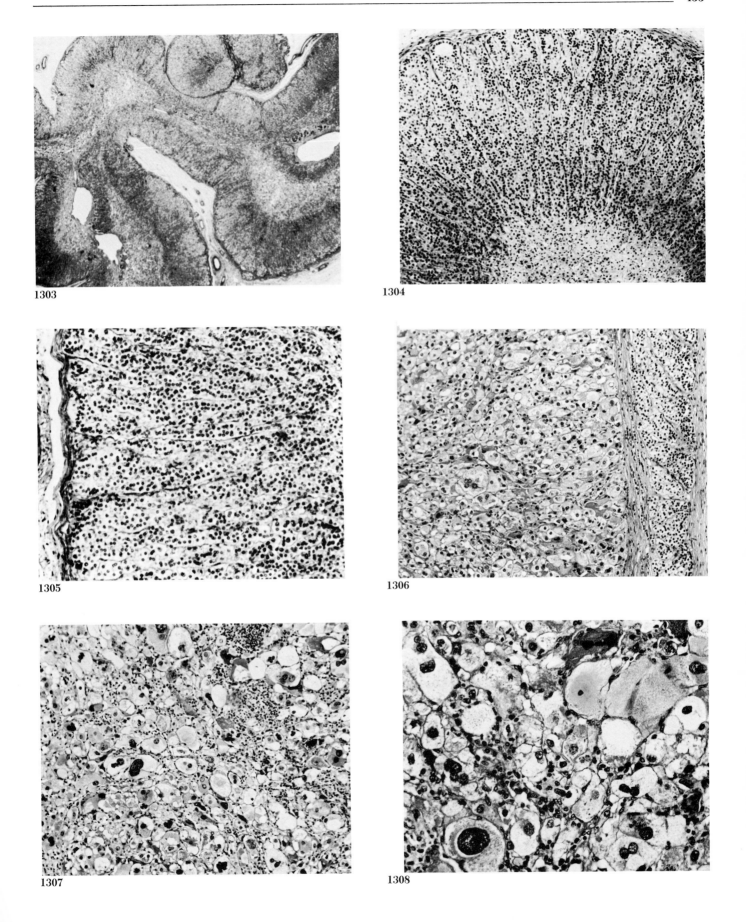

1303

1304

1305

1306

1307

1308

11

Placentation and Morphologic Alterations Encountered in Pregnancy

1309 Decidua of pregnancy
The uterine mucosa is thickened 4 to 10 times its normal size. Coiled arterioles extend to the surface, and straight venules return blood. After an early phase of hypersecretion, the endometrial glands become exhausted, even slitlike, and are lined by a flat epithelium. (H&E. ×15)

1310 Decidua of pregnancy (compacta)
High magnification of Fig. 1309. Note the exhausted gland and the characteristic increase in cytoplasmic volume of endometrial stromal cells. These polyhedral stromal cells assume an epithelioid appearance, are arranged in a pavement or mosaic pattern, and are the characteristic target cells of the decidual reaction. (H&E. ×110)

1311 Decidua of pregnancy (spongiosa)
High magnification of Fig. 1309. During the phase of glandular hypersecretion, dense eosinophilic spherules appear within the lumens representing concentrated glandular secretion. The clearly defined cell membranes of the decidualized stromal cells are well shown. (H&E. ×150)

1312 Decidua of pregnancy
Infiltration of the decidua by leukocytes is a regular concomitant of aborted products of conception, but it is less well known that similar infiltration may be found in the decidua of a normal pregnancy, as shown here, albeit usually quantitatively less impressive. (H&E. ×75)

1313 Decidua of pregnancy showing Arias-Stella phenomenon
Note the hypersecretion and accentuated plication of endometrial glands with atypical endometrial epithelium. The nuclei of glandular epithelial cells are often relatively large and hyperchromatic. (H&E. ×125)

1314 Decidua of pregnancy with Arias-Stella phenomenon
The large hyperchromatic nuclei in the glandular epithelium often exhibit a degree of pleomorphism which suggests neoplasia to the uninitiated. This effect is seen in the endometrium of ectopic as well as intrauterine pregnancy. It is also observed with hydatidiform mole and choriocarcinoma. Presumably, it is an endocrine effect, possibly related to chorionic gonadotropin or progesterone-estrogen ratio changes. (H&E. ×125)

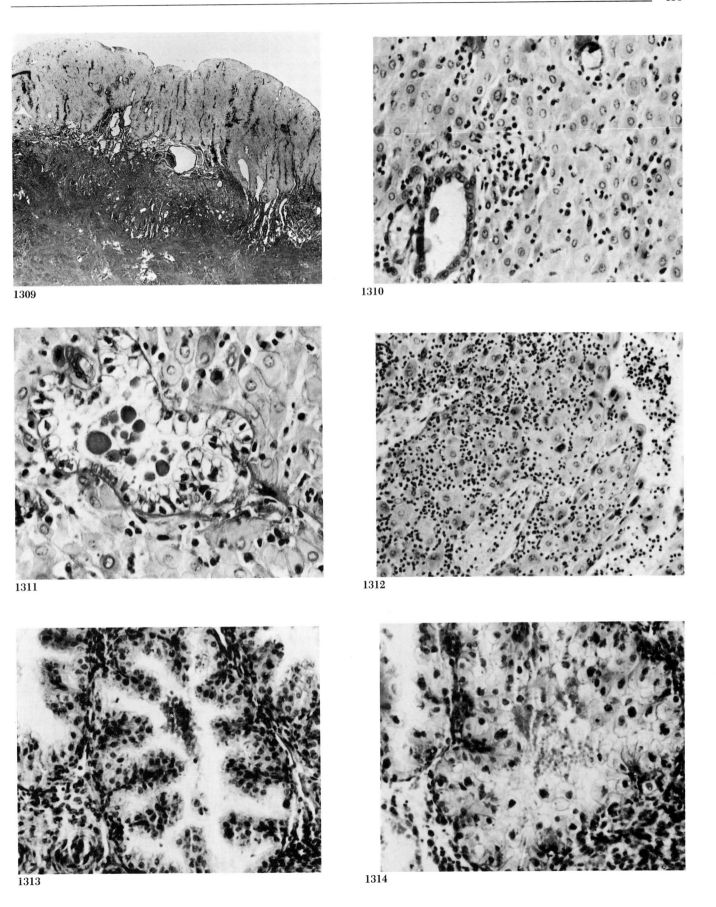

1309

1310

1311

1312

1313

1314

1315   Peridecidual degeneration of reticulum fibers

Degeneration and fragmentation of reticulum fibers around decidual cells occur occasionally, giving the misleading impression of intracellular granules or inclusions. This degenerative process occurs chiefly during the fifth month of gestation. (Bielschowsky silver impregnation. ×700)

1316   Ovum 10 days old

This abnormal ovum was recovered during endometrial biopsy in a supposedly infertile patient before the period was missed. The germ disk is absent. Cytotrophoblasts are markedly deficient, and degenerative changes are seen in the syncytiotrophoblasts. (H&E. ×90)

1317   Placental site, 1 to 2 weeks implantation age

Chorionic villi have not formed. A plaque of cytotrophoblasts is invading endometrial stroma with an early decidual reaction. Syncytiotrophoblastic plasmodia are likewise in contact with maternal tissue. (H&E. ×200)

1318   Placental site, 3 to 4 weeks implantation age

Well-formed chorionic villi are present, and the anlage of fetal blood vessels is seen, but nucleated red blood cells are not in evidence. The ovum has been entirely embedded into the decidua. (H&E. ×50)

1319   Placental villi, 5 to 10 weeks

The villi are covered by a double layer of trophoblasts. Early budding of the outer layer of syncytiotrophoblasts is seen. The villous stroma is loose and contains poorly defined, peripherally situated, capillary primordia as well as Hofbauer cells. (H&E. ×125)

1320   Placental villi, 10 to 16 weeks

The double layer of trophoblasts persists. The stroma is loose, and capillaries are well defined, containing nucleated fetal erythroid cells. (H&E. ×150)

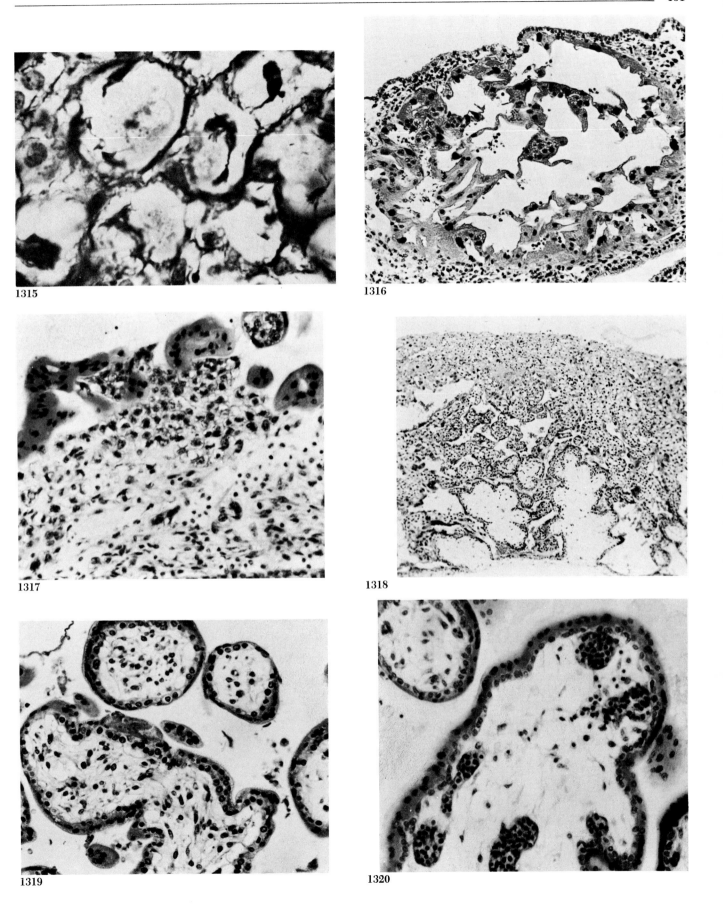

1315

1316

1317

1318

1319

1320

1321   Placental villi over 16 weeks
Collagenization of the stroma has begun. Nucleated erythroid cells have disappeared, and non-nucleated erythrocytes fill capillary lumens. The trophoblastic layers are somewhat attenuated. (H&E. ×621)

1322   Hyperplasia of Hofbauer's cells
Placental villi, 5 months. The stroma contains a relatively large amount of fibrous tissue, and in this particular instance there is hyperplasia of the Hofbauer cells which form nests and cords. The significance of this phenomenon is unknown. (H&E. ×150)

1323   Placental villi at term
The double layer of trophoblast is no longer visible as such. Syncytial knots are abundant. The villous stroma is often densely fibrous. (H&E. ×60)

1324   Placental villi at term
High magnification of Fig. 1323. The stroma is dense. Focal areas in which a double layer of trophoblasts persists are shown. (H&E. ×120)

1325   Placenta at term
This section through the chorionic plate shows an intact amniotic lining, intermediary layer, the fibrous membrane of the chorion with deposition of fibrinoid and disappearance of trophoblasts. The small villi are characteristic of this stage. (H&E. ×24)

1326   Placenta at term
This section through the basal (maternal) plate shows the fibrin stria of Nitabuch intervening between the fetal portion and decidual layers of the placenta. Focal calcification of villus is present. (H&E. ×24)

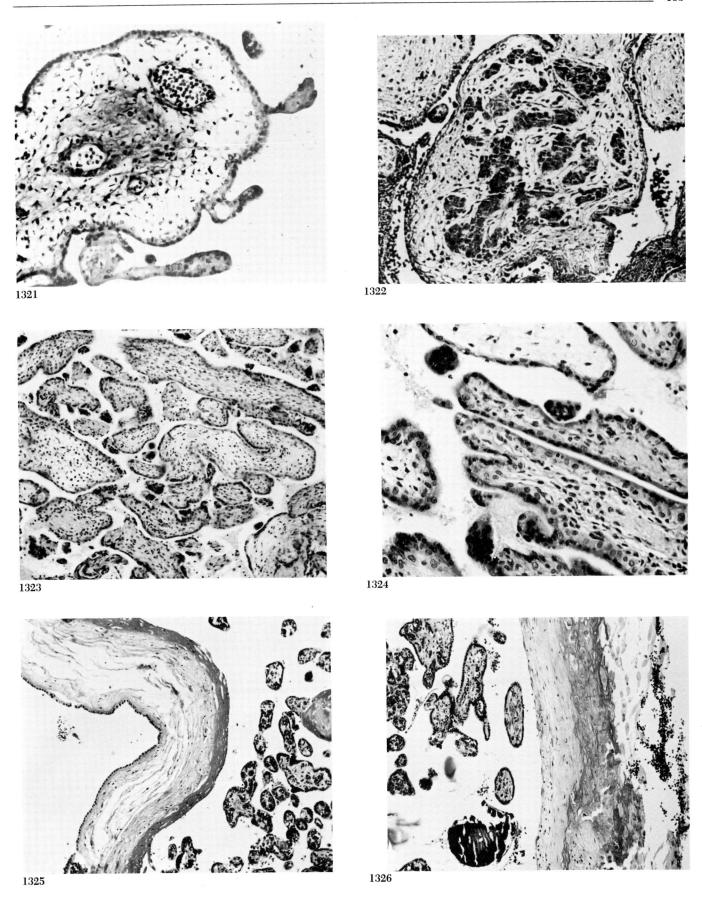

1321

1322

1323

1324

1325

1326

1327   Syncytial endometritis
This term is applied to an exaggeration of the physiologic response at the placental site in which multinucleated cells wander freely into the decidua and subjacent myometrium. The giant cell response is often exaggerated in molar pregnancies and may persist, giving rise to symptoms. It should not be confused with choriocarcinoma. (H&E. ×160)

1328   Syncytial myometritis
Even in normal pregnancy, multinucleated cells may be found fairly deep in the myometrium, often situated along fibrous septums between muscle bundles. Although most of the multinucleated cells represent detached buds of syncytiotrophoblast, some are derived from decidua and others may be derived from uterine smooth muscle. (H&E. ×160)

1329   Syncytial myometritis
Minor degrees of inflammation are often present. The multinucleated cell along the left upper border suggests origin from smooth muscle; the one at the upper right is presumably derived from syncytiotrophoblast. (H&E. ×160)

1330   Corpus luteum of pregnancy, 6 to 8 weeks gestation
This general view shows the relative size of this transient endocrine gland at the peak of its functional capacity. (H&E. ×8)

1331   Corpus luteum of pregnancy, 6 to 8 weeks gestation
High magnification of Fig. 1330. A narrow margin of theca lutein cells separates the plump polyhedral granulosa lutein cells from the ovarian stroma. The latter cells comprise the bulk of the structure. (H&E. ×50)

1332   Corpus luteum of pregnancy, 6 to 8 weeks gestation
High magnification of Fig. 1330. Trabeculae of granulosa lutein cells with a rich network of thin-walled capillaries are seen. Focal calcification is present, a finding which, when present, is seen only in the corpus luteum of pregnancy or in a luteoma. (H&E. ×110)

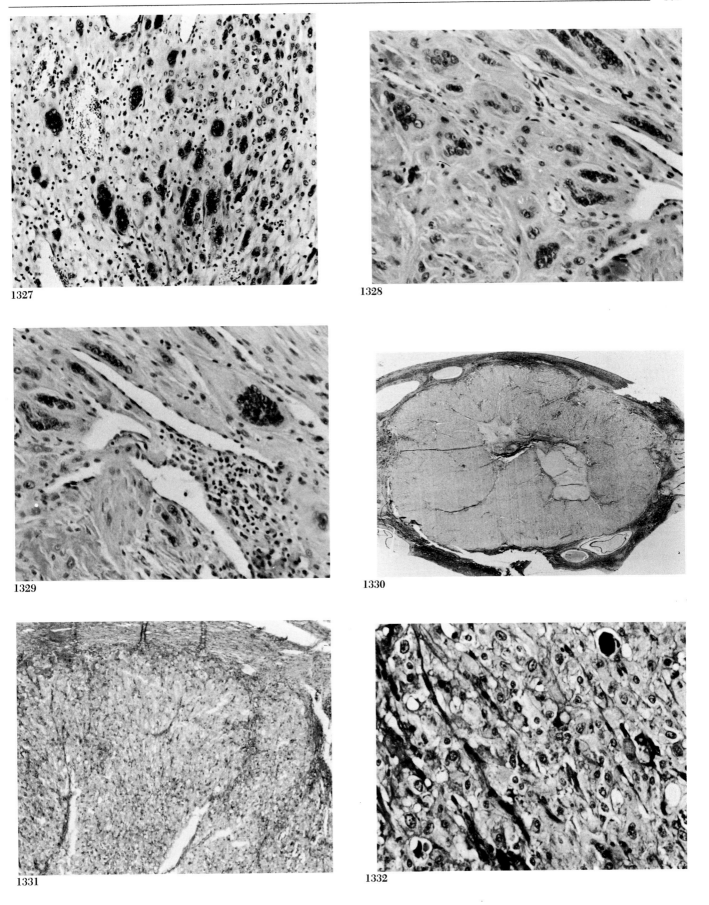

1327

1328

1329

1330

1331

1332

1333   Corpus luteum of pregnancy, 6 to 8 weeks gestation
High magnification of Fig. 1330. Intracytoplasmic hyaline bodies, single or multiple, are present and serve to distinguish this corpus luteum from one in a nonpregnant patient. (H&E. ×260)

1334   Ovary in pregnancy
Hyperplasia of the theca interna and externa surrounds the atretic follicles. A minute decidual reaction is present beneath the coelomic surface. (H&E. ×10)

1335   Endocervix at term gestation
The glands are filled with inspissated secretion. The stroma is edematous and the vascularity is increased. (H&E. ×19)

1336   Endocervix at term gestation
High magnification of Fig. 1335. Note the loose edematous stroma and the rich plexus of capillaries. The endocervical epithelium shows signs of exhaustion. (H&E. ×70)

1337   Endocervix intrapartum
The surface has been eroded, and there is focal hemorrhage into the stroma. (H&E. ×50)

1338   Myometrial changes associated with pregnancy
Fibers seen in cross section are swollen by hydrops and simulate nests of epithelium. This phenomenon seems restricted to the inner half of the uterine wall. (H&E. ×62)

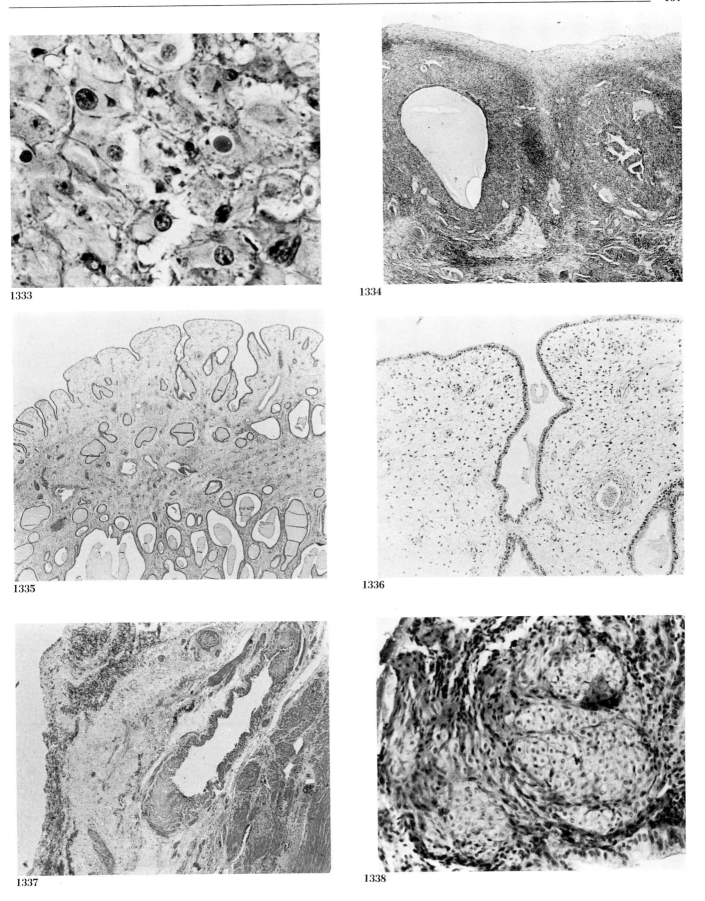

1333

1334

1335

1336

1337

1338

1339 Myometrial changes associated with pregnancy
High magnification of Fig. 1338. The clear perinuclear zone of hydropic smooth muscle fibers is emphasized. (H&E. ×180)

1340 Tubal mucosa at term
The epithelium is in the resting phase. Ciliated cells, secretory cells, and intercalated cells are present in normal proportions, and there is no evidence of secretion but rather a secretory exhaustion. (H&E. ×200)

1341 Ovarian decidual reaction in pregnancy
The subcoelomic surface of the ovary is coated by a thick layer of richly vascularized tissue derived from the subcoelomic mesenchymal elements and shows massive decidual reaction. (H&E. ×12)

1342 Ovarian decidual reaction in pregnancy
Intact, thinned coelomic surface (serosa) and nests of pale, plump decidual cells extend downward into the ovarian cortex. (H&E. ×45)

1343 Ovarian decidual reaction in pregnancy
The reaction may form relatively discrete nests as well as diffuse alterations. (H&E. ×50)

1344 Ovarian decidual reaction in pregnancy
High magnification of Fig. 1343. (H&E. ×120)

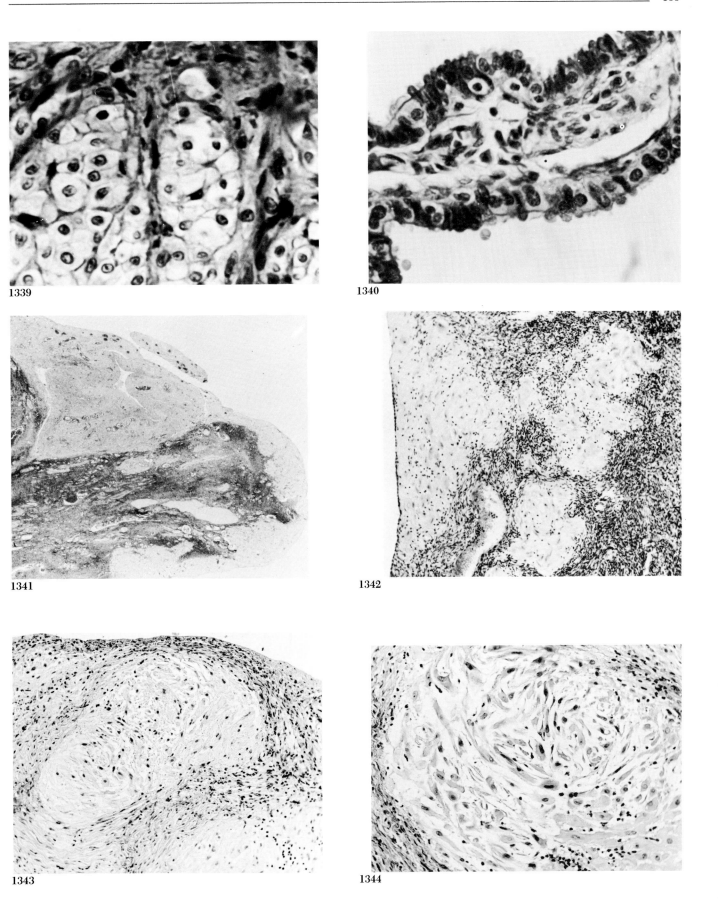

1339

1340

1341

1342

1343

1344

1345   Focal, cortical decidual reaction of the ovary in pregnancy
A focal subserosal decidual reaction is seen. (H&E. ×180)

1346   Decidual reaction of endometriosis of the ovary in pregnancy
Note the ectopic decidual reaction in the stroma of an endometrial "implant." (H&E. ×50)

1347   Decidual reaction of an endocervical polyp in pregnancy
Decidual reaction is seen in the stroma of an endocervical polyp removed during pregnancy. (H&E. ×50)

1348   Decidual reaction in adenomyosis uteri in pregnancy
Decidual reaction of a minor degree surrounds a gland in adenomyosis uteri during pregnancy. (H&E. ×165)

1349   Decidual reaction in adenomyosis uteri in pregnancy
Decidual reaction of extensive degree surrounds atrophic glands in adenomyosis uteri during pregnancy. (Compare with the preceding figure.) (H&E. ×120)

1350   Decidual reaction of the oviduct in pregnancy
Decidual reaction is seen in the endosalpinx during pregnancy. In this instance, the reaction is diffuse. (H&E. ×120)

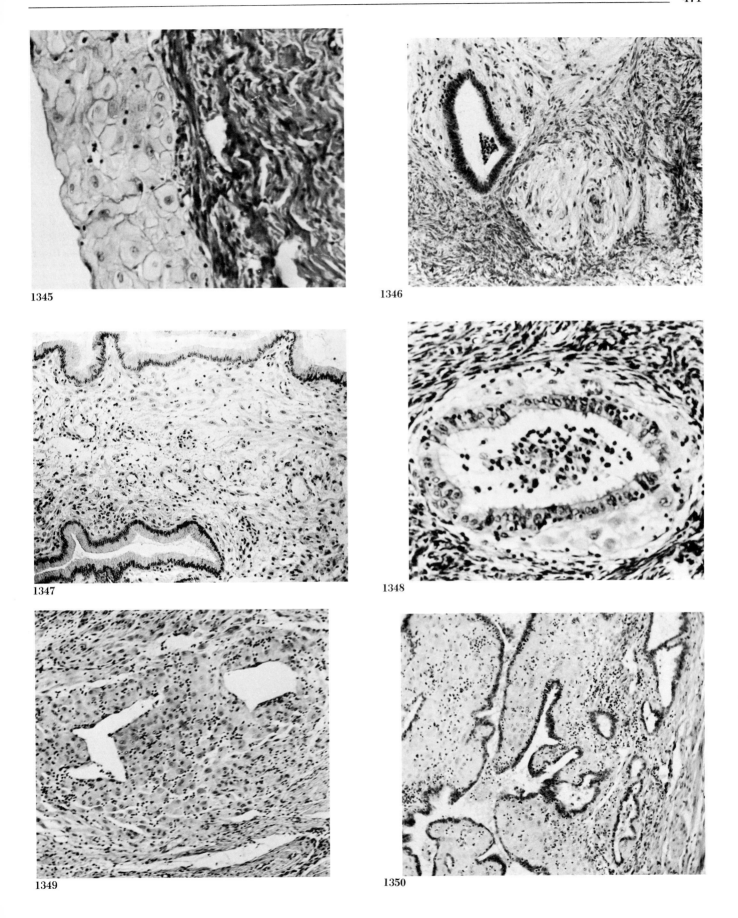

1345

1346

1347

1348

1349

1350

1351   Decidual reaction of the oviduct in pregnancy

Decidual reaction is seen in the endosalpinx during pregnancy. The reaction may be focal and isolated. The tubal epithelium covering the decidual plaque is thinned. (H&E. ×40)

1352   Decidual reaction in the oviduct associated with tuberculous salpingitis

Decidual reaction abuts a tuberculous granuloma in the wall of the oviduct in a case of tuberculous salpingitis and ectopic pregnancy. (H&E. ×45)

1353   Decidual reaction of the parietal pelvic peritoneum in pregnancy

(H&E. ×90)

1354   Decidual reaction in the septum of a pelvic lymph node in pregnancy

(H&E. ×80)

1355   Decidual reaction in the stroma of endometriosis of the vermiform appendix in pregnancy

(H&E. ×15)

1356   Decidual reaction in the stroma of endometriosis of the vermiform appendix in pregnancy

High magnification of Fig. 1355. The atrophic endometrial gland is surrounded by a collar of decidual cells. (H&E. ×50)

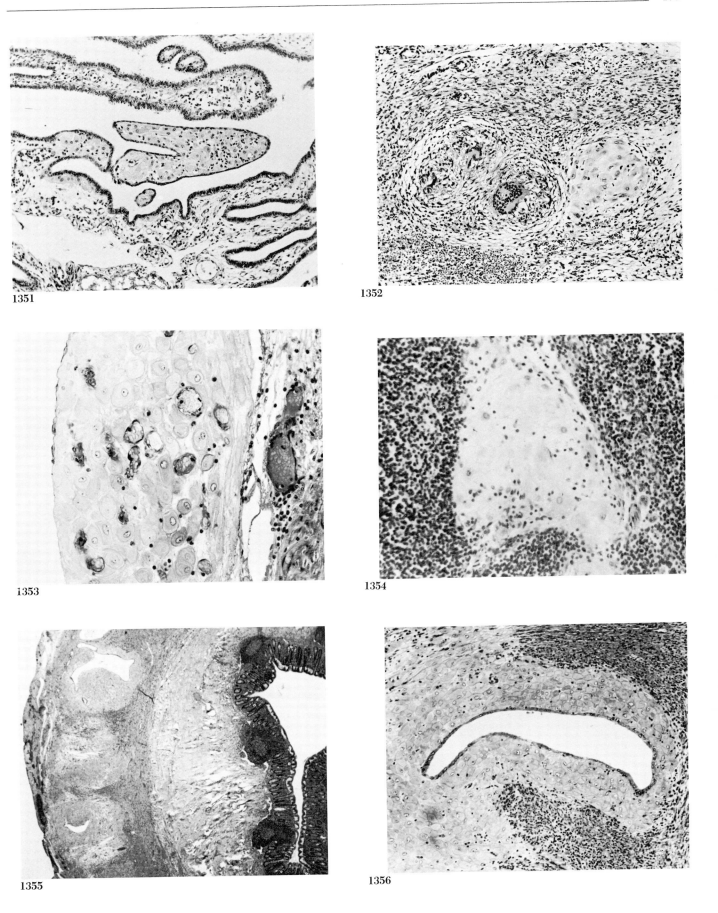

1351

1352

1353

1354

1355

1356

1357 Normal pituitary gland at full-term pregnancy
The anterior lobe is enlarged to about twice normal size. Even at low magnification the lateral lobes contain ill-defined islands of darker staining cells. (H&E. ×10)

1358 Normal pituitary gland at full-term pregnancy
High magnification of Fig. 1357. There is a numerical increase of beta-basophilic cells. (Aldehyde fuchsin. ×50)

1359 Normal pituitary gland at full-term pregnancy
High magnification of Fig. 1357. Note the focus of hyperplasia of beta-basophilic cells. Gonadotropin elaboration has been assigned to basophilic cells, and their increase may be related to some of the "cushingoid" features sometimes found in pregnant women. (Aldehyde fuchsin. ×150)

1360 Pituitary normal at full-term pregnancy
High magnification of Fig. 1357. Note the appearance of beta-basophilic cells (lower left), alpha-eosinophilic cells (right), and chromophobe cells (upper center). (Aldehyde fuchsin. ×120)

1361 Ovary, 2 days post partum
Persistence of the corpus luteum of pregnancy and a few atretic follicles can be seen. (H&E. ×4)

1362 Endometrium at the time of the first menstruation post partum
There is no evidence of glandular secretion or predecidual reaction in the stroma; over 30 per cent of these first cycles are anovulatory. Note also the moderate epithelial hyperplasia and cystic glandular pattern in the regenerated endometrium. (H&E. ×100)

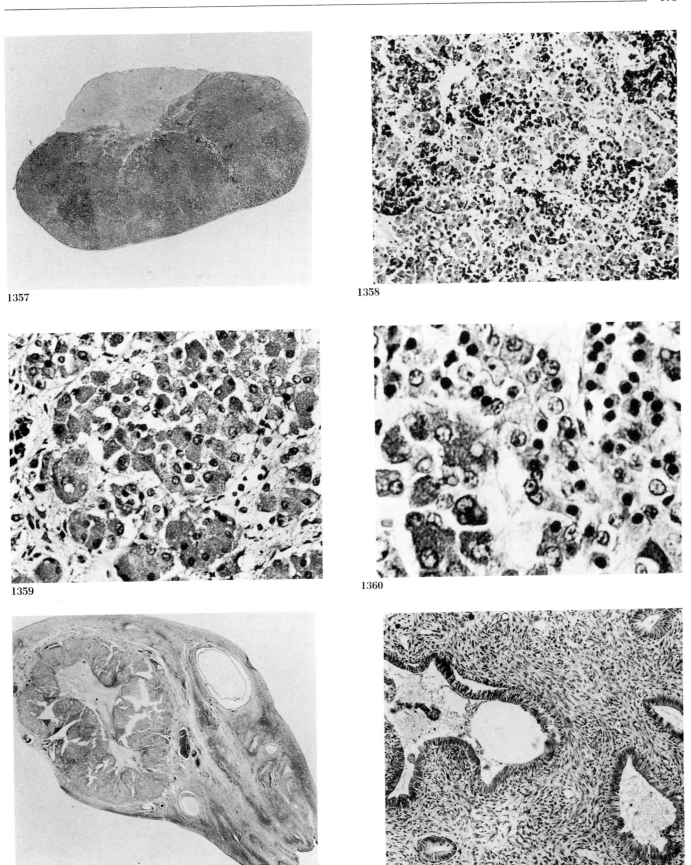

1357

1358

1359

1360

1361

1362

12

Abortion, Puerperal Infection, and Ectopic Pregnancy

1363   Blighted ovum
This general view shows an intact ovisac, an absent germ disk, and relative hypoplasia of the chorionic villi. (H&E. ×10)

1364   Hydropic degeneration of chorionic villi associated with a blighted ovum
The villous stroma is avascular and edematous; the trophoblast layer is thinned over the distended stroma. (H&E. ×60)

1365   Hydropic degeneration of chorionic villi associated with an aborted blighted ovum
Trophoblastic proliferation from the surface of anchoring villi is found. Such changes are frequently seen in early intrauterine and ectopic pregnancies. The edematous villi are not to be confused with hydatidiform mole. (H&E. ×62)

1366   Advanced hydropic degeneration of chorionic villus in an aborted placenta
This is not to be labeled a hydatidiform villus unless the villus is grossly visible as a separate unit. (H&E. ×50)

1367   Hemorrhagic mole (Breus's mole, subchorionic tuberous hematoma)
A partly autolyzed embryonic structure lies in the amniotic cavity. The chorion is stuffed (infarcted) with blood in the intervillous space forming confluent hematomas with varying degree of thrombosis. Decidual venous sinuses are also thrombosed. (H&E. ×10)

1368   Retained incomplete abortion, curetted for completion
Fibrosis and hyalinization of villous stroma, denudation of trophoblasts and large amount of intervillous fibrin clot point to intrauterine death of the conceptus some time before symptoms necessitated curettage. (H&E. 90)

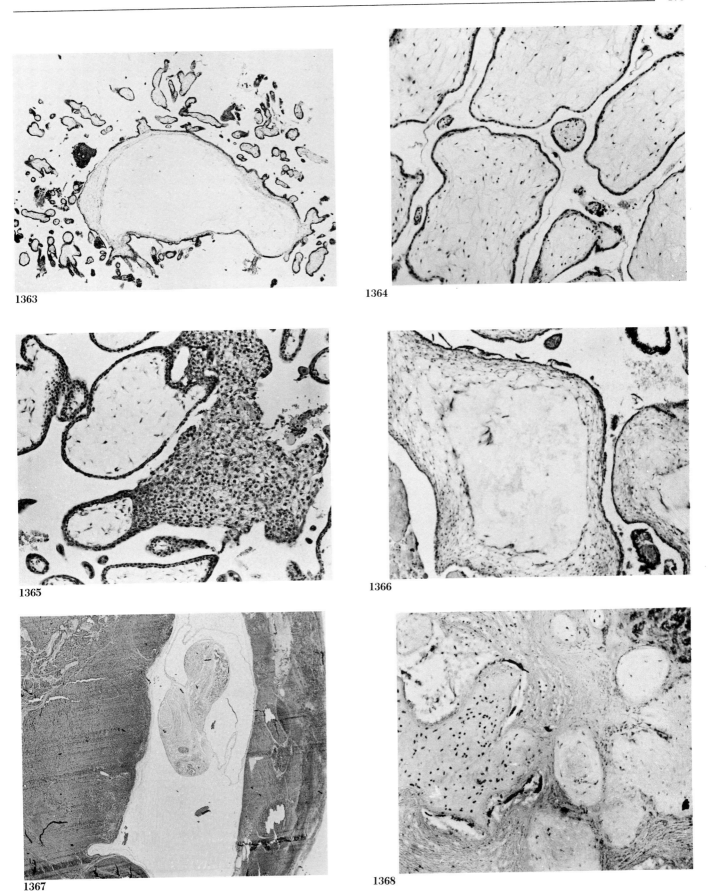

1363

1364

1365

1366

1367

1368

1369 Decidua from curettings to complete abortion
Degenerative changes create an appearance which simulated chondroid tissue. (H&E. ×250)

1370 Incomplete abortion, curetted for completion, showing fragments of necrotic fetal bone
If sufficient time elapses between partial expulsion of the abortus and the curettage, decidua may be absent and inflammation minimal. The two fragments of endometrium at the right and left corners showed an essentially normal secretory endometrium. (H&E. ×24)

1371 Placental polyp in situ
The uterine cavity is filled with a hemorrhagic mass in which a few term chorionic villi remain, often attached to the myometrium as a focal accretion. (H&E. ×2)

1372 Placental polyp curettings
Term chorionic villi, some well preserved, others as "ghost villi" are found admixed with clotted blood at curettage several weeks post partum. (H&E. ×45)

1373 Postabortal endometritis
Islands of partly hyalinized decidua, often perivascular in position, are found in a regenerating endometrium which is infiltrated by leukocytes. (H&E. ×85)

1374 Postabortal endometrium showing complete regeneration of the mucosa with an intact surface and slightly irregular gland pattern
Islands of hyalinized decidua remain in the stroma. Inflammatory reaction may be minimal. (H&E. ×75)

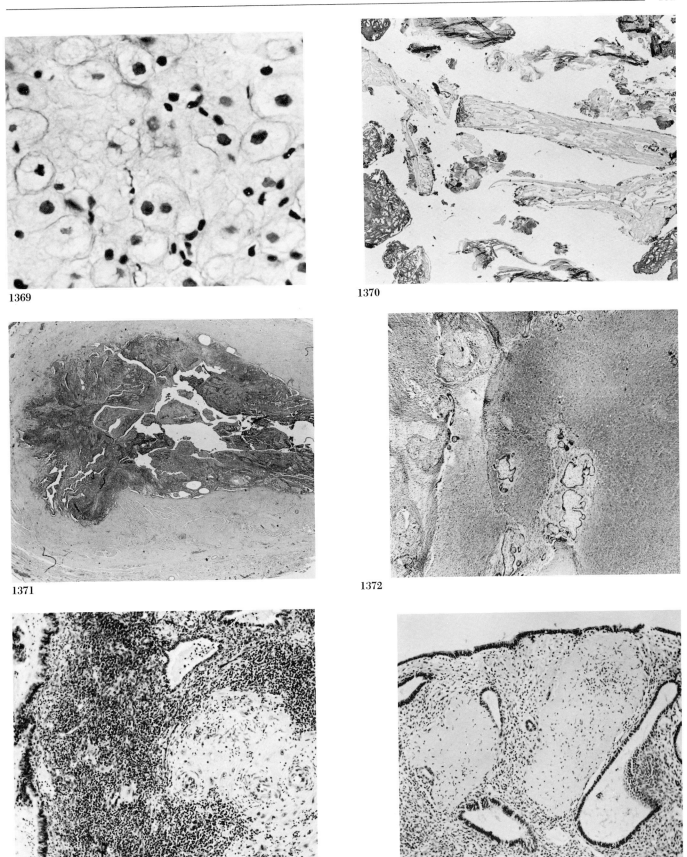

1369

1370

1371

1372

1373

1374

1375 Postabortal decidual "polyp" with massive hyalinization

The fragment of retained secundines is presented as a structure loosely attached to the uterine fundus. (H&E. ×50)

1376 Postabortal diffuse, massive hyalinization of residual decidual tissue
(H&E. ×50)

1377 Postabortal fibrinoid nodule in the endometrium

No longer definitely identifiable as decidual in origin, such isolated nodules may be the only finding in curettings after an almost complete abortion. (H&E. ×50)

1378 Postabortal fibrinoid nodule in the endometrium

High magnification of Fig. 1377. Amorphous eosinophilic material is shown surrounded by regenerating stroma and containing trapped leukocytes. Decidual cell outlines are no longer visible. (H&E. ×100)

1380 Postabortal endometritis showing the phenomenon of "helle Drüsen"

Residual glands with relatively clear cytoplasm are located in the stratum basalis. The clear cytoplasm and occasional hyperchromatic nuclei suggest a relationship to the Arias-Stella phenomenon. Their presence indicates a preexisting pregnancy which has terminated. A normal-appearing endometrial gland is present in the upper center for comparison. (H&E. ×50)

1379 Postabortal hyalinized decidual tissue surrounding an endometrial venule or sinusoid

The vessel wall cannot collapse; hence continuous uterine hemorrhage may ensue. (H&E. ×50)

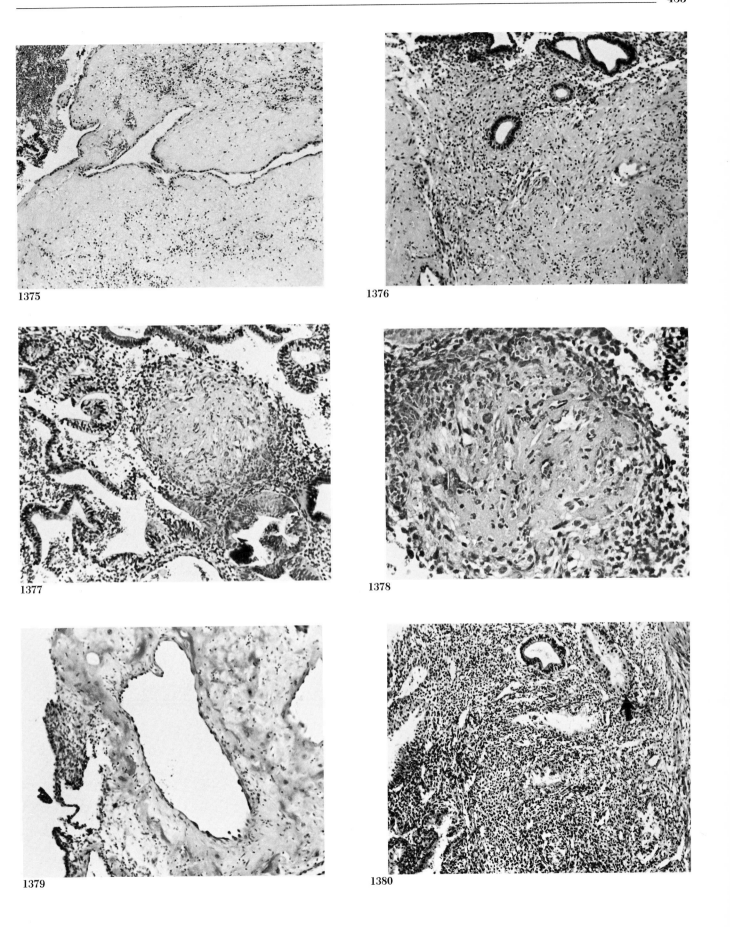

1375

1376

1377

1378

1379

1380

1381 Induced abortion
Marked degeneration and autolysis of chorionic villi (4 months placenta) may suggest induction by instillation of hypertonic saline or glucose. (H&E. ×50)

1382 Induced abortion
High magnification of Fig. 1381. Edema and degeneration of cells in the villous stroma are present. (H&E. ×115)

1383 Uterus from a septic abortion with endotoxin shock
There are diffuse thromboses in the vessels of the uterine wall. (H&E. ×24)

1384 Uterus from a septic abortion with endotoxin shock
High magnification of Fig. 1383. Necrosis, hemorrhage, and deposition of fibrin, all nonspecific features, are found at the site of the primary injury. (H&E. ×125)

1385 Endotoxin shock: fibrin thrombi in the lung
The pulmonary capillaries contain multiple small fibrin thrombi. (H&E. ×62)

1386 Endotoxin shock: fibrin thrombi in the lung
High magnification of Fig. 1385. A well-formed fibrin thrombus is seen in a small pulmonary artery. These thrombi are not embolic but are formed *in loco*. (H&E. ×125)

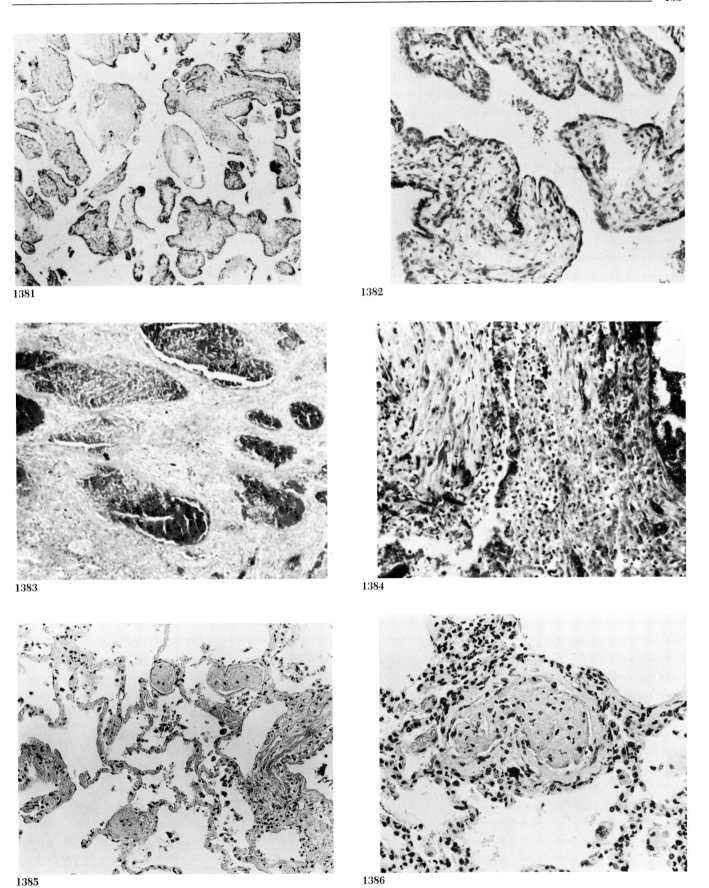

1381

1382

1383

1384

1385

1386

1387   Kidney in endotoxin shock
Note the fibrin thrombus in a glomerulus with ischemic changes of the subtended capillary loop. (H&E. ×150)

1388   Cervix uteri in puerperal sepsis
The mixed *Escherichia coli* and streptococcus infection is accompanied by necrosis of the myometrium and massive thrombosis of the cervical vessels. (H&E. ×24)

1389   Myometrium in puerperal sepsis
Same case as shown in Fig. 1388. Note the necrosis of uterine muscle and the acute inflammatory exudate. (H&E. ×50)

1390   Myometrium in puerperal sepsis
Same case as shown in Figs. 1388 and 1389. Note the thrombosis and necrosis of small arteries in the uterine wall and an inflammatory exudate. (H&E. ×90)

1391   Post-partum pseudomembranous endometritis
In this variety of puerperal sepsis, the exudate forms a pseudomembrane over the necrotic uterine wall. (H&E. ×35)

1392   Soap-intoxication syndrome
Induced abortion with soap intoxication. Coagulation necrosis of the chorionic villi and uterine wall is produced by the alkali. (H&E. ×50)

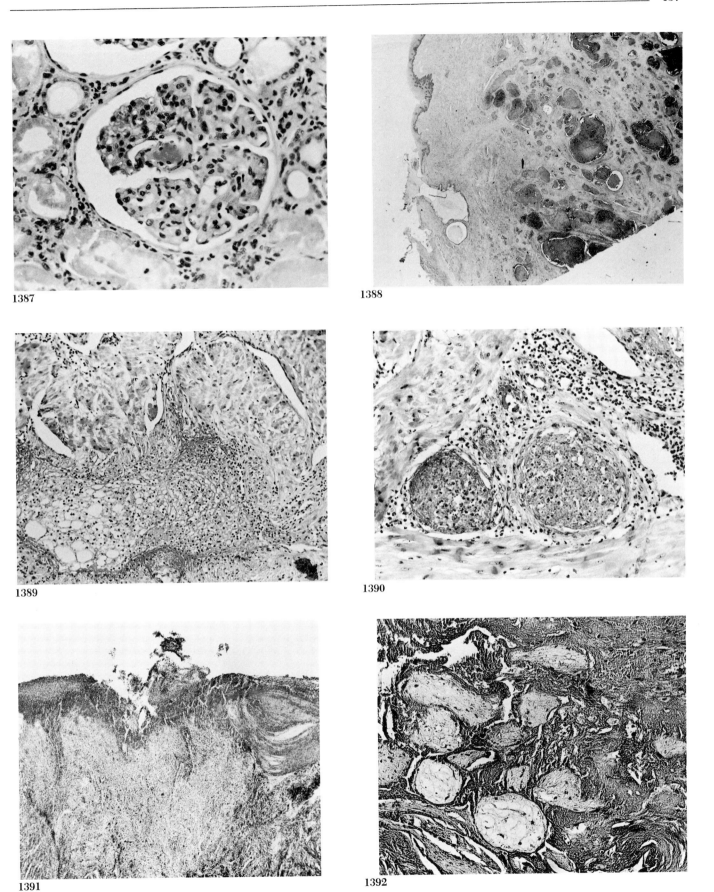

1387

1388

1389

1390

1391

1392

1393   Soap-intoxication syndrome
Thrombosis of the ovarian vein is produced as the chemical panmetritis and perimetritis spread to adjacent structures. (H&E. ×50)

1394   Soap-intoxication syndrome
Healing acute tubular necrosis is found in the kidneys. (H&E. ×150)

1395   Soap-intoxication syndrome
High magnification of Fig. 1394. Casts are seen in the renal tubules lined by regenerating epithelium. Death may result from renal failure or from other complications. (H&E. ×200)

1396   Soap-intoxication syndrome
A secondary infection is present here. Monilial infection involving the lung (attacking bronchial cartilage) is shown. The mycosis developed against a background of antibiotics, steroids, and bone marrow damage. (H&E. ×62)

1397   Soap-intoxication syndrome
Hypoplasia of the bone marrow is evidence of systemic toxicity. (H&E. ×125)

1398   Intact ectopic tubular pregnancy
The fetus is absent, and the amniotic cavity is filled with blood, but the immature placenta is attached to the endosalpinx and has invaded the wall of the tube. (H&E. ×2)

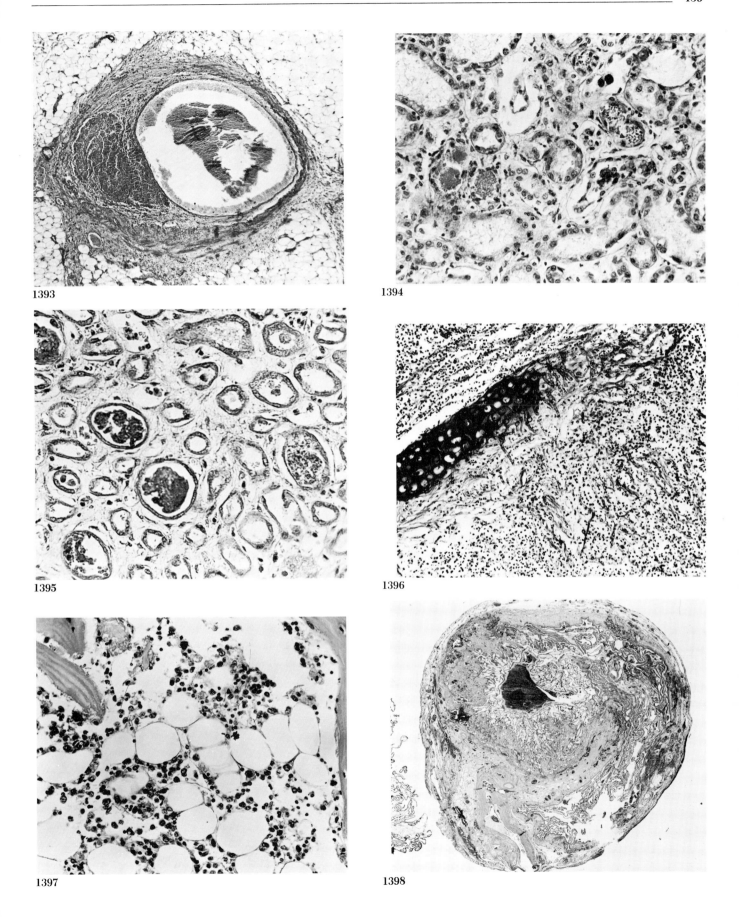

1393

1394

1395

1396

1397

1398

1399 Intact ectopic tubal pregnancy
The arrows point to the poorly developed decidua (left) and to the trophoblastic proliferation at the tips of the young anchoring villi (lower center). (H&E. ×62)

1400 Hydropic degeneration of chorionic villi in an ectopic tubal pregnancy
(H&E. ×50)

1401 Ectopic pregnancy at the fimbriated end of the tube
Chorionic villi are attached to edematous tips of fimbrias by a blood clot. (H&E. ×50)

1402 Ovarian pregnancy
Chorionic villi are shown penetrating a corpus luteum of pregnancy. (H&E. ×50)

1404 Proliferative endometrium associated with ectopic pregnancy
Endometrial biopsy or curettage is helpful in the diagnosis of ectopic pregnancy only if it reveals decidua, as it may in up to 40 per cent of cases. However, the majority of patients with ectopic pregnancy will have an endometrium inappropriate for gestation, about 30 per cent in the secretory phase, about 30 per cent in the proliferative phase of the cycle. (H&E. ×120)

1403 Secretory endometrium associated with ectopic tubal pregnancy
(H&E. ×120)

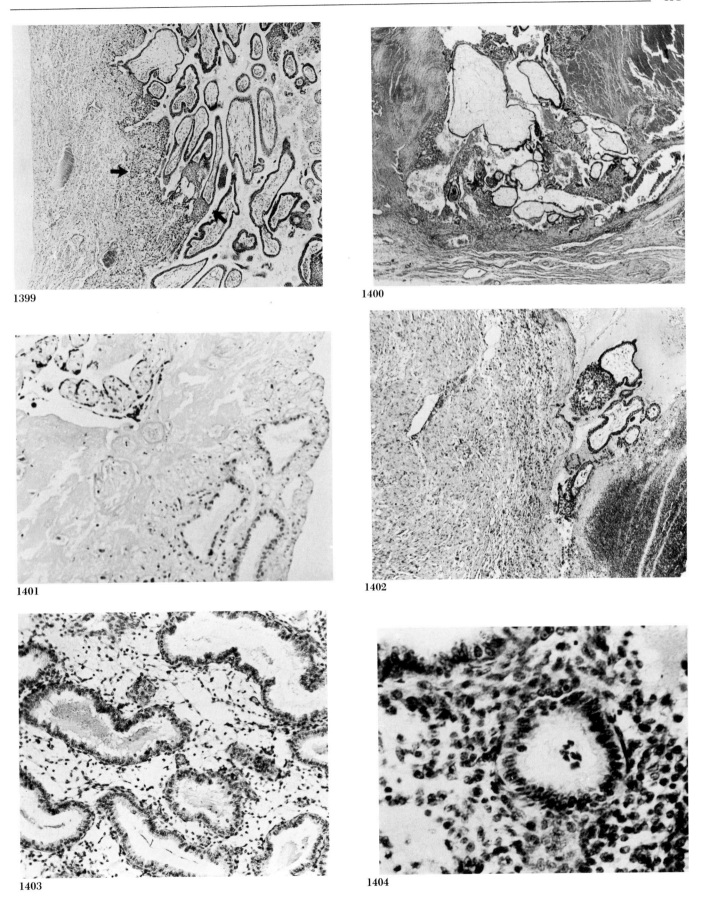

1399

1400

1401

1402

1403

1404

13

Diseases of the Placenta and Membranes

1405 Placenta membranacea
This section through the chorionic plate reveals a thin fibrous membrane, heavily collagenized, lined by a flattened amnion and a thin chorionic epithelium without villi. (H&E. ×50)

1406 Full-term extrauterine placenta
This section through the chorionic plate shows edema and considerable deposition of Langhans' fibrinoid. (H&E. ×50)

1407 Placenta membranacea
This section through the thinned placenta shows small, fibrotic, avascular villi and hyalinization of trophoblastic overgrowths. (H&E. ×50)

1408 Full-term extrauterine placenta
The small chorionic villi show syncytiotrophoblastic knots and a normal vascular pattern. There is little difference in the villi themselves from those in a term intrauterine placenta. (H&E. ×50)

1409 Placenta membranacea
This section through the basal plate shows thin, somewhat degenerate decidua, condensation of the fibrin stria of Nitabuch, and atrophic villi as shown in Fig. 1407. (H&E. ×50)

1410 Full-term extrauterine placenta
This section through the basal plate shows absence of decidual cells. Anchoring villi are attached to the tubal wall and ovary. Nitabuch's fibrinoid is massively deposited on tubal walls. The placenta is from a term tubo-ovarian pregnancy. (H&E. ×50)

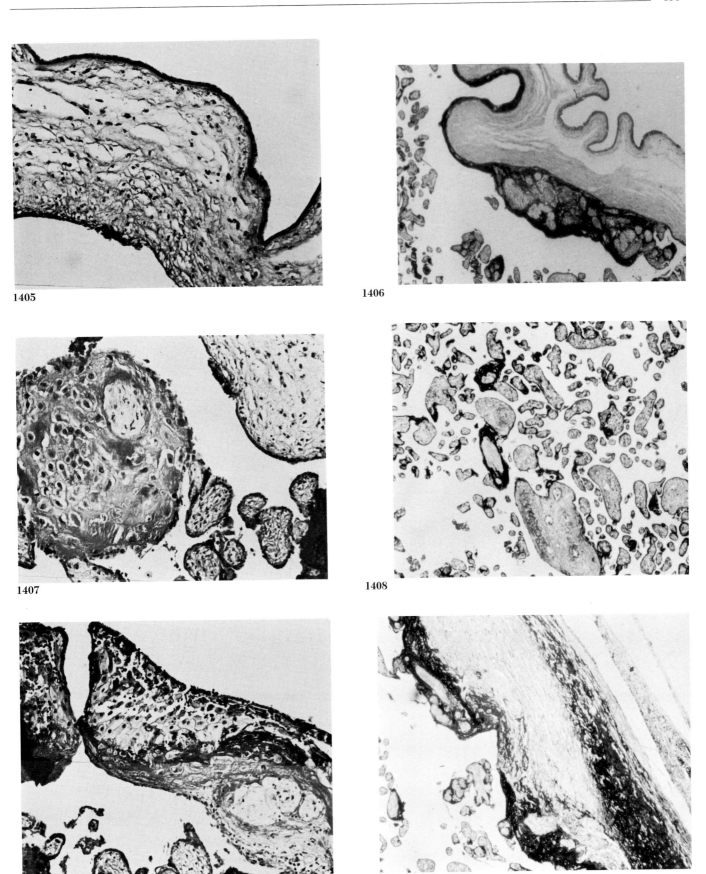

1405

1406

1407

1408

1409

1410

1411 Placenta in interstitial pregnancy, 3d month

The compressed placental tissue shows very few preserved intervillous spaces. Chorionic villi show fusion and a marked degree of fibrosis. Premature aging of the placenta characterized by disappearance of cytotrophoblasts and syncytial knots is becoming apparent. (H&E. ×62)

1412 Placenta accreta

Term villi with fibrotic stroma are plastered against the myometrium without intervening decidua. The fibrin stria of Nitabuch is absent in this field, but there is intervillous fibrin deposition. (H&E. ×62)

1414 Localized clostridial chorioamnionitis

The chorionic plate is heavily infiltrated by acute inflammatory cells. Focal areas of necrosis are present. The remaining placental tissue is free of inflammatory infiltration. Evacuation of the uterus was followed by rapid recovery. (H&E. ×70)

1413 Placenta increta

Chorionic villi have penetrated the myometrium at term. (H&E. ×62)

1415 Acute necrotizing placentitis in a septic abortion with *Clostridium perfringens* infection

Coagulation necrosis of the placenta is seen. Septic abortion at the third month resulted in a fatal outcome. (H&E. ×50)

1416 Acute chorioamnionitis with early placentitis

Polymorphonuclear leukocytes are seen diffusely infiltrating the amnion and chorion and to a lesser extent the chorionic villi. (H&E. ×45)

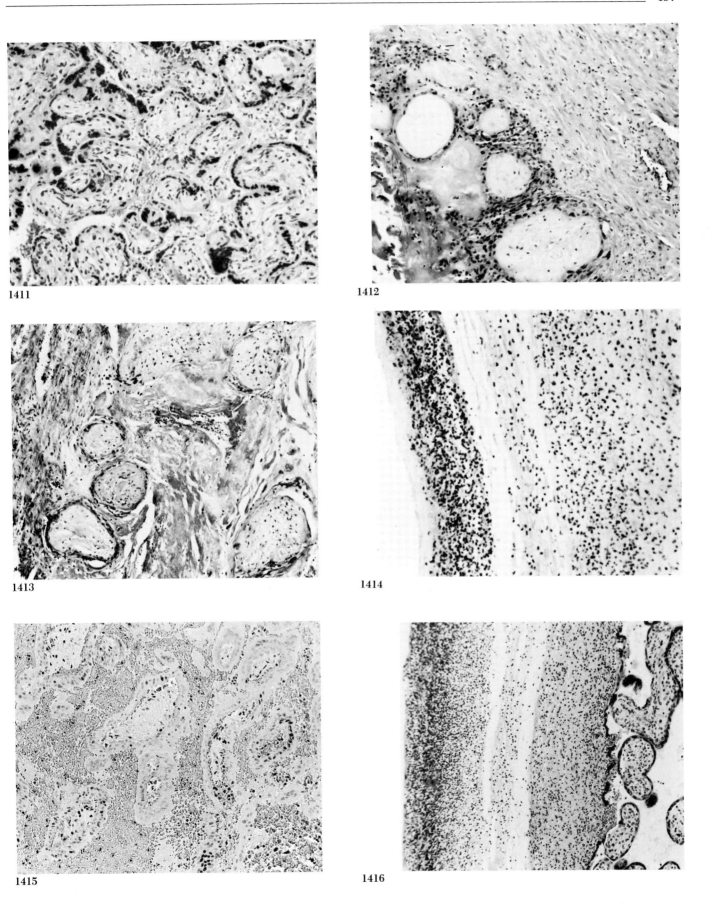

1411

1412

1413

1414

1415

1416

1417   Advanced acute placentitis
Intense exudation of polymorphonuclear leukocytes infiltrates the fetal membranes, the villi, and the intervillous space. (H&E. ×50)

1418   Tuberculous placentitis
Granulomatous inflammation involving chorionic villi is seen in a case of widely disseminated tuberculosis of the mother. (H&E. ×50)

1419   Listeriosis of the placenta
Foci of acute granulomatous inflammation with central necrosis involve mature chorionic villi and intervillous spaces. (H&E. ×80)

1420   Listeriosis of the placenta
The myriad of small microorganisms *Listeria monocytogenes* is shown in a foci of granulomatous inflammation by a silver impregnation–Levaditi stain. (×510)

1421   Syphilis of the placenta
This section through the basal plate shows a normal decidua and fibrotic chorionic villi with degeneration of trophoblasts. (H&E. ×62)

1422   Syphilis of the placenta
Concentric vascular fibrosis is seen occurring in the connective tissue stroma of villi. Occasional villi show stromal hypercellularity. (H&E. ×125)

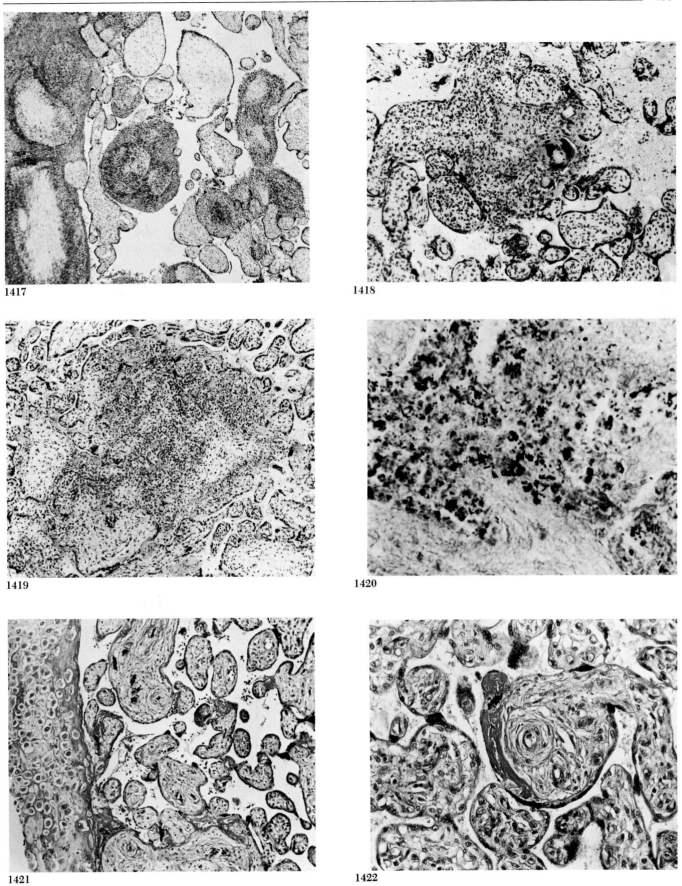

1417

1418

1419

1420

1421

1422

1423 Syphilis of the placenta
Pronounced obliterative endarteritis is seen in the vessels of the cotyledon. (H&E. ×180)

1424 Coccidioidomycosis of the placenta
A broad zone of necrotizing granulomatous inflammation is shown. (H&E. ×65)

1425 Coccidioidomycosis of the placenta
A granuloma formed by giant cells and epithelioid cells involves the chorionic villi and intervillous spaces. (H&E. ×220)

1426 Coccidioidomycosis of the placenta
A single spore is shown in a fibrin-filled intervillous space. (H&E. ×180)

1427 Coccidioidomycosis of the placenta
Endospores are seen within the capsule of the fungus. (H&E. ×450)

1428 Malaria of the placenta
The intervillous space contains maternal erythrocytes with parasites (seen as small black dots). (H&E. ×80)

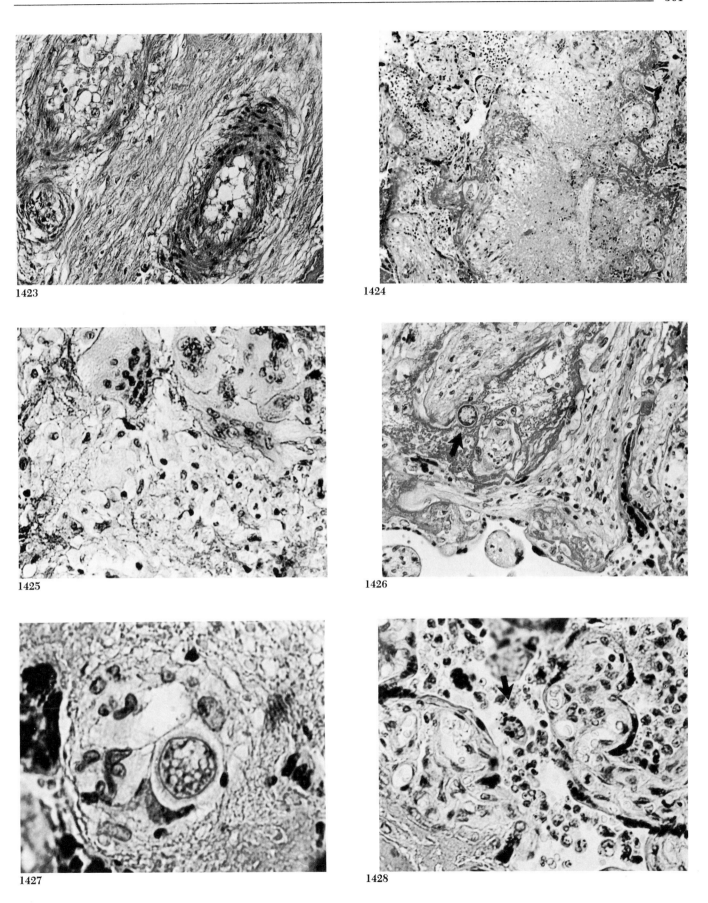

1423

1424

1425

1426

1427

1428

1429   Malaria of the placenta
The trophoblastic cells contain malarial parasites and parasitized erythrocytes in the intervillous spaces. (H&E. ×150)

1430   Malaria of the placenta
Erythrocytes in the intervillous space contain malarial parasites in different stages of development. (H&E. ×400)

1431   Placenta in diabetes mellitus
Pronounced edema of villous stroma is seen. Hypermaturation of the trophoblastic layer is another nonspecific feature. (H&E. ×50)

1432   Placenta in diabetes mellitus
Small intravillous thrombi with hyalinization are also found. (H&E. ×50)

1433   Placenta in sickle cell anemia
Sickled erythrocytes are seen in the intervillous space. The villous architecture is normal. (H&E. ×50)

1434   Placenta in sickle cell anemia
Bridges of fibrinohyaline material connect chorionic villi. Degeneration of the trophoblast adjacent to the bridges is striking. (H&E. ×125)

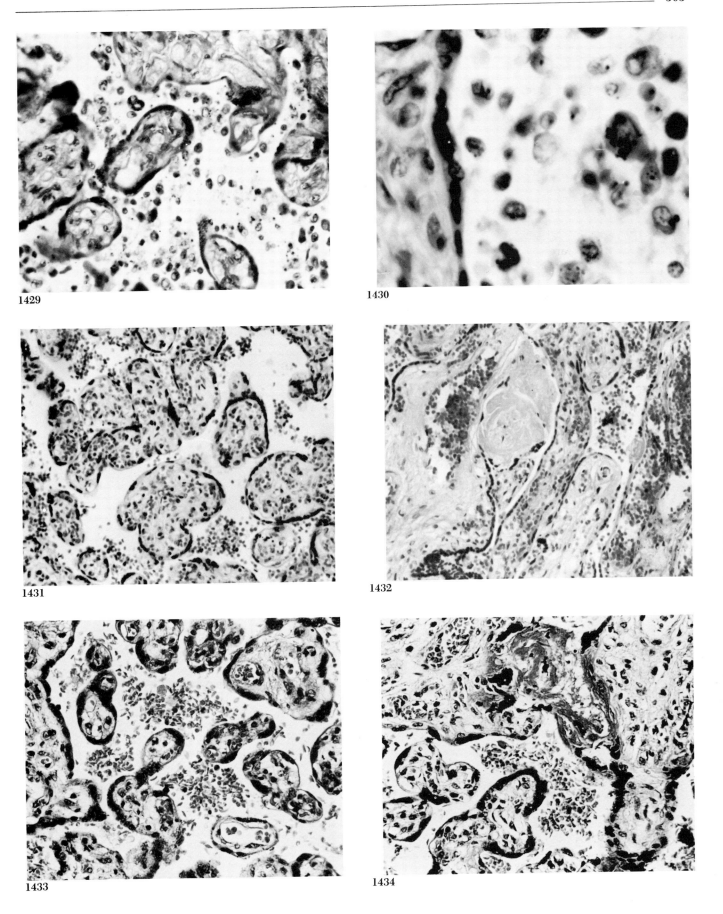

1429

1430

1431

1432

1433

1434

1435 Placenta in sickle cell anemia. Detail showing the variety of forms assumed by sickled erythrocytes
Note that the fetal erythrocytes in the villous capillaries are not sickled. (H&E. ×180)

1436 Placenta in erythroblastosis fetalis (isoimmunization disease)
The villi are edematous, hypercellular, and covered by relatively immature trophoblasts for a given age. Many nucleated erythroid cells (normoblasts and erythroblasts) distend the villous capillaries. (H&E. ×180)

1437 Placenta in erythroblastosis fetalis (isoimmunization disease)
Placental edema is shown by the looseness of stroma in the villous stalks at (or near) term. (H&E. ×90)

1438 Placenta in erythroblastosis fetalis (isoimmunization disease)
This detail shows the tip of an edematous villus and a capillary distended by nucleated red cells (normoblasts and erythroblasts). (H&E. ×350)

1439 Placenta in toxemia of pregnancy
The changes are nonspecific. Chorionic villi are close together and agglomerated but, not infarcted. (H&E. ×50)

1440 Placenta in toxemia of pregnancy
High magnification of Fig. 1439. Deposition of fibrinohyaline material is seen within both the villi and the intervillous space. (H&E. ×150)

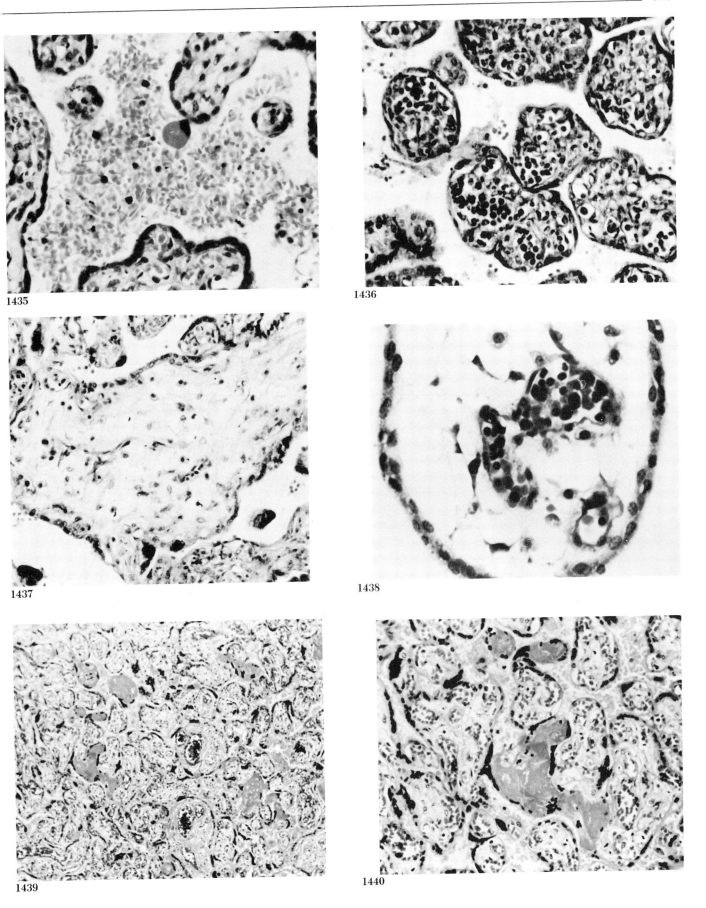

1435

1436

1437

1438

1439

1440

1441   Placenta in toxemia of pregnancy
The intervillous space is markedly narrowed. Fibrinohyaline deposits are present in villous stroma, trophoblastic layer, and intervillous space. (H&E. ×150)

1442   Placenta in toxemia of pregnancy
Accentuated deposition of fibrin at the basal plate is sometimes found. (H&E. ×125)

1443   Placenta in toxemia of pregnancy
Acute fibrinoid necrosis is seen in the wall of a large decidual vessel. In general, lesions of toxemia are more prominent in the mother's tissues than in the placenta. (H&E. ×125)

1444   Thrombosis of the marginal sinus of the placenta
The marginal sinus and its tributaries are distended by a fresh thrombus. (H&E. ×7)

1445   Early infarct of the placenta
A clear line of demarcation by early deposition of fibrin separates the zone of coagulation necrosis (upper center and right) from the undamaged placenta. Agglomeration of villi is evident in the infarcted zone. (H&E. ×7)

1446   Early infarct of the placenta
The outline of the villi is well preserved, but they are conglomerated to each other by diffuse deposition of intervillous fibrin. (H&E. ×50)

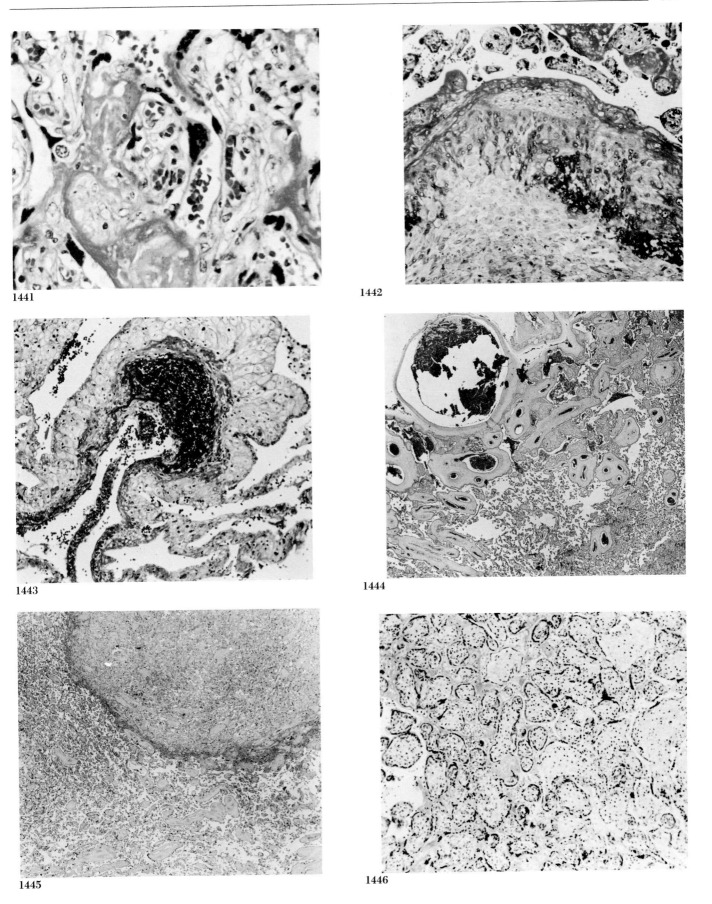

1441

1442

1443

1444

1445

1446

1447   Early infarct of the placenta
High magnification of Fig. 1446. There is focal necrosis of the villous stroma (left) and a diffuse network of intervillous fibrin. Occasional necrotic trophoblastic buds are seen, but most of the trophoblasts are still undamaged. (H&E. ×125)

1448   Old infarct of the placenta
The infarcted area contains ghost villi in a bed of fibrin. The infarcted zone is sharply separated from viable placenta by a zone of fibrin with leukocytes, the latter being absent in the deeper part of the infarct. (H&E. ×20)

1449   Old infarct of the placenta
Only occasional viable trophoblastic elements are seen; most of the trophoblasts are necrotic. Intervillous fibrin is increased when compared with the early stages of infarction. The architectural outline of villi is preserved, but the stroma is necrotic. (H&E. ×50)

1450   Old infarct of the placenta
Syncytial knots are prominent, being the last cellular element to undergo necrosis. (H&E. ×50)

1451   Subchorionic fibrosis of the placenta
This section through the chorionic plate shows a broad zone of diffuse fibrosis without other cellular reaction. Focal calcific deposits are seen in the subjacent placental tissue. (H&E. ×12)

1452   Nonspecific fibrosis of the placenta
The intervillous space is obliterated, and there is diffuse collagenization of chorionic villi without other evidence of cellular reaction. The lesion may be diffuse or focal. (H&E. ×50)

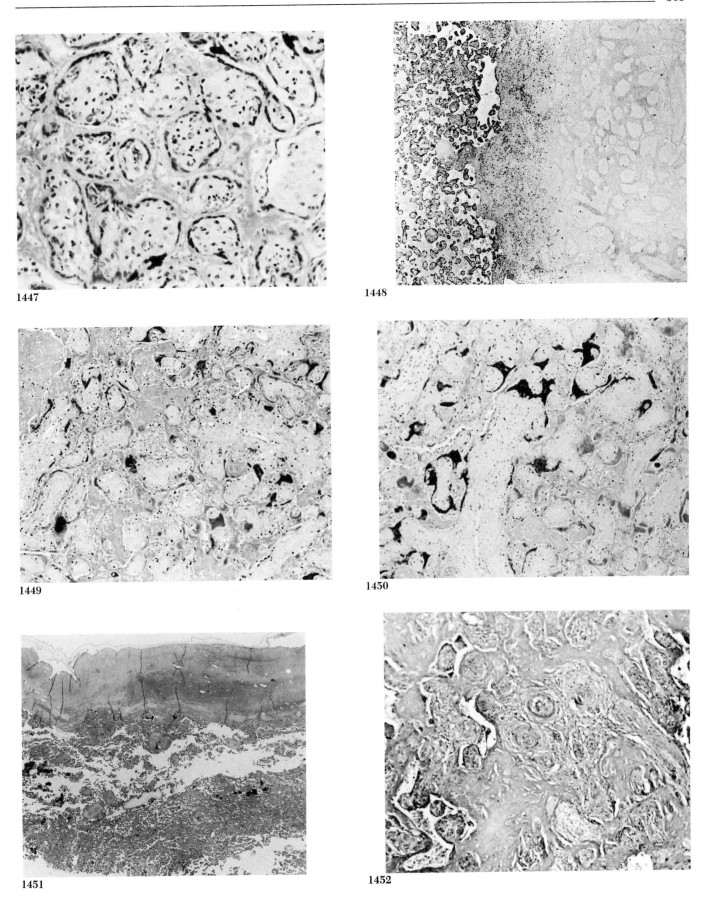

1447

1448

1449

1450

1451

1452

1453   Calcification of chorionic villi in a term placenta
This nonspecific change is found in both normal term placentas and in a variety of associated pathologic states. (H&E. ×30)

1454   Amniotic placental cyst
A thin-walled cyst lined by amniotic epithelium is found on the fetal surface of the placenta. (H&E. ×6)

1455   Placental cyst, not otherwise defined
A thin-walled cyst lined by a flat, nondescript lining is attached to the chorionic plate. (H&E. ×5)

1456   Chorioangioma of the placenta
A tumor arising within the chorionic plate is composed of numerous vascular spaces lined by plump endothelial cells. (H&E. ×50)

1457   Chorioangioma of the placenta
High magnification of Fig. 1456. Proliferated endothelial cells form vascular spaces as in hemangiomas. (H&E. ×125)

1458   Chorioangioma of the placenta
Note the clearly defined vascular spaces and somewhat flatter endothelial cells. (H&E. ×125)

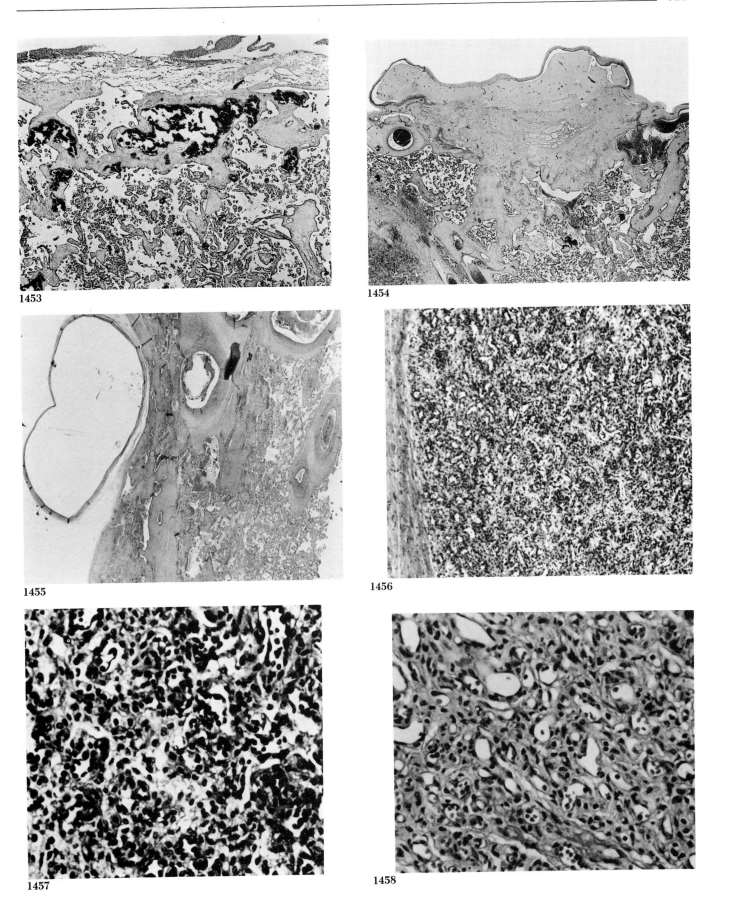

1453

1454

1455

1456

1457

1458

1459   Chorioangioma of the placenta
This tumor is composed of capillary structures.
(H&E. ×260)

1460   Teratoma of the placenta
Attached to the placenta was a solid tumor covered by mature skin and well-differentiated, mature skin appendages. (H&E. ×25)

1461   Teratoma of the placenta
Glomerulus-like structures and tubular structures irregularly disposed in a fibromuscular stroma suggest a renal anlage. A different area of the tumor shown in Fig. 1460. (H&E. ×50)

1462   Malignant melanoma of the skin metastatic to the placenta
A nest of neoplastic polyhedral cells containing melanin is found in the intervillous space of a term placenta. (H&E. ×50)

1463   Malignant melanoma of the skin metastatic to the placenta
High magnification of Fig. 1462. Note the neoplastic features of the melanoma cells, the density of pigment, and detached tumor cells circulating in the intervillous space. (H&E. ×100)

1464   Melanosis of the placenta
Phagocytosed melanin pigment is found in the stroma of villous stalks and villi as well as in trophoblastic cells. (This patient had widely disseminated malignant melanoma, but there were no metastases as such to the placenta. The placenta was grossly discolored dark brown.) (H&E. ×125)

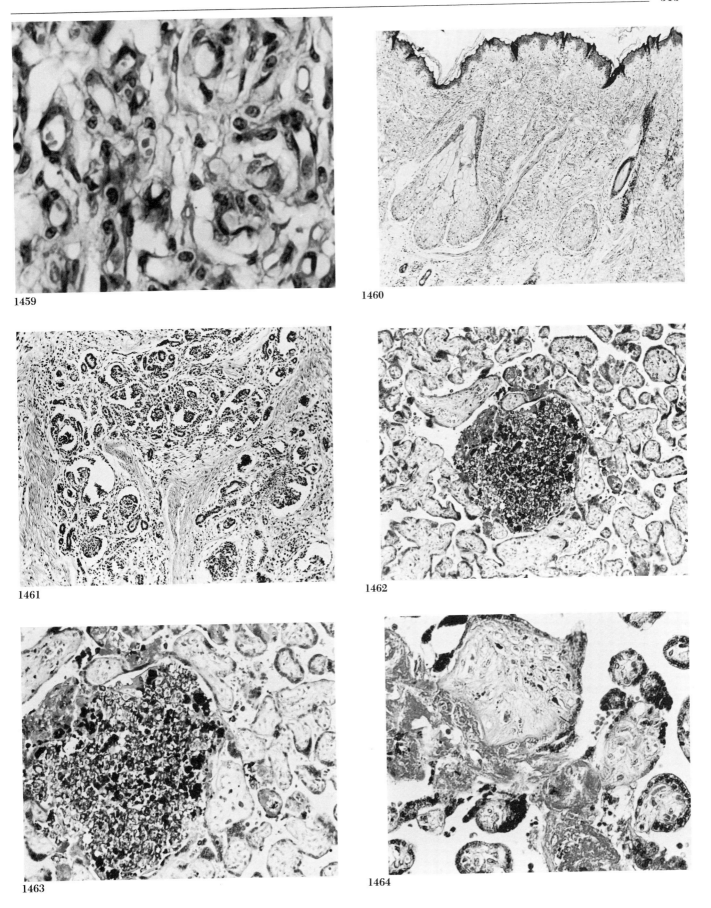

1459

1460

1461

1462

1463

1464

1465 Congenital granulocytic leukemia of the placenta
The chorionic plate is essentially intact, but the villi are stuffed with leukemic cells. (H&E. ×50)

1466 Congenital granulocytic leukemia of the placenta
Diffuse infiltration of the villous stalk and villi by fetal leukemic cells is seen. (H&E. ×50)

1467 Congenital granulocytic leukemia of the placenta
High magnification of Fig. 1466. The large number of immature granulocytes in the stroma of chorionic villi obliterate their architecture. Note the trophoblastic bridging between villi. (H&E. ×125)

1468 Congenital granulocytic leukemia of the placenta
This section through the maternal plate shows occasional leukemic cells in between decidual cells, as well as involvement of chorionic villi. (H&E. ×50)

1469 Congenital neuroblastoma of the placenta
Clumps of small, dark neoplastic cells fill irregularly the vascular channels of chorionic villi. (H&E. ×125)

1470 Congenital neuroblastoma of the placenta
High magnification of Fig. 1469. Rosettes typical of neuroblastoma are seen within villous capillaries. The tumor cells are typically nondescript with dark nuclei and scanty cytoplasm. (H&E. ×320)

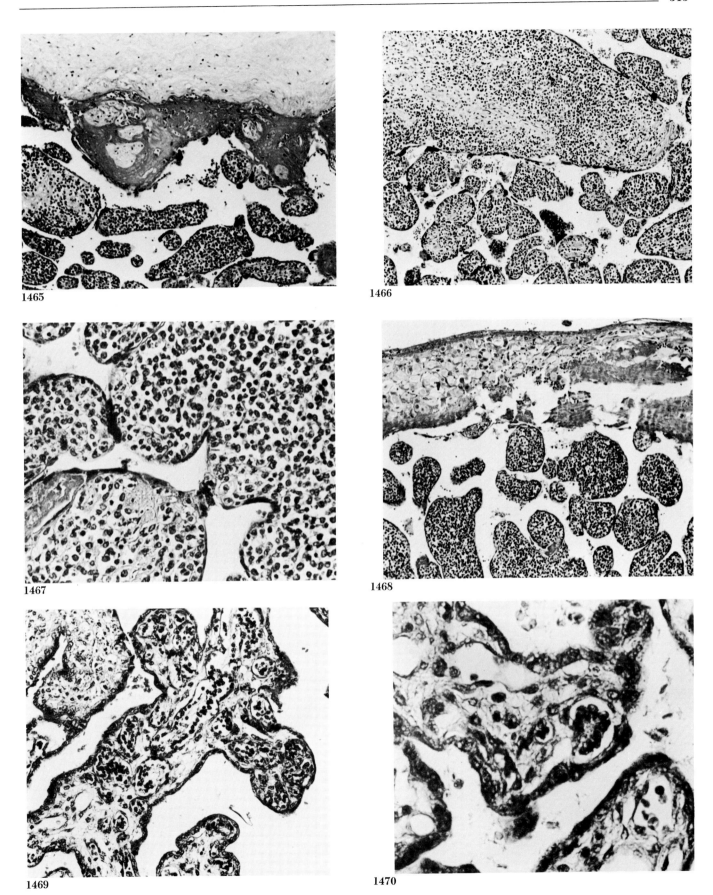

1465

1466

1467

1468

1469

1470

1471 Carcinoma of the breast metastatic to a term placenta
Sheets of neoplastic epithelium occupy much of the intervillous space. Occasional acinic spaces are seen in the metastatic neoplasm. (H&E. ×72)

1472 Normal amniotic membrane
A regular cuboidal epithelium lines a thin membrane composed of fibroblasts and collagen fibers arranged in parallel lamellas. (H&E. ×125)

1473 Diamniotic, dichorionic twin fetal membranes
Two separate fetal compartments, each lined internally by an amnion (upper and lower layers), are apposed to each other by their chorions (middle layers). There is a narrow space between the two chorions. (H&E. ×70)

1474 Diamniotic, monochorionic twin fetal membranes
(H&E. ×70)

1475 Amnion nodosum
A nodular, plaquelike structure composed of partly degenerated epithelial cells and keratin debris lies in close apposition to the amnion. There is no inflammation in the anmiotic membrane. The degree of apposition of the plaque varies from being almost free to densely adherent. (H&E. ×50)

1476 Amnion nodosum
Note the keratin structure of the plaque in proximity to a normal amnion. The lesion is often associated with oligohydramnios. Degenerated squamous epithelium composes the plaque or nodule. (H&E. ×125)

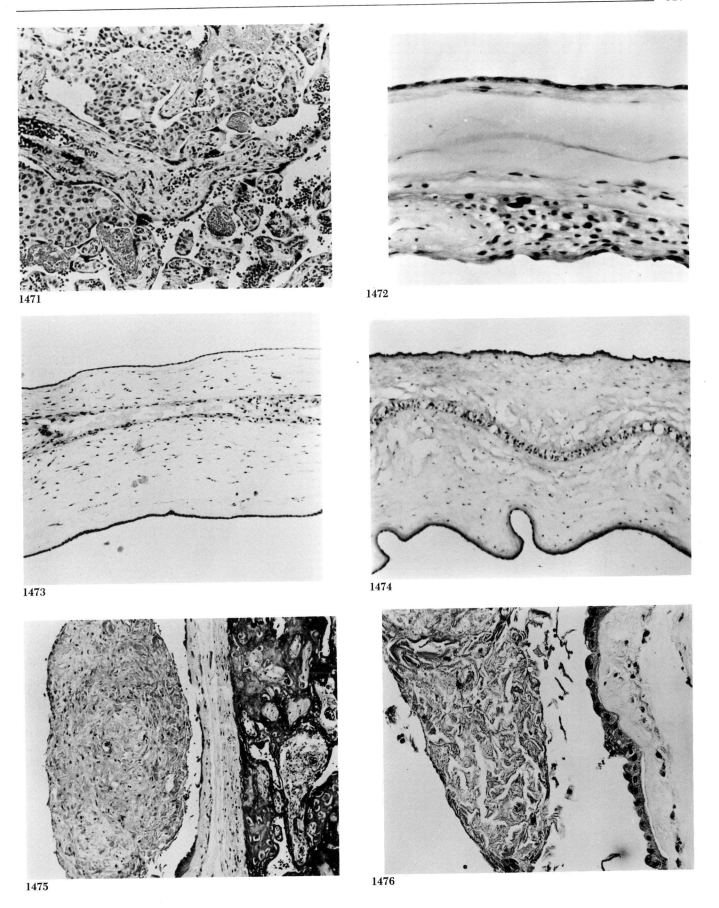

1471

1472

1473

1474

1475

1476

14

Diseases of the Umbilical Cord

1477 Normal umbilical cord
Two arteries and one vein are surrounded by Wharton's jelly. (H&E. ×10)

1478 Agenesis of the umbilical artery
Only one artery and one vein are seen. (H&E. ×8)

1479 Thrombosis of the umbilical vein
The vein is distended by a fresh thrombus. (H&E. ×5)

1480 Acute funisitis
Umbilical artery is thrombosed and the wall is diffusely infiltrated with acute inflammatory cells. (H&E. ×50)

1481 Angiomyxoma of the umbilical cord
The tumor, formed by proliferation of the myxoid stroma with many tiny blood vessels, creates a discrete nodular mass within the cord. (H&E. ×24)

1482 Angiomyxoma of the umbilical cord
High magnification of Fig. 1481. Myxoid stroma and numerous thin-walled blood vessels are seen. (H&E. ×50)

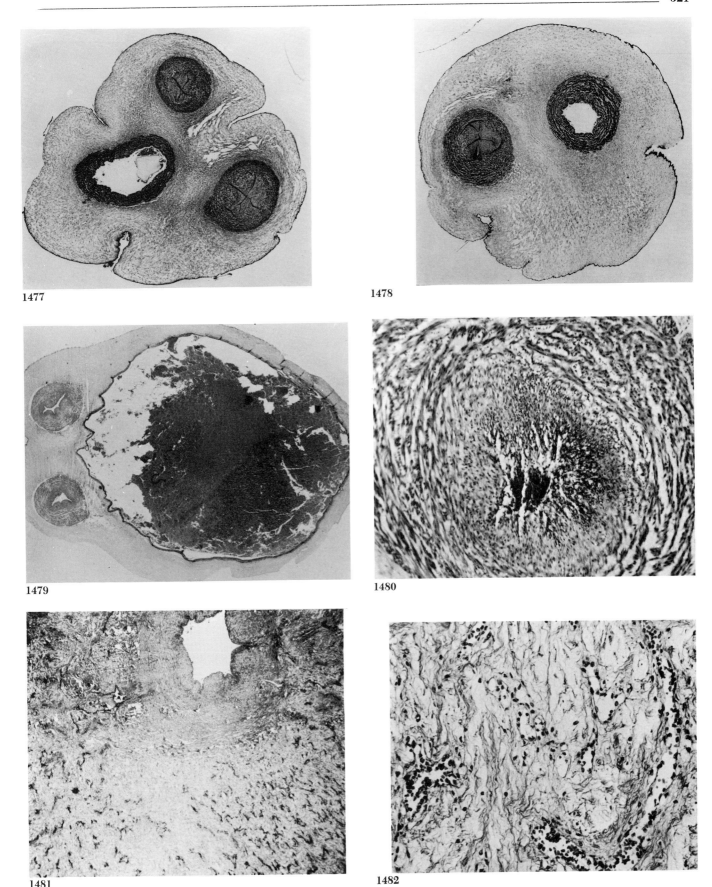

1477

1478

1479

1480

1481

1482

15

Hydatidiform Mole, Chorioadenoma Destruens, and Choriocarcinoma

1483 Hydatidiform mole in situ
Molar villi are seen attached to normal decidua. Blood and blood clot are present in the intervillous space. (H&E. ×6)

1484 Hydatidiform mole with slight trophoblastic overgrowth
About 1 per cent of patients with this degree of trophoblastic activity develop choriocarcinoma. (H&E. ×50)

1485 Hydatidiform mole with slight trophoblastic overgrowth and minor degree of nuclear hyperchromasia
About 1 per cent of patients with this degree of trophoblastic activity develop choriocarcinoma. (H&E. ×50)

1486 Hydatidiform mole with slight trophoblastic overgrowth, minor nuclear hyperchromasia, and cellular pleomorphism
About 1 per cent of patients with this degree of trophoblastic activity develop choriocarcinoma. (H&E. ×50)

1487 Hydatidiform mole with slight trophoblastic overgrowth and bizarre degenerating cells
About 1 per cent of patients with this degree of trophoblastic activity develop choriocarcinoma. (H&E. ×50)

1488 Hydatidiform mole with slight trophoblastic hyperplasia, degenerative changes, and focal necroses
About 1 per cent of patients with this degree of trophoblastic activity develop choriocarcinoma. (H&E. ×50)

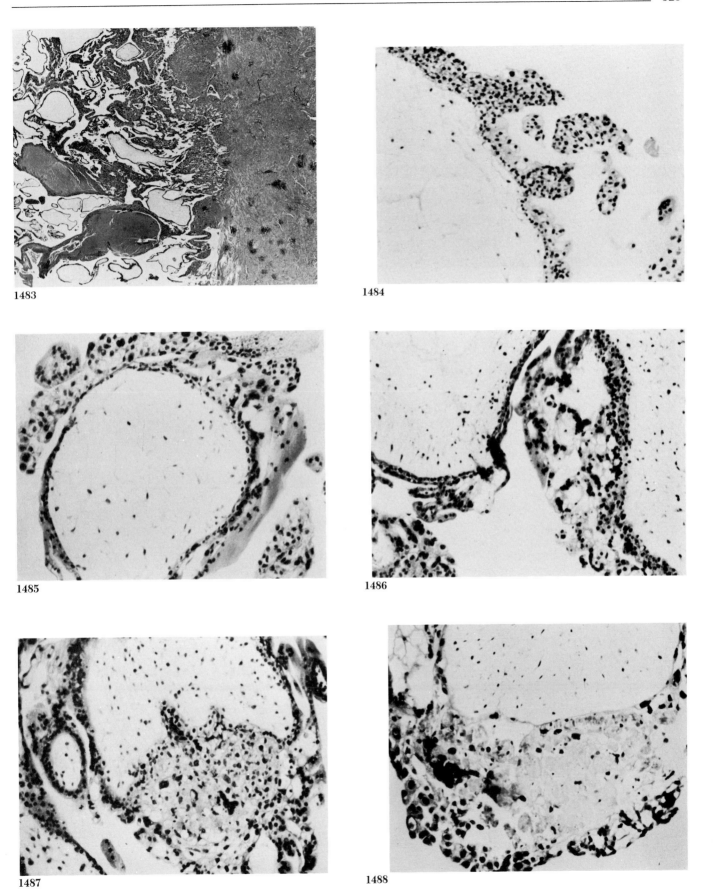

1483

1484

1485

1486

1487

1488

1489 Hydatidiform mole with moderate degree of trophoblastic hyperplasia
About 5 per cent of patients with this degree of trophoblastic activity develop choriocarcinoma. (H&E. ×35)

1490 Hydatidiform mole with moderate trophoblastic hyperplasia, chiefly of cytotrophoblast
About 5 per cent of patients with this degree of trophoblastic activity develop choriocarcinoma. (H&E. ×50)

1491 Hydatidiform mole with moderate degree of trophoblastic hyperplasia and cellular hyperchromasia
About 5 per cent of patients with this degree of trophoblastic activity develop choriocarcinoma. (H&E. ×50)

1492 Hydatidiform mole with moderate degree of trophoblastic hyperplasia, nuclear hyperchromasia, and cellular pleomorphism
About 5 per cent of patients with this degree of trophoblastic activity develop choriocarcinoma. (H&E. ×50)

1493 Hydatidiform mole with moderate degree of trophoblastic hyperplasia and occasional degenerative cellular changes
About 5 per cent of patients with this degree of trophoblastic activity develop choriocarcinoma. (H&E. ×50)

1494 Hydatidiform mole with moderate degree of trophoblastic hyperplasia and occasional degenerative cellular changes
About 5 per cent of patients with this degree of trophoblastic activity develop choriocarcinoma. (H&E. ×110)

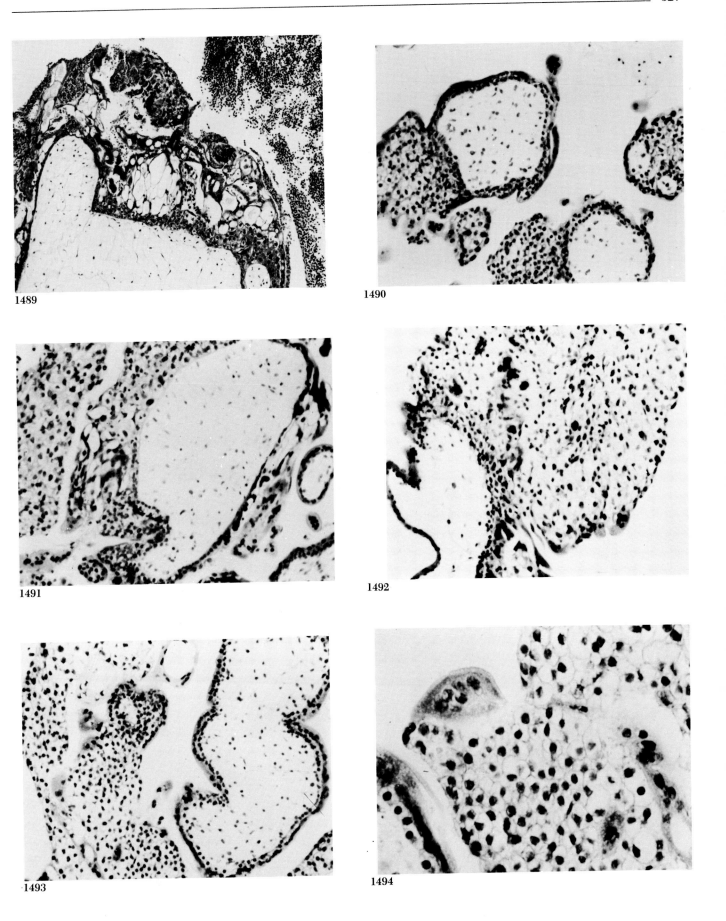

1489

1490

1491

1492

1493

1494

1495 Hydatidiform mole with marked tropho-blastic hyperplasia
About 10 per cent of patients with this degree of trophoblastic activity develop choriocarcinoma. (H&E. ×70)

1496 Hydatidiform mole with marked tropho-blastic hyperplasia, nuclear hyper-chromasia, and cellular pleomorphism
About 10 per cent of patients with this degree of trophoblastic activity develop choriocarcinoma. (H&E. ×8)

1497 Hydatidiform mole with marked tropho-blastic hyperplasia and pleomorphism in proliferated cytotrophoblast
About 10 per cent of patients with this degree of trophoblastic activity develop choriocarcinoma. (H&E. ×80)

1498 Hydatidiform mole with marked tropho-blastic hyperplasia and cellular pleomorphism
About 10 per cent of patients with this degree of trophoblastic activity develop choriocarcinoma. (H&E. ×80)

1499 Hydatidiform mole with marked tropho-blastic hyperplasia and cellular pleomor-phism
About 10 per cent of patients with this degree of trophoblastic activity develop choriocarcinoma. (H&E. ×125)

1500 Hydatidiform mole with marked tropho-blastic hyperplasia and cellular pleomor-phism
High magnification showing cellular detail. About 10 per cent of patients with this degree of trophoblastic activity develop choriocarcinoma. (H&E. ×250)

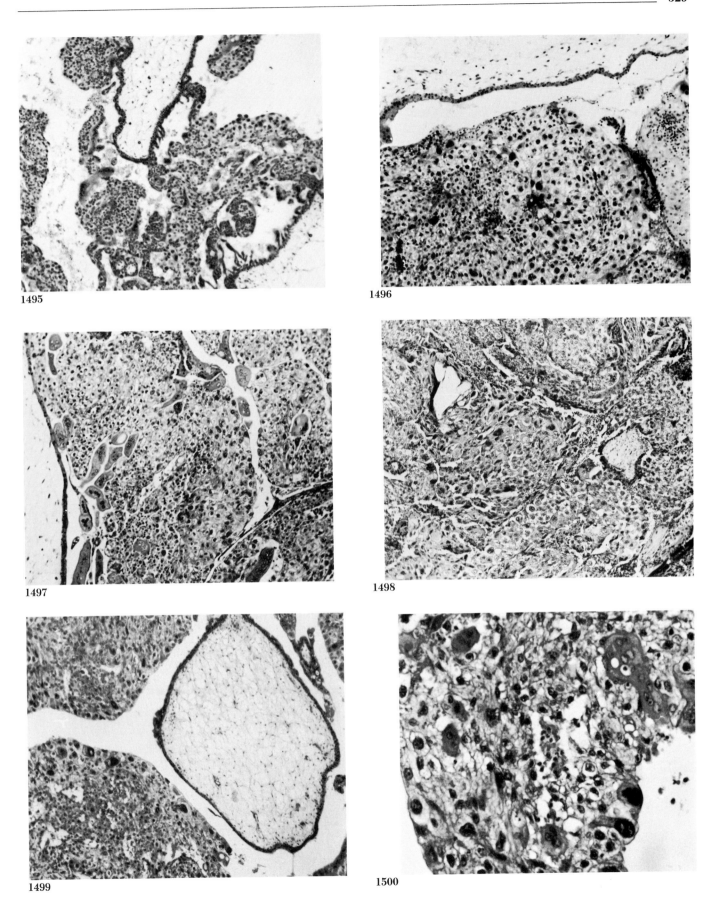

1495

1496

1497

1498

1499

1500

1501   Chorioadenoma destruens
The basic morphologic unit consists of molar villi invading myometrium with some degree of trophoblastic overgrowth and vascular invasion. (H&E. ×25)

1502   Chorioadenoma destruens
Molar villi with moderate trophoblastic hyperplasia have invaded uterine veins. (H&E. ×35)

1503   Chorioadenoma destruens
There is attachment and organization of the invading villus to the vascular lining by fibrin. (H&E. ×72)

1504   Chorioadenoma destruens invading the broad ligament
The lumen of the fallopian tube is seen at 1 o'clock. The veins of the broad ligament are filled with molar villi surrounded by proliferated trophoblast. (H&E. ×8)

1505   Chorioadenoma destruens with massive myometrial invasion
Hydatidiform villi and trophoblasts penetrate deep into the myometrium. (H&E. ×50)

1506   Retained hydatidiform mole
The degenerating villus and its surrounding proliferated trophoblasts lay superficial to the endomyometrial junction. (Detail of Color Fig. 111, Plate XIX.) (H&E. ×50)

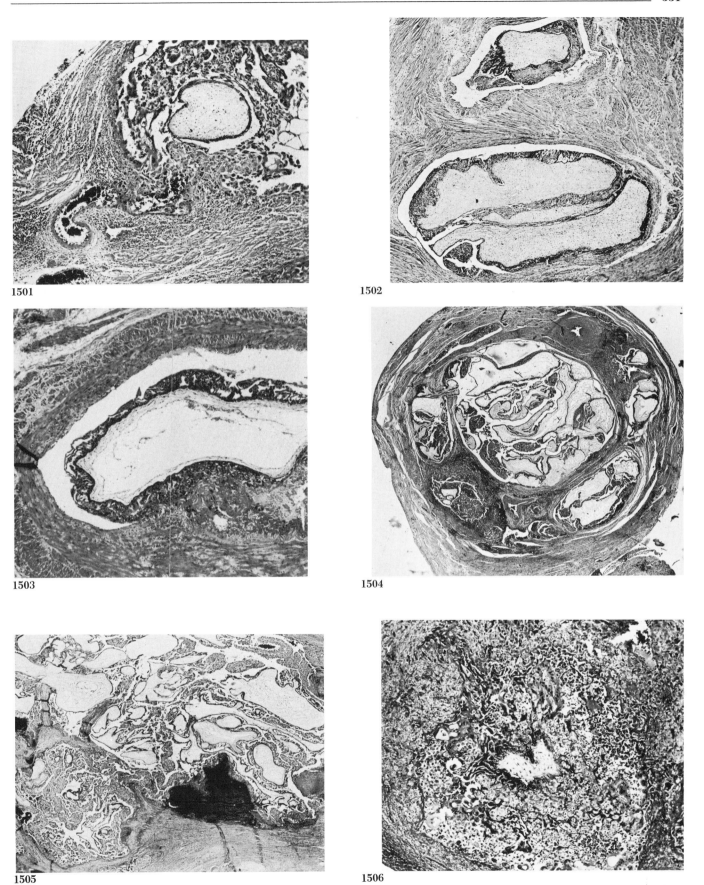

1501

1502

1503

1504

1505

1506

1507 Syncytiotrophoblasts in a lymphatic channel
Two buds of syncytiotrophoblast are seen within the lumen of a myometrial lymphatic in a case of hydatidiform mole. (H&E. ×90)

1508 Cytotrophoblasts in lymphatic channel
Cytotrophoblastic cells are seen in the lumen of a myometrial lymphatic in a case of hydatidiform mole. (H&E. ×100)

1509 Uterine curetting diagnostic of choriocarcinoma
There is marked proliferation of immature cytotrophoblast and syncytiotrophoblast intimately admixed in the absence of chorionic villi. (H&E. ×13)

1510 Uterine curettings diagnostic of choriocarcinoma
The degree of cellular atypia is striking even for such embryonic tissue as a trophoblast. No chorionic villi were found. (H&E. ×80)

1511 Uterine curetting diagnostic of choriocarcinoma
Large fragments of friable myometrium invaded by trophoblasts were removed with the curette. (H&E. ×24)

1512 Uterine curettings diagnostic of choriocarcinoma
High magnification of Fig. 1511. Sheets of trophoblasts are seen invading the myometrium. A modest inflammatory reaction is present, chiefly lymphocytic. (H&E. ×80)

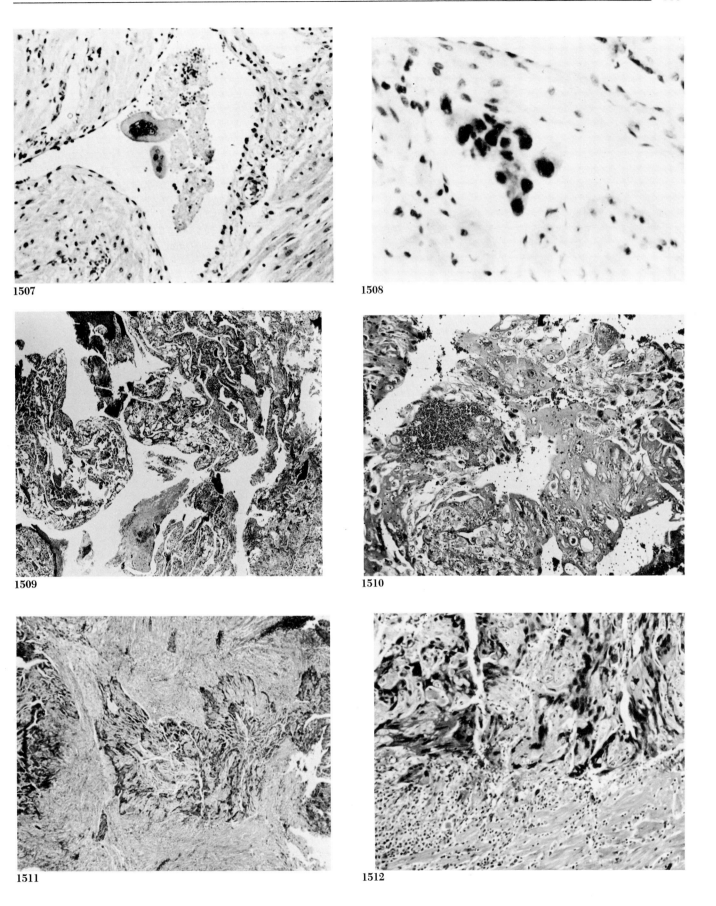

1507

1508

1509

1510

1511

1512

1513 Choriocarcinoma permeating vascular spaces in the decidual endometrium
(H&E. ×45)

1514 Choriocarcinoma permeating vascular spaces in decidual endometrium
High magnification of Fig. 1513. Islands of choriocarcinoma are present in an endothelial-lined channel resembling a lymph vessel. Note the decidua of pregnancy. (H&E. ×125)

1515 Choriocarcinoma diffusely invading the myometrium and myometrial vessels
(H&E. ×50)

1516 Choriocarcinoma uteri
Cords of cytotrophoblasts are capped by thinned layers of syncytiotrophoblasts which form apparent "vascular spaces," recapitulating thereby the function of syncytiotrophoblasts as the lining of the intervillous space in the normal placenta. (H&E. ×65)

1517 Choriocarcinoma uteri
The mixture of cytotrophoblast and syncytiotrophoblast is relatively even. The cytotrophoblast tends to form cords and clumps. The syncytiotrophoblast forms ribbons and occasional sheets with cytoplasmic vacuoles. (H&E. ×65)

1518 Choriocarcinoma uteri
The tumor is composed chiefly of cytotrophoblasts with only occasional syncytiotrophoblastic elements. (H&E. ×150)

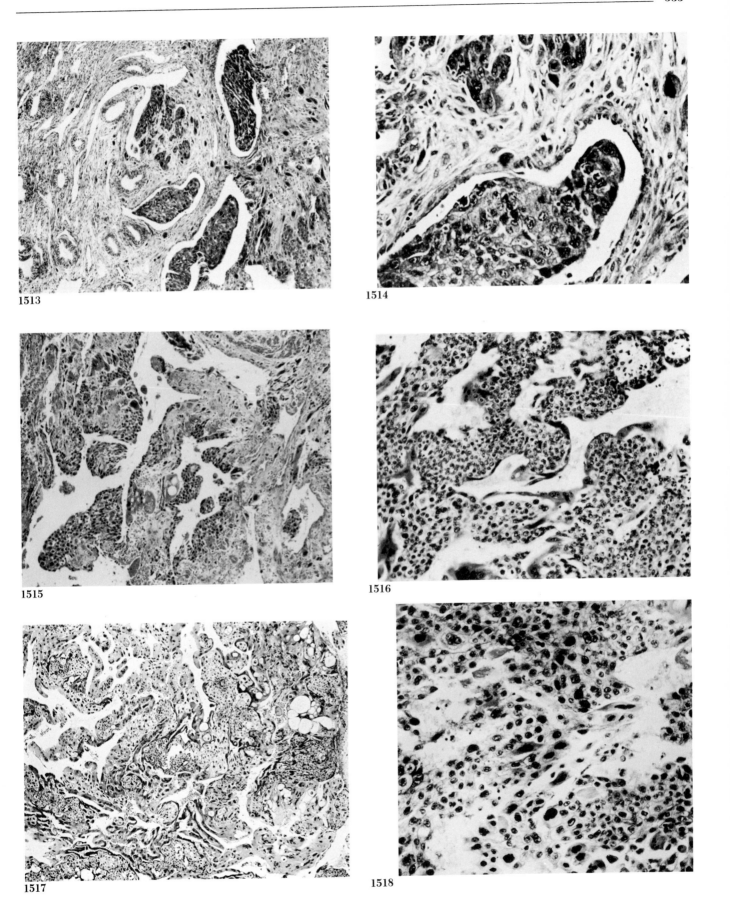

1513

1514

1515

1516

1517

1518

1519 Choriocarcinoma embolic to the lung
The trophoblastic emboli are entirely intra-vascular, and the pulmonary parenchyma is not invaded. Such patients may develop chronic cor pulmonale; chest films are usually negative for metastatic tumor. (H&E. ×17)

1520 Choriocarcinoma embolic to the lung
High magnification of Fig. 1519. An embolic trophoblast is seen within a medium-sized pulmonary artery twig. There is an inflammatory reaction in and around the vessel wall which has been construed as morphologic evidence of a mechanism which restrains parenchymal invasion, possibly an "immune" mechanism. (H&E. ×90)

1521 Choriocarcinoma metastatic to the lung
There is deposition of choriocarcinoma in the lung. The tumor is formed by cytotrophoblasts compressing a bronchiolus. (H&E. ×50)

1522 Choriocarcinoma metastatic to the lung
Lung tissue is compressed by a metastatic nodule composed of cytotrophoblasts, syncytiotrophoblasts, and extensive areas of hemorrhagic necrosis. (H&E. ×50)

1523 Choriocarcinoma metastatic to the liver
There is usually more hemorrhage as the trophoblasts tap the hepatic sinusoidal circulation; the picture is from a histologically preserved area. (H&E. ×70)

1524 Choriocarcinoma invading the veins of the broad ligament
The thin fibrovascular membrane and its vessels are markedly distorted by large cords of invasive neoplasm. (H&E. ×6)

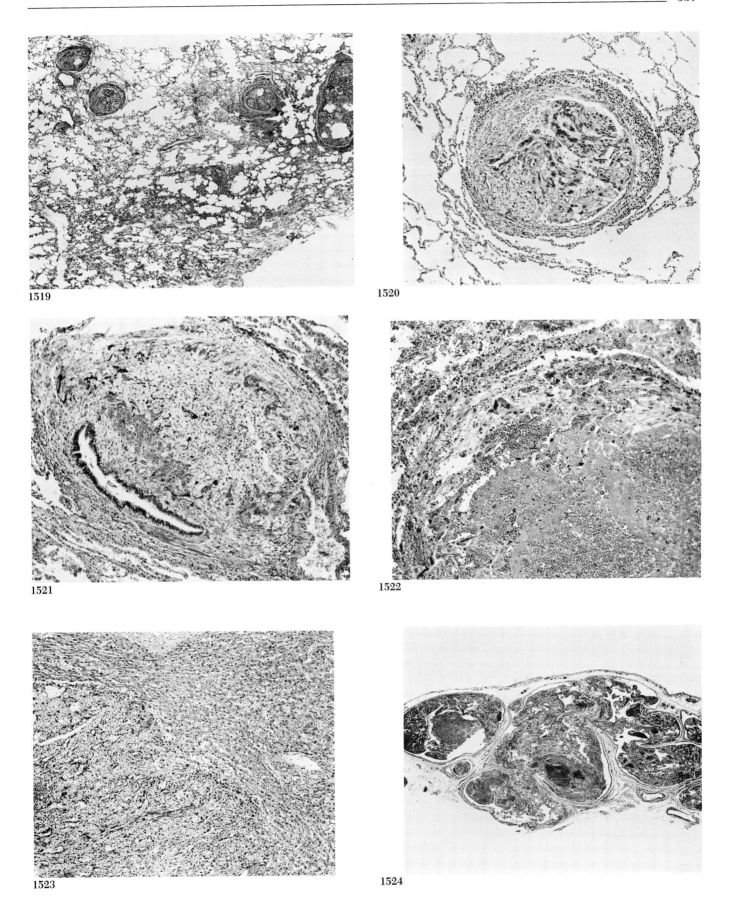

1519

1520

1521

1522

1523

1524

1525 Choriocarcinoma metastatic to the cerebellum
(H&E. ×25)

1526 Multicystic ovary associated with choriocarcinoma
Some of the features of the micropolycystic ovary in the Stein-Leventhal syndrome are reproduced, as chorionic gonadotropin stimulates the ovaries in much the same way as pituitary LH. (H&E. ×8)

1527 Lining of theca lutein cysts in the ovary of a patient with choriocarcinoma
The luteinization is of the theca interna. Only rarely does one see luteinization of granulosa cells in this context. (H&E. ×90)

1528 Hyperplasia of breast tissue in choriocarcinoma
The intrinsic lobular stroma is principally affected, but there is proliferation of ducts and lobules as well. (H&E. ×10)

1529 Choriocarcinoma primary in the oviduct
This cross section shows a largely necrotic mass in the lumen of the tube, hemorrhage and vascular thromboses in the wall. Viable tumor is not visible at this power. There was no primary tumor in the uterus or elsewhere. (H&E. ×5)

1530 Choriocarcinoma primary in the oviduct
High magnification of Fig. 1529. A few fragments of identifiable viable trophoblast are seen invading the wall of the fallopian tube. (H&E. ×60)

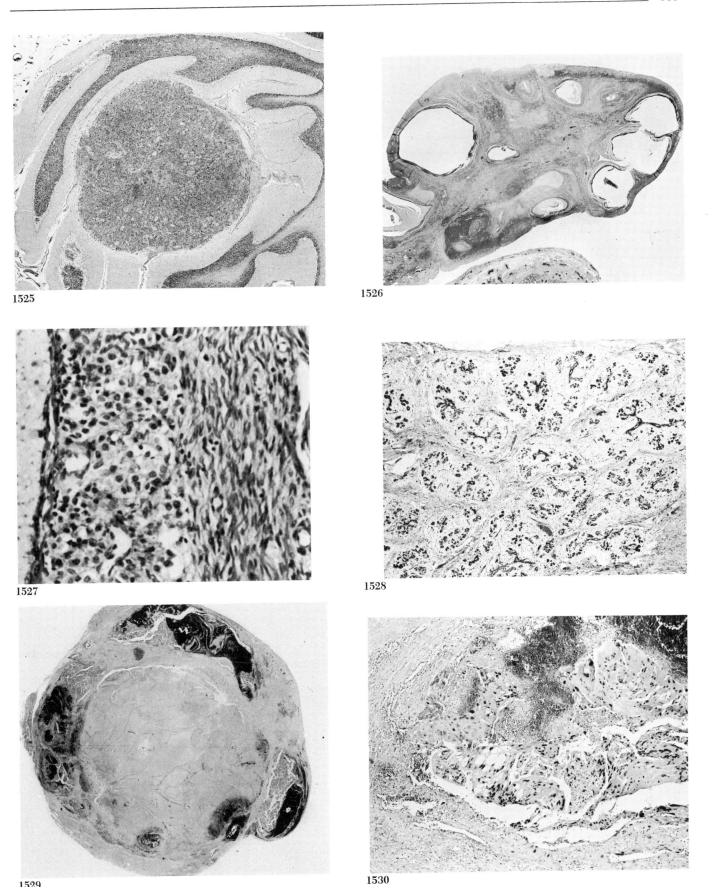

1525

1526

1527

1528

1529

1530

16

Complications of Pregnancy

1531   Amniotic fluid embolism
Pulmonary arterioles and capillaries are distended by squamous and keratin debris from the amniotic fluid admixed with leukocytes. (H&E. ×200)

1532   Amniotic fluid embolism
Pulmonary vessels may contain relatively large amounts of amniotic fluid and only a few formed elements. (H&E. ×280)

1533   Fatty metamorphosis of the liver in pregnancy
The central two-thirds of every lobule shows extensive intracytoplasmic fatty vacuolation. (H&E. ×24)

1534   Fatty metamorphosis of the liver in pregnancy
There is no necrosis of liver parenchyma and no inflammatory exudate. (H&E. ×75)

1536   Viral hepatitis in pregnancy
Hepatocellular trabeculae are disrupted, and liver cell necrosis is accompanied by an inflammatory exudate of lymphoid and mononuclear cells. There is no fatty metamorphosis. (H&E. ×200)

1535   Viral hepatitis in pregnancy
A diffuse infiltrate disrupts the lobular architecture of the liver. (H&E. ×130)

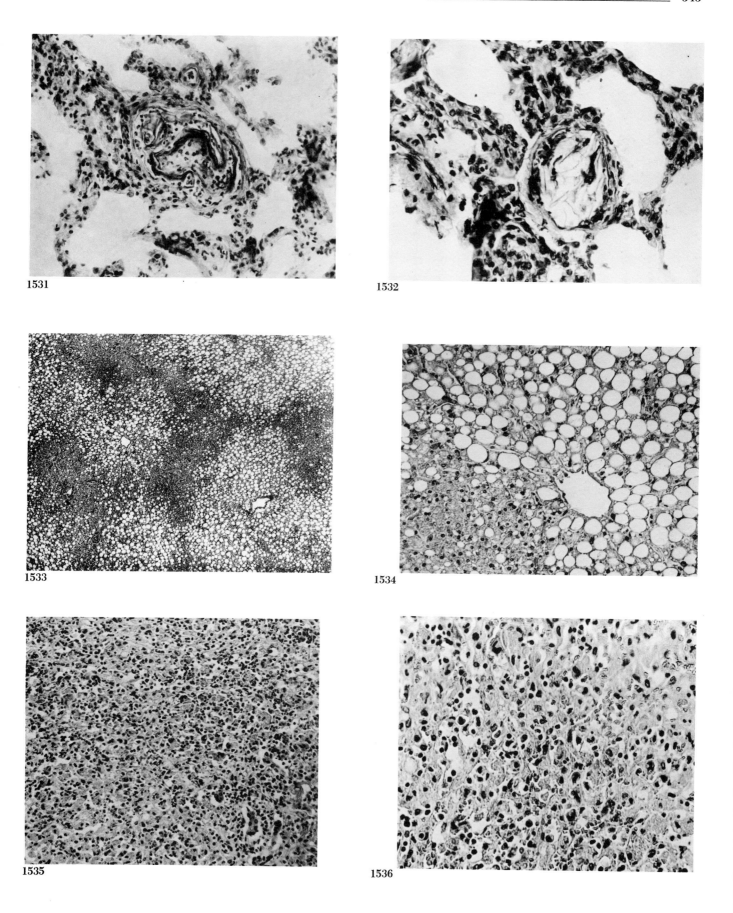

1531

1532

1533

1534

1535

1536

1537 Intrapartum pituitary necrosis
Acute ischemic necrosis of almost the entire anterior lobe is evident. (H&E. ×24)

1538 Intrapartum pituitary necrosis
High magnification of Fig. 1537. Only a few scattered pituitary cells remain identifiable at the periphery of the gland. (H&E. ×50)

1539 Post-partum pituitary necrosis
Diffuse necrosis without conspicuous inflammatory reaction involves more than 80 per cent of the anterior lobe parenchyma. (H&E. ×24)

1540 Post-partum pituitary necrosis
High magnification of Fig. 1539. The spared rim of viable pituitary tissue is seen as a continuous marginal zone, almost a pseudocapsule around the necrotic area. (H&E. ×50)

1541 Post-partum pituitary scarring associated with Sheehan's syndrome
Distinct areas of loss of substance are seen in a general view of the anterior lobe. (H&E. ×10)

1542 Post-partum pituitary scarring associated with Sheehan's syndrome
High magnification of Fig. 1541. Hyalinized collagen fibers with a rich capillary network have replaced the foci of damage to the parenchyma. The abutting parenchyma is of normal cell population. (H&E. ×50)

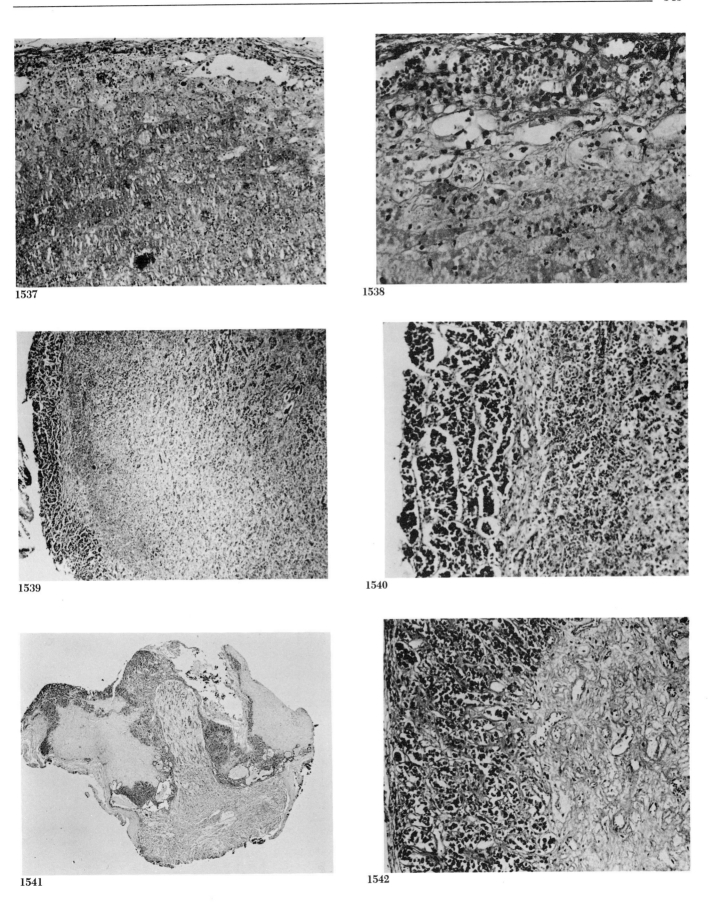

1537

1538

1539

1540

1541

1542

1543   Vaginitis emphysematosa in pregnancy
Frequent complication of pregnancy. The cause is undetermined. (H&E. ×80)

1544   Erosive vaginitis in pregnancy
The vaginal mucosa shows degenerative changes and is ulcerated. A mixed inflammatory exudate and vascularized granulation tissue underlies the epithelium, and the exudate pours out into the lumen. (H&E. ×60)

1545   Cervicitis with basal cell hyperplasia (dysplasia) during pregnancy
A general view of the endocervix shows conversion of mucus-secreting glandular epithelium to a squamous epithelial covering. (H&E. ×12)

1546   Cervicitis with basal cell hyperplasia (dysplasia) during pregnancy
High magnification of Fig. 1545. Nonglycogenated squamous epithelium covers the endocervical surface and extends into an endocervical gland. The basal cell layer is thickened. Numerous mitoses are present. (H&E. ×50)

1547   Cervicitis with basal cell hyperplasia (dysplasia) during pregnancy
High magnification of Fig. 1545. The thickened layer of basal cells is seen with the long axes of their nuclei perpendicular to the basement membrane. Mitotic figures are seen as high as the middle of the epithelial layer. The maturation of cells is preserved. (H&E. ×250)

1548   Cervicitis with basal cell hyperplasia (dysplasia) during pregnancy
Parakeratotic maturation is present on the surface, and there is a moderate degree of cellular pleomorphism and hyperchromatism as well as loss of polarity in the thickened basal layers. (H&E. ×100)

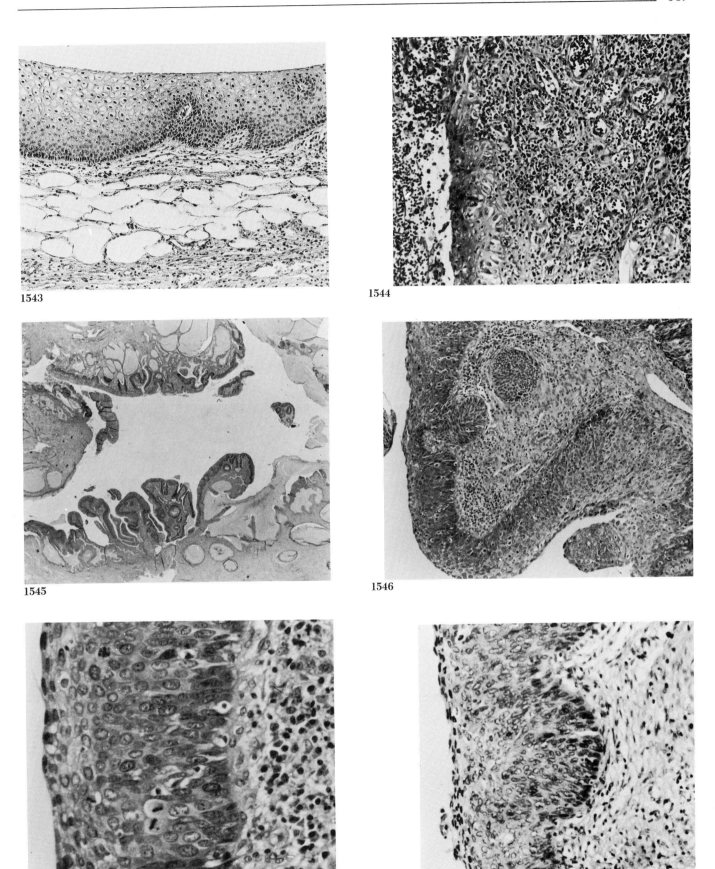

1543

1544

1545

1546

1547

1548

1549   Cervicitis with basal cell hyperplasia (dysplasia) during pregnancy
Proliferated cells derived from basal layer are spindle-shaped rather than squamous and polyhedral, possibly as the result of cellular crowding as reparative epithelial growth is stimulated. Minimal glycogenization is seen in isolated cells in the upper layers. There is little surface maturation. (H&E. ×200)

1550   Intraepithelial carcinoma (carcinoma in situ) during pregnancy
Complete loss of epithelial polarity, pronounced immaturity of spindle-shaped epithelial cells, intense hyperchromasia, and excessive pleomorphism are characteristic findings. (H&E. ×125)

1551   Post-partum renal cortical necrosis
A general view shows pallor and necrosis of most of the cortex. Only a thin spared rim at the capsular surface and another abutting the level of the arcuate arteries can be seen. (H&E. ×20)

1552   Post-partum renal cortical necrosis
High magnification of Fig. 1551. Coagulation necrosis involves both glomeruli and tubules. Fresh thrombi are seen in intralobular vessels. (H&E. ×100)

1553   Post-partum renal cortical necrosis
High magnification of Fig. 1551. A fresh thrombus snakes its way into a glomerular tuft which is necrotic. (H&E. ×100)

1554   Post-partum renal cortical necrosis
An afferent arteriole is occluded by a fresh thrombus and the glomerulus is infarcted. The surrounding tubular epithelium is also pale staining and necrotic secondary to larger vascular occlusions in other fields. (H&E. ×160)

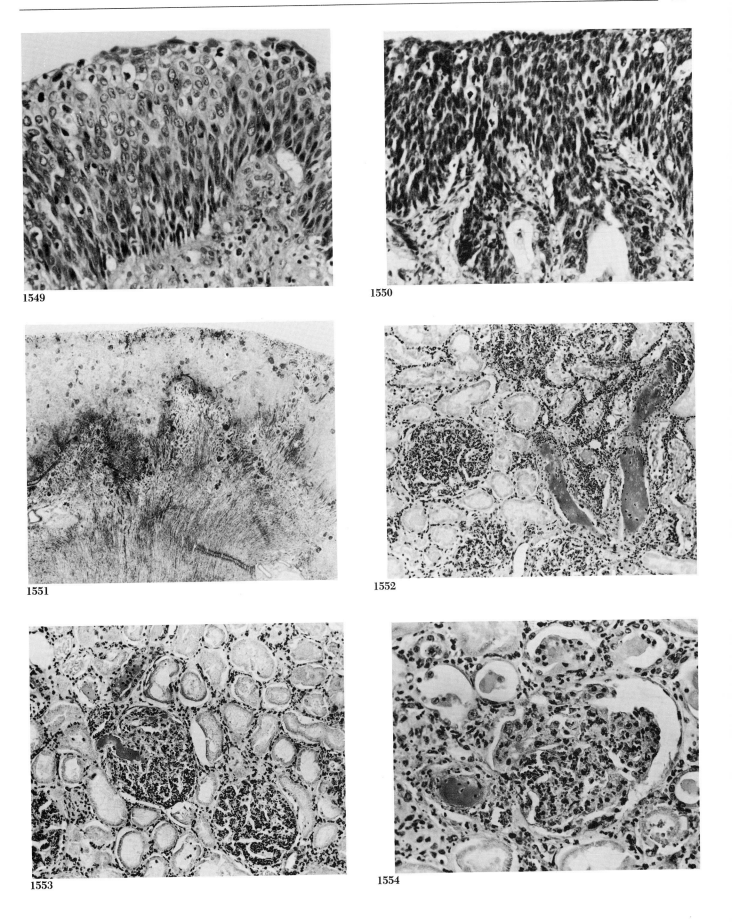

1549

1550

1551

1552

1553

1554

1555 Acute pyelonephritis in pregnancy
There is destruction of renal parenchyma by acute exudative inflammation, originating in the renal pelvis. Small to medium-sized abscesses from gram-negative bacilli are commonly found in severe cases. (H&E. ×60)

1556 Nephrosclerosis associated with pregnancy
The intima of arcuate and interlobular arteries shows concentric thickening by fibrohyaline lamellas. Bearing a facultative relationship to hypertension, this lesion may sometimes be found in young women with hypertensive toxemia of pregnancy. (H&E. ×100)

1557 Chronic glomerulonephritis associated with pregnancy
The connective tissue stroma shows marked infiltration with lymphocytes. There is atrophy of the tubuli; some show protein casts. Advanced hyalinization of glomeruli is seen. (H&E. ×50)

1558 Kidney in toxemia of pregnancy
The glomeruli are ischemic and swollen; the tubules are intact. (H&E. ×100)

1559 Kidney in toxemia of pregnancy
High magnification of Fig. 1558. The glomerulus is relatively ischemic. There is neither epithelial nor endothelial proliferation, but the basement membrane and capillary wall seem thickened. Periglomerular edema is present. (H&E. ×310)

1560 Kidney in toxemia of pregnancy
High magnification of Fig. 1558. The capillary walls of the glomerulus are thick, but whether this is intrinsic thickening of the basement membrane or represents material deposited on it cannot be ascertained by light microscopy. (H&E. ×320)

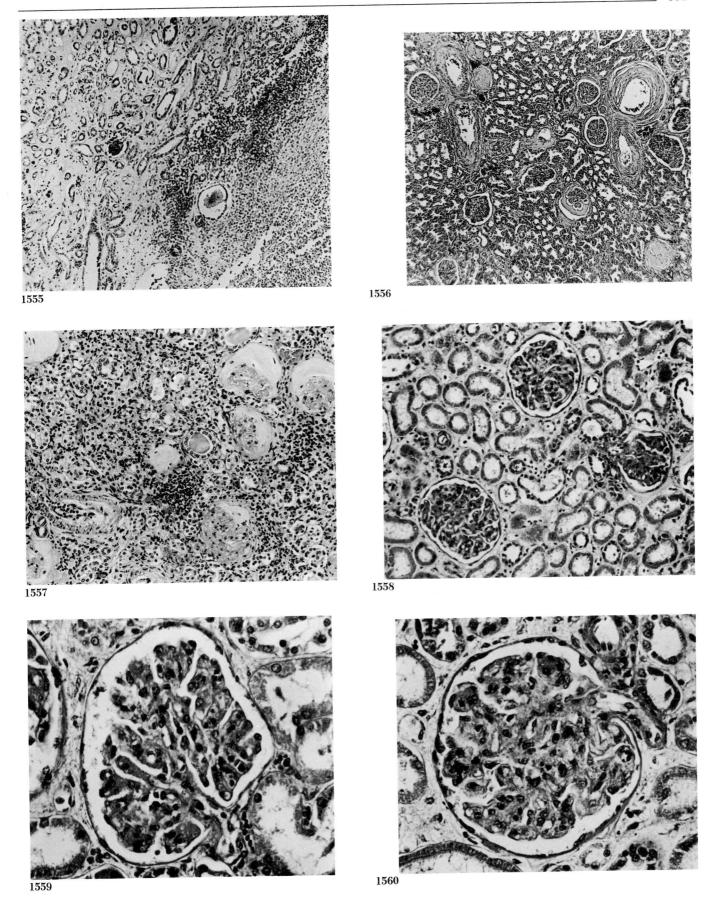

1555

1556

1557

1558

1559

1560

1561   Liver in toxemia of pregnancy
Petechial hemorrhage and focal necrosis, mid-zonal or random in distribution, is shown. (H&E. ×50)

1562   Liver in toxemia of pregnancy
Irregular patches of necrosis, neither centrilobular nor portal, may be found. (H&E. ×50)

1563   Liver in toxemia of pregnancy
High magnification of Fig. 1562. There is deposition of fibrin thrombi in the sinusoids and necrosis of nearby liver cells. (H&E. ×120)

1564   Brain in toxemia of pregnancy
Intense congestion and multiple petechial hemorrhages are shown. (H&E. ×70)

1565   Leiomyoma uteri in pregnancy
This tumor often becomes hypercellular with an increase in the size of individual cells. Central liquefaction or "red degeneration" may also occur. Nuclear hyperchromatism is present. There is edema of interstitial tissue. (H&E. ×125)

1566   Placental site vessels showing hyalinization, 1 month post partum
The uterine mucosa has regenerated normally, and none of the vessels is gaping or patulous. Many have been recanalized by a small central channel surrounded by a thick, scalloped hyaline wall. (H&E. ×8)

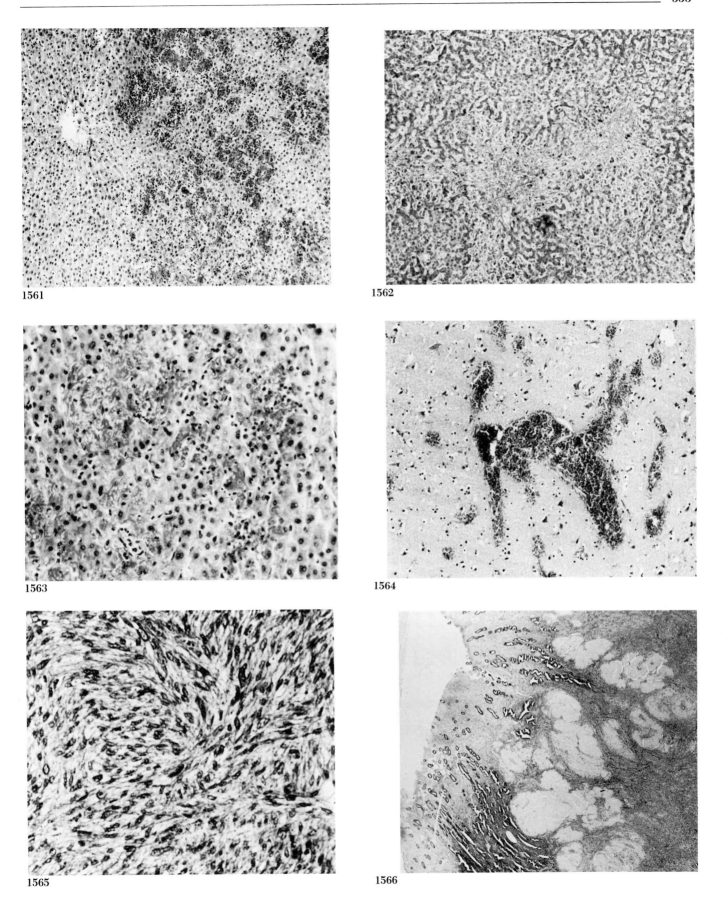

1561

1562

1563

1564

1565

1566

1567 Placental site vessel, 1 month post partum
High magnification of Fig. 1566. The thick hyaline wall surrounding a central zone of loose collagen fibers is admixed with a few foam cells. (H&E. ×100)

1568 Placental site vessels, 3 months post partum
There is no substantial difference between this picture and Fig. 1566 taken a 1 month post partum. (H&E. ×13)

1569 Placental site vessels, 3 months post partum
Demonstration of elastic fibers. (Verhoeff's elastica stain. ×13)

1570 Subinvolution of placental site vessels, 4 weeks post partum
Despite efforts of the endometrium to regenerate around it, an intraendometrial vessel remains patulous, filled with thrombotic material, and has a thin hyaline wall. (H&E. ×15)

1571 Subinvolution of uterus, 1 month post partum
Medium-sized arteries deep within the myometrium are dilated and filled with blood and blood clot. Damage to their walls prevents normal closure. (H&E. ×25)

1572 Subinvolution of uterus
Same case as shown in Fig. 1571. The muscular coats of vessel walls are hyalinized and a varying degree of collagen fiber deposition thickens the intima; however, the lumens of such vessels are partly open, partly closed. (Masson's trichrome stain. ×40)

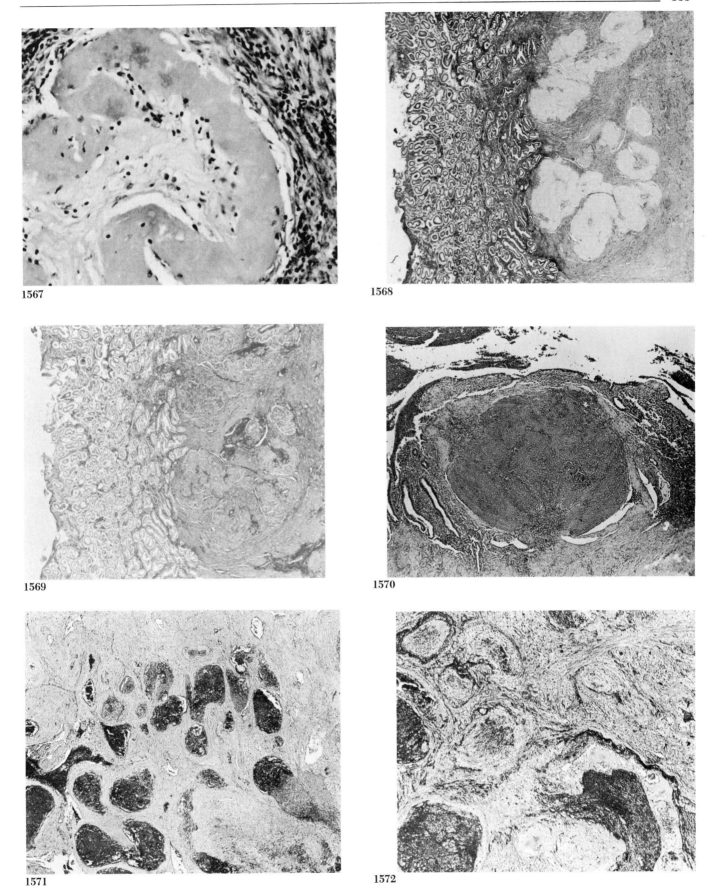

1567

1568

1569

1570

1571

1572

COLOR PLATES
Chapter 16
Complications of Pregnancy
Plates 18, 19, and 20

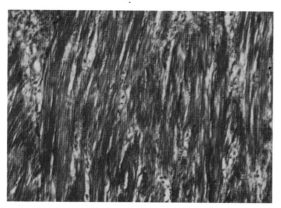

103 Myometrium in pregnancy A calculation based on multiple blocks studied with Specht trichrome stain indicates that the myometrium of pregnancy is composed of 42.0 ± 3.9 per cent of smooth muscle fibers, the remainder being collagen and blood vessels. (Specht's trichrome stain. ×120)

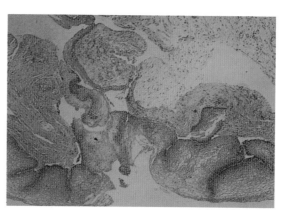

104 Decidual reaction in laparotomy scar (H&E. ×50)

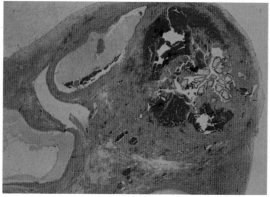

105 Ovarian pregnancy The ovum has implanted in the ovary; no villi were found in the tube. Chorionic villi and patchy areas of hemorrhage are shown. (H&E. ×10)

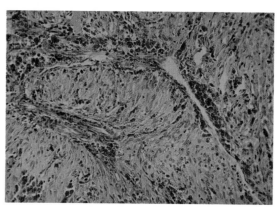

106 Chronic ectopic pregnancy (peritubal hematoma with organization) Tissue from the periphery of the tubal mass shows proliferation of fibroblasts and extensive phagocytosis of hemosiderin pigment. (H&E. ×110)

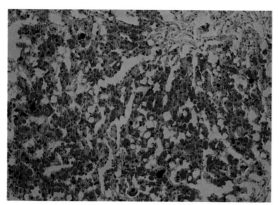

107 Soap-intoxication syndrome following criminal abortion Fatty metamorphosis and cholestasis are seen in the liver. (H&E. ×72)

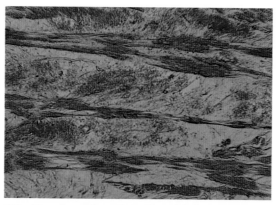

108 Uteroplacental apoplexy (Couvelaire's uterus) Myometrial fibers are dissected by extravasated blood under pressure from the retroplacental space. (Mallory's stain. ×60)

Plate 18

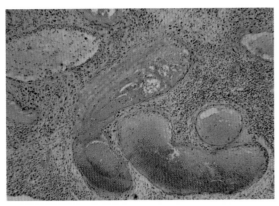

109 Subinvolution of placental site vessels, 2 weeks post-abortal Decidual vessels are maintained as ectatic channels by hyalinization of their walls. Organization is deficient. (H&E. ×60)

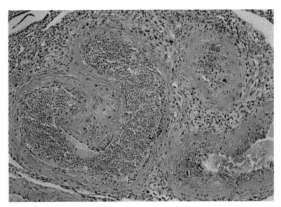

110 Subinvolution of placental site vessels, 4 weeks post partum A spiral arteriole within the regenerated endometrium maintains a tortuous, dilated configuration. The arteriolar wall is a collar of hyalinized decidua which extends up to the endothelial lining. Vascular thrombosis is minimal; there is no organization. (H&E. ×75)

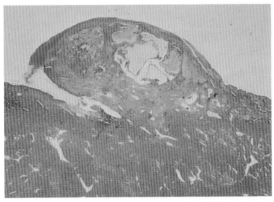

111 Retained hydatidiform mole (See Fig. 1506 for detail.) A polypoid structure composed of a few molar villi and proliferated trophoblasts projects above the endomyometrial junction. When this 22-year-old patient developed uterine bleeding 2 weeks after the mole was passed and curetted, a hysterectomy was done without further investigation or a second curettage. (H&E. ×15)

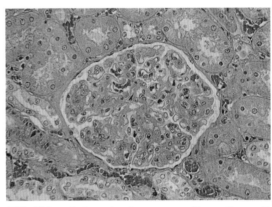

112 Kidney in toxemia of pregnancy The capillary wall and basement membrane of the glomerulus are thickened and increased in substance. Capillary lumens are narrowed, and the glomerular tuft is relatively ischemic. With H&E preparations, one cannot distinguish between actual thickening of the basement membrane and deposition of a new substance between the capillary endothelial cells and the membrane. (H&E. ×200)

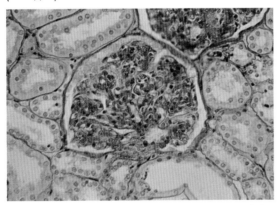

113 Kidney in toxemia of pregnancy Thickening of the basement membrane and capillary wall structure are shown in a section stained with periodic acid–Schiff. Again, one cannot distinguish between the capillary wall and the basement membrane. Patient 20 years old, para I. (PAS. ×200)

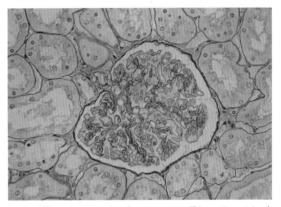

114 Kidney in toxemia of pregnancy This section stained with periodic acid–Schiff and then digested with diastase reveals a relatively thin basement membrane, suggesting that a deposited material has been enzymatically removed. (PAS stain with diastase digestion. ×200)

Plate 19

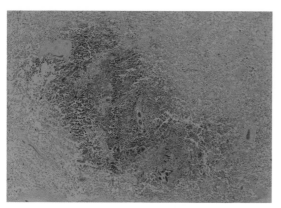

115   Placenta, full term, with "red infarct"   (H&E. ×36)

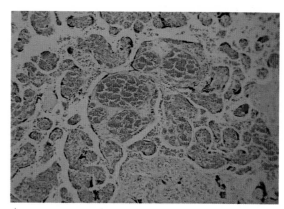

116   Placenta, full term, with "red infarct"   High magnification of Fig. 115. There is dilatation of fetal capillaries, congestion, and stasis. The intervillous spaces are narrowed and compressed. See Fig. 34A. (H&E. ×100)

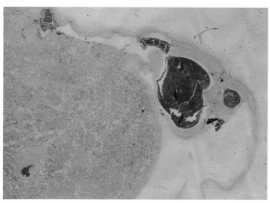

117   Rupture of the marginal sinus, full term placenta (H&E. ×7)

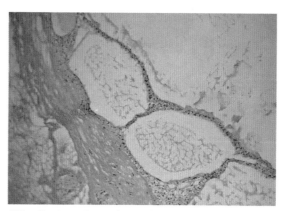

118   Chorionic placental cyst   (H&E. ×90)

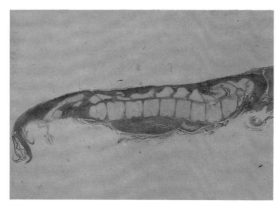

119   Fetus papiraceus   The fetus papiraceus was located plastered in amniochorionic membrane in a twin pregnancy. (H&E. ×4)

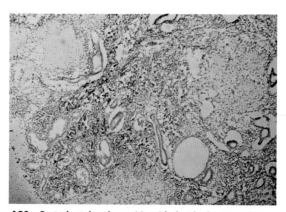

120   Post abortal endometritis with decidual rests and massive stromal hemosiderin deposition   Hemosiderin deposition in endometrial tissue is highly suspicious for an abortion. (H&E. ×50)

Plate 20

Part 3 *Chromosomal Aberrations in Gynecology*

by

Horst Naujoks, M.D.

Department of Obstetrics and Gynecology
University of Frankfurt am Main, Germany

17

Chromosomes and Their Aberrations

HUMAN CHROMOSOMES

The diploid chromosome set of somatic cells in man consists of 46 chromosomes. Two of these are gonosomes or sex chromosomes; in the female there are two X chromosomes, in the male there is one X and one Y chromosome. The 44 autosomes or non-sex chromosomes exist in 22 homologous pairs.

Chromosomes are best observed during the metaphase of the mitotic cycle when they are condensed. Cells of several tissues, including bone marrow, skin, and embryonic tissue, have been examined for their chromosomes. The most frequent currently used method is the analysis of chromosomes in white blood cells of the peripheral venous blood.

Chromosomal aberrations concern autosomes and sex chromosomes. They can be numerical (monosomy, trisomy, triploidy) or structural ones (deletion, translocation, isochromosome formation, inversion).

Numerical aberrations may be produced by disturbances during meiosis and mitosis. Nondisjunction and anaphase lag may lead to cells with an excess or loss of chromosomal material. The union of gametes with an irregular chromosome number results in an organism which may show a chromosomal defect in all its cells. The disturbance of chromosome distribution may also arise during early cleavage divisions, thus causing a chromosomal mosaic with two or more different chromosome sets in the cells of this organism. In man, the number of cells with aneuploidy will increase with age.[16]

Structural aberrations are consequences of chromosome breaks. These points of fracture show a tendency to stick to similarly broken ends. Several variations of structural anomalies are possible in this way and are also found in man.

Numerical aberrations of the X chromosome can be indicated by the number of sex chromatin bodies. In a normal diploid set the number of X chromosomes is one more than the number of sex chromatin bodies; thus two sex chromatin bodies would point to the existence of three X chromosomes. Structural aberrations of the X chromosome could be predicted by the size of the sex chromatin body, small ones indicating a deleted X chromosome, large ones an isochromosome X. Low sex chromatin counts may point to a case with sex chromosome mosaicism.

CHROMOSOMAL ABERRATIONS

Chromosomes in Metaphase

1 Air-dried metaphase plate of a human leukocyte culture, stained with May-Grünwald-Giemsa. Below the middle of the picture two small autosomes are overlapping slightly. The cells which go into mitosis under the influence of the bean extract phytohemagglutinin are most probably intermediate lymphocytes.

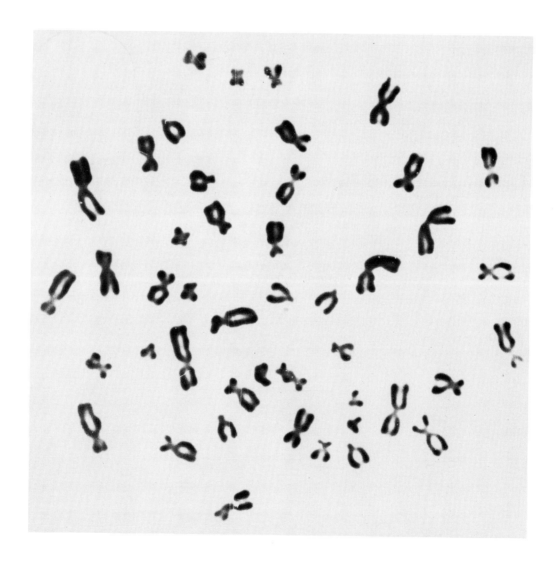

The Normal Karyotype

The normal human karyotype consists of 44 autosomes and two sex chromosomes. The 44 autosomes are paired according to their length and the seat of the centromere. The 22 pairs of autosomes are usually subdivided into seven groups A–G[28] since distinction between certain pairs is most difficult.

In the normal female chromosomal complement, there are two X chromosomes, whereas in the normal male, there is one X and one Y chromosome.

The Y chromosome corresponds in its size with the small acrocentric autosomes 21 and 22, but frequently shows more parallel long arms.

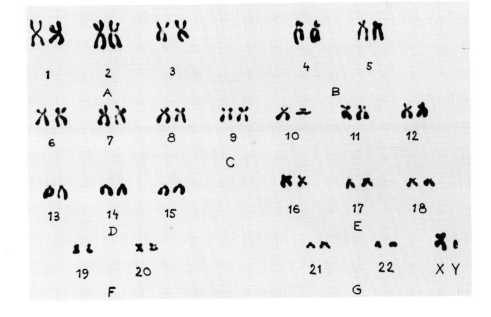

2   Female karyotype.

3   Male karyotype.

Numerical and Structural Aberrations

The main numerical chromosomal aberration is trisomy. The best-known example is trisomy of autosome 21 in Down's syndrome (mongolism). Less frequently encountered are trisomy of an autosome in group D (13–15) and trisomy of an autosome in group E (17–18). Both of the latter trisomies are seen in cases with multiple somatic anomalies (Patau's syndrome[27] and Edwards' syndrome[9]). Trisomy 22, trisomy 19, and trisomy 16 have also been described on rare occasions.

Cases with structural aberrations include those with translocation, deletion, inversion, or duplication of chromosomal segments. Translocation is the best-known example of a structural chromosome anomaly in man, because it is most easily identified. Down's syndrome which shows translocation between autosome 15 and the third autosome 21 (15/21 translocation) is an example of translocation.

4 Karyotype with a translocation chromosome in the normal mother of a translocation mongol. There are 45 chromosomes; autosome 15 and autosome 21 form the translocation chromosome. The chromosome set is genetically balanced, no autosome is missing, none is in excess

5 Karyotype of a newborn with multiple anomalies. There are 47 chromosomes due to trisomy in group E (17–18).

X Chromosome and Sex Chromatin

According to the standard of nomenclature of human mitotic chromosomes proposed by the Denver Study Group,[14] "the X chromosome resembles the longer chromosomes in group 6–12, especially chromosome 6 from which it is difficult to distinguish." One can assess the number of X chromosomes by determining the number of sex chromatin bodies (Barr bodies) in nuclei of the buccal or vaginal mucosa cells or in cells of the skin or of other somatic tissues. One Barr body indicates the presence of two X chromosomes, one of which forms the sex chromatin. A missing Barr body in the nuclei of these cells points to a chromosome set with only one X chromosome, this may be either a male karyotype (XY) or a deficient one, as in Turner's syndrome with 45 chromosomes due to the presence of only one sex chromosome, an X chromosome (XO).

By autoradiography it has been shown that each X chromosome in excess of one will present a late replicating pattern ("hot" X chromosome). This X chromosome is thought to form the sex chromatin. More refined techniques have shown that other X chromosomes ("cold" X chromosomes) may be also distinguished from the autosomes by a heavy labeling pattern of the long arms at the same time.[35]

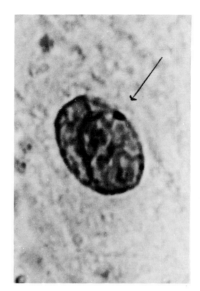 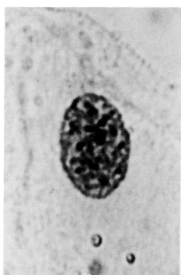

6 Sex chromatin–positive cell. (Cresyl violet)

7 Sex chromatin–negative cell. (Cresyl violet)

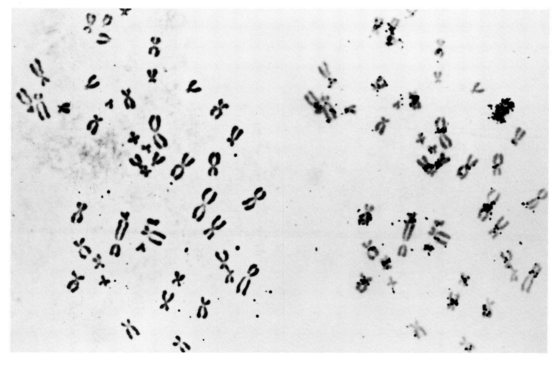

8 Female cell in metaphase, showing on the right the findings after autoradiography. The cell had begun to take up tritiated thymidine less than 5 hr before entering metaphase. The late replicating "hot" X chromosome is on the upper right.

Turner's Syndrome (XO)

Patient 28 years old.

Primary amenorrhea, short stature, multiple somatic anomalies, sex chromatin negative.

History. First medical consultation at 10 years of age because of short stature.

Findings. No breast development. Webbed neck. Low implantation of hair. Pigmented nevi. Coarctation of aorta. Thoracic kyphoscoliosis. Shortened fourth metacarpal bones. Diminished intelligence. Sparse pubic and axillary hair. External genitalia female, but infantile labia and vagina. Clitoris not enlarged. Uterus small. The 17-ketosteroid and estrogen excretion low. Gonadotropin excretion elevated.

The first description of this chromosome anomaly was given in C. E. Ford et al., A sex chromosome anomaly in a case of gonadal dysgenesis (Turner's syndrome), *Lancet,* 1: 711, 1959.

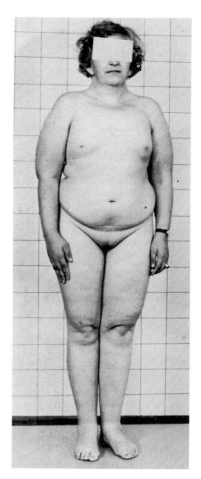

9 Patient with Turner's syndrome, described by Lindsten.

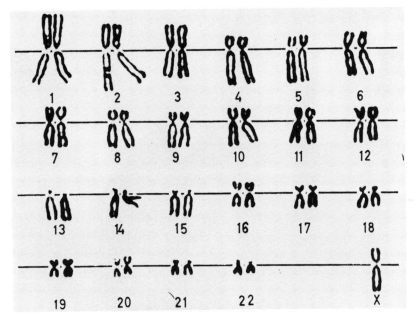

10 Karyotype of the patient. 45 chromosomes due to a missing sex chromosome (XO).

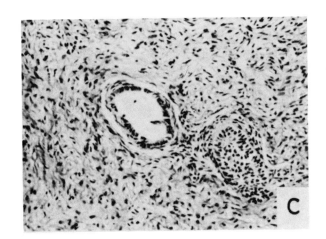

11 Gonadal tissues in an XO case. Remnants of mesonephric ducts are found in the inner layer of the connective tissue. (×150)

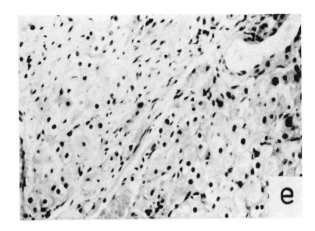

12 Same case as in Fig. 11. Cluster of hilar cells. (×190)

Turner's Syndrome (XO/XX isochromosome Mosaicism)

Patient 17 years old.

Primary amenorrhea. Short stature. Sex chromatin positive.

History. Normal mental development. Short stature since infancy. First medical consultation at age 14 because of short stature. Estrogen therapy started at that time.

Findings. Height 1.42 m; weight 42 kg. No webbing of neck; low hairline in neck. Strabismus of left eye. Pigmented nevi. Bilateral perceptive hearing impairment. Short fourth metacarpal and metatarsal bones. Breast development and growth of pubic and axillary hair only after estrogen therapy. Infantile labia, clitoris, vagina, and uterus. The 17-ketosteroid excretion in low normal range, gonadotropin excretion normal, estrogen excretion low.

The first description of the XX isochromosome constitution was given in M. Fraccaro et al., A new type of chromosomal abnormality in gonadal dysgenesis, *Lancet*, 2: 1144, 1960.

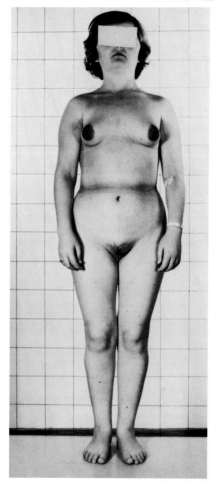

13 Patient after 3 years of estrogen therapy, described by Lindsten.

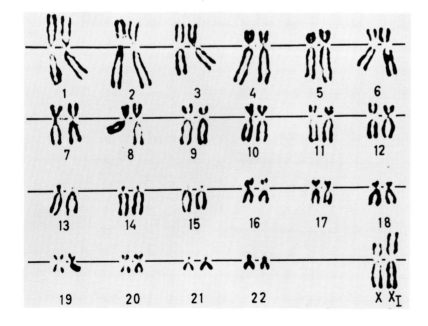

14 Karyotype of an XX isochromosome cell of the patient.

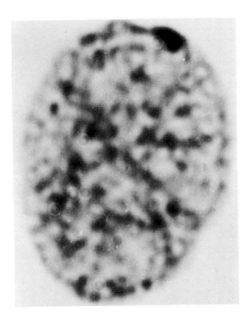

15 Distinct sex chromatin in a cell of this patient. In XX isochromosome cases, the sex chromatin may be larger than in XX cells.

16 Microscopic view of gonadal tissue in an XO/XX isochromosome case. Ectopic adrenal cortex found in a streak gonad. Outside a thin capsule, indicated by the arrow, cells of the type found in the hilar region of normal ovaries. (×40)

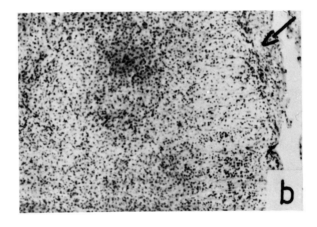

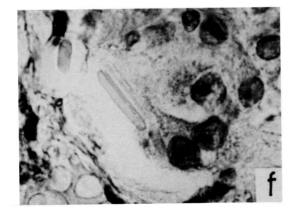

17 Higher magnification of these hilar cells. Crystalloids of the Reinke type of testicular Leydig cells are seen. (×820)

Triple-X Female (XXX)

Patient 16 years old.

Oligomenorrhea. Obesity. Feeble-mindedness and instability. No somatic anomalies.

Findings. Female appearance, with well-developed breasts. Obesity with striae. Sparse pubic hair. No axillary hair. Narrow vagina. Small uterus and inconspicuous adnexal regions. Normal excretion of gonadotropins, 17-ketosteroids, and corticoids.

Sex chromatin

Buccal smear
   Chromatin-negative cells: 38.67 per cent
   Chromatin-positive cells
      One Barr body: 44.67 per cent
      Two Barr bodies: 16.66 per cent
Leukocyte test
   One drumstick: 8 per 500 leukocytes
   Two drumsticks: 1 per 2,000 leukocytes

The first description of the XXX syndrome was given in P. A. Jacobs et al., Evidence for the existence of the human "super female," *Lancet*, 2: 423, 1959.

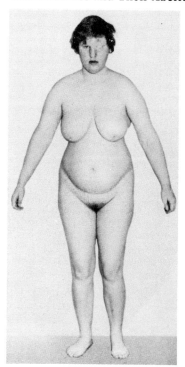

18 Patient with three X-Chromosomes.

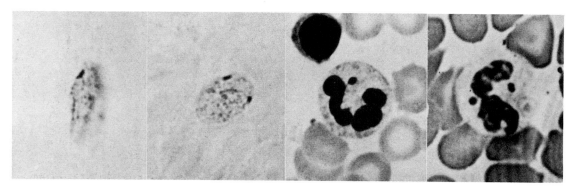

19 Sex chromatin pattern and drumsticks in the same case. Single and double Barr bodies and drumsticks. (×1,800)

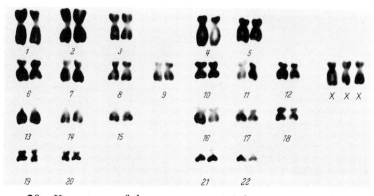

20 Karyotype of the same case. 47 chromosomes, due to three X chromosomes.

Triple-X Female (XXX) (with fertility)

Patient 60 years old.

Gravida I, para I (32-year-old son). No somatic anomalies.

History. Patient is tenth of 11 siblings. Finished school and later worked in factories. Married and became pregnant at 27 years. Has been a patient in a mental institution for the last 5 years. Increasing dementia probably due to cerebral atrophy.

Findings. Female appearance. Obesity. No external anomalies. Female genitalia.

Sex chromatin

Buccal smear

   Chromatin-negative cells : 50.50 per cent

   Chromatin-positive cells

      One Barr body : 37.50 per cent

      Two Barr bodies : 12.00 per cent

Leukocyte test

   One drumstick : 7 per 500 leukocytes

   Two drumsticks : 0 per 500 leukocytes

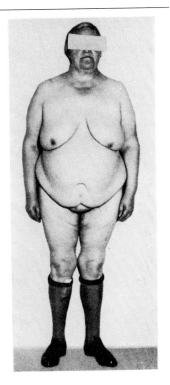

21 Patient with three X-Chromosomes, described by Hienz et al.

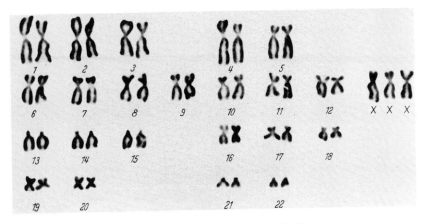

22 Karyotype of the same patient. 47 chromosomes, due to three X chromosomes.

Ring Chromosome in Gonadal Dysgenesis

Patient 20 years old.

Primary amenorrhea. Small stature. Chromatin positive.

History. Premature, with a birth weight 2,000 Gm. Medical consultation at 16 years of age because of primary amenorrhea and small stature. Hormonal therapy started at that time.

Findings. Short broad neck. No webbing. Deep hairline. Micrognathia. Moderate bilateral ptosis. High palate. No breast development. Small nipples far apart. Sparse pubic and axillary hair. Scoliosis of thoracic spine due to unilateral flattening of fourth and fifth vertebra. Pigmented nevi. Osteoporosis. Uterus very small. Vagina infantile and short.

Course. Following hormone therapy, some development of breasts, pubic and axillary hair, and growth of vagina and uterus. Increase in height of 3 cm within 2 years; at 19 years of age epiphyseal lines of radius and ulna still open. Persistent apophysis of iliac bone and ischium.

Sex chromatin

Buccal smears: 9 per cent chromatin-positive cells (2 per cent with markedly small Barr body).

Vaginal smear: 3 per cent chromatin-positive cells. No drumsticks.

Chromosome analysis

Karyotype	45/XO	45/X+ ring	46/XX	46/X+ ring	46/XX+ fragment
Number of cells	61	1	14	5	2

The first description of the ring form of an X chromosome was given in J. Lindsten and K. G. Tillinger, Self-perpetuating ring chromosome in a patient with gonadal dysgenesis, _Lancet_, 1: 593, 1962.

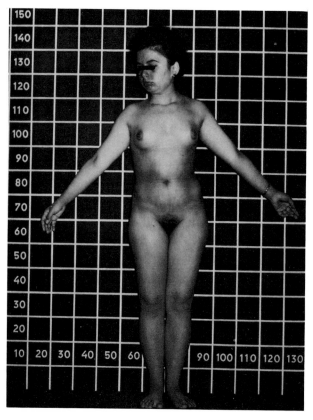

23 Patient with mosaicism and ring chromosomes, described by Lüers et al., after hormone therapy.

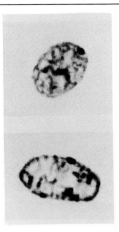

24 Sex chromatin–positive cells of the buccal mucosa.

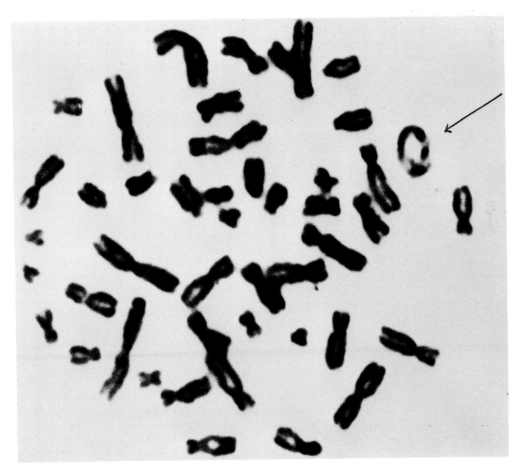

25 Metaphase plate with the ring chromosome (*arrow*).

Deleted X Chromosome (Xx)

Patient 21 years old.

Primary amenorrhea.

Findings. Normal female distribution of body hair. Poor breast development only after long-lasting hormone treatment. Slight retardation of skeletal maturation. Inconspicuous external genitalia. Uterus hypoplastic. Ovaries not felt on palpation. Excretion of hypophyseal gonadotropin markedly reduced.

Sex chromatin

Buccal smear: 8.5 per cent chromatin-positive cells, of which about one-half showed considerably smaller Barr bodies.

Chromosome analysis

Karyotype	46/XX	46/Xx
Number of cells	32	22

The first description of a deleted X chromosome was given in P. A. Jacobs et al., Abnormalities involving the X-chromosome in women, *Lancet*, 1: 1213, 1960.

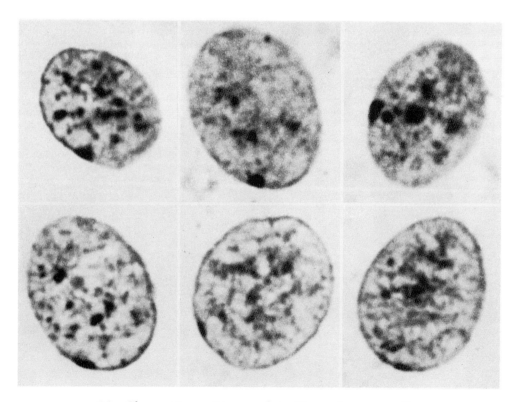

26   Chromatin-positive nuclei of buccal smear cells. The three cell nuclei in the upper row show distinct Barr bodies, the three nuclei in the lower row contain very small Barr bodies. (×4,400)

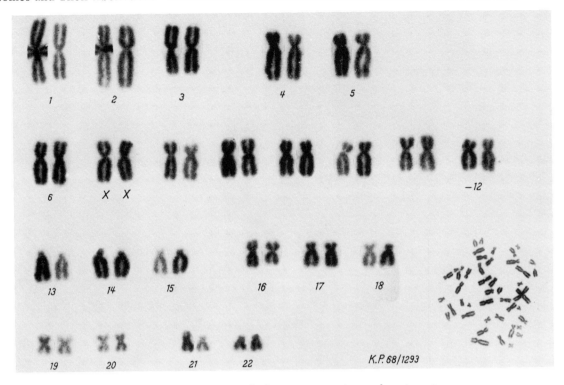

27 A karyotype of the same patient showing two inconspicuous X chromosomes.

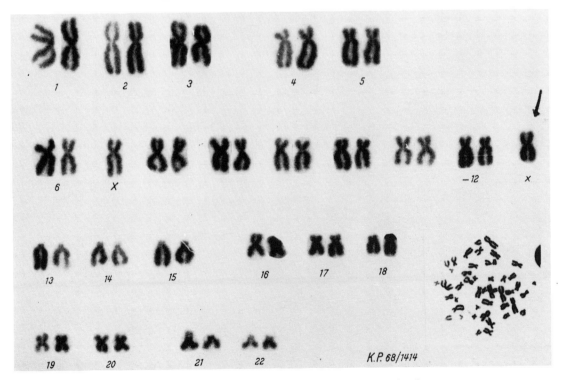

28 A karyotype of the same patient which shows beside one regular X chromosome another chromosome which is thought to present the other X chromosome with a deletion of the long arms. The cell line with a deleted X chromosome can explain the occurrence of cell nuclei with small Barr bodies.

Testicular Feminization (XY)

Patient 21 years old, not married.

Primary amenorrhea. Sex chromatin negative.

History. During childhood two small tumors had been observed in the inguinal region. They enlarged to the size of a pigeon's egg. At age 16 an operation for bilateral inguinal hernia was performed. At this time probably the tumors were placed in the abdomen because sexual development had continued with breast development which had started at age 13. Growth of some pubic hair. Axillary hair missing.

Findings. Infantile labia minora. Clitoris not enlarged. Length of vagina 7 to 8 cm. Cervix and uterine fundus not felt on palpation. A tumor measuring 2 by 2 cm present on left side in small pelvis. Excretion of 17-ketosteroids and gonadotropins in normal range, excretion of estrogens in lower normal range.

Pedigree. Two sisters, two aunts, one great-aunt, one cousin with the syndrome.

The first description of this chromosome anomaly was given in P. A. Jacobs et al., Chromosomal sex in the syndrome of testicular feminization, *Lancet*, 2: 591, 1959.

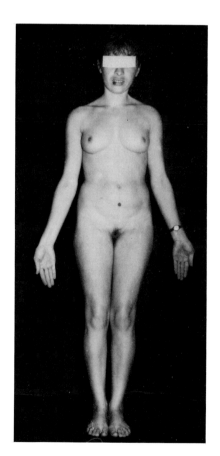

29 Patient with testicular feminization, described by Rabau et al.

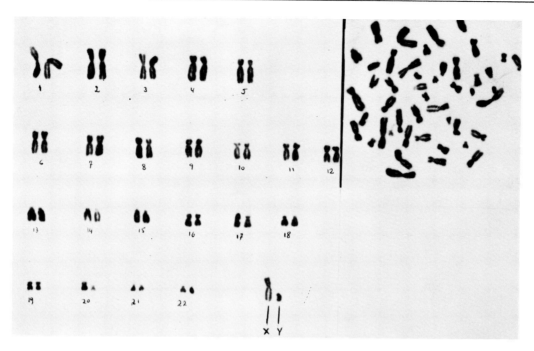

30 Karyotype of the case, with one X and one Y chromosome.

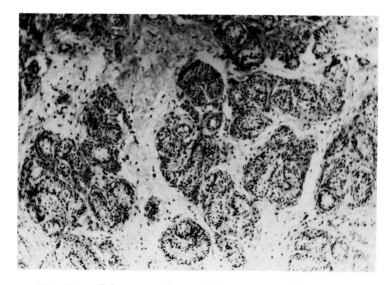

31 Gonadal tissue of one of the sisters of this patient. The seminiferous tubules without signs of spermatogenesis. Hypertrophied Sertoli cells. Interstitial cells correspond to Leydig cells. (H + E. ×45)

Vestigial Pelvic Organs, Absent Gonads and XY

Patient 17 years old.

Primary amenorrhea. Chromatin negative.

Findings. Height 1.65 m. Minimal breast development with poor and rather widely spaced nipples. Sparse pubic and axillary hair. Normal sized clitoris. Minute blind pit in region of vaginal introitus. Labia majora not well developed. Labia minora appeared to be fused in midline.

Laparotomy. No gonads and no internal genital organs, except tiny remnants on lateral pelvic wall on each side.

Histology. Each of the two strips composed of a small tubular structure, morphologically resembling an immature uterine horn, and of a part of fibromuscular tissue with tubules of Wolffian duct type.

Hormone assay. Estriol 8 μg per day; estrone 5 μg per day; estradiol 3 μg per day; gonadotropins 135 mouse units per day; 17-ketosteroids 7.1 mg per day; 17-ketogenic steroids 18.7 mg per day.

Chromosome analysis

Karyotype	45	46/XY	47
Number of cells	2	58	1

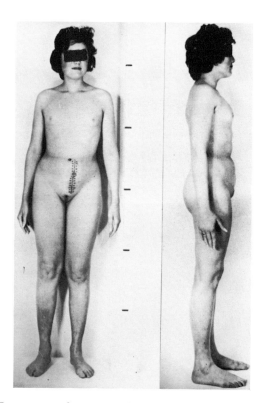

32 Patient with minimal breast development and sparse pubic hair. No virilization. Described by Dewhurst, et al.

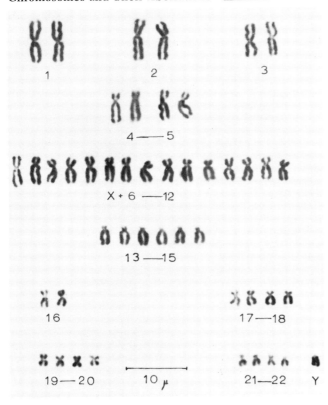

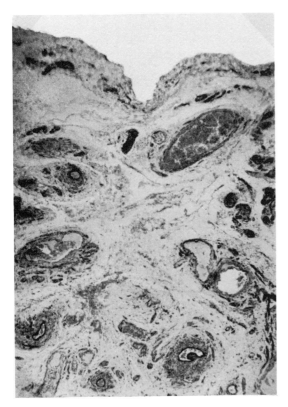

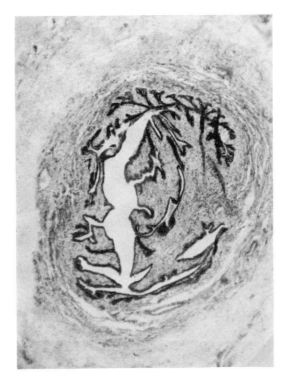

33 Karyotype of the same patient with one X and one Y chromosome.

34 Microscopic view of the tiny remnants. Small tubules of mesonephric duct origin. (H + E. ×30)

35 Microscopic view of the tiny remnants. A tubular structure of Müllerian duct origin, resembling an immature uterine horn. (H + E. ×30)

Klinefelter's Syndrome (XXY)

Patient 22 years old.

Slight gynecomastia, small testicles, female distribution of hair. Sex chromatin positive.

Findings. Height 1.71 m. Scanty beard hair. Normal axillary hair. Pubic hair with female distribution. Male external genital organs. Left testicle in inguinal canal. Right testicle of bean size. Male voice.

Drumsticks: 27 of 1,000 polymorphonuclear leukocytes with one drumstick.

Gonadotropins: not demonstrable.

The first description of this chromosome anomaly was given in P. A. Jacobs and J. A. Strong, A case of human intersexuality having a possible XXY sex-determining mechanism, *Nature*, 183: 302, 1959.

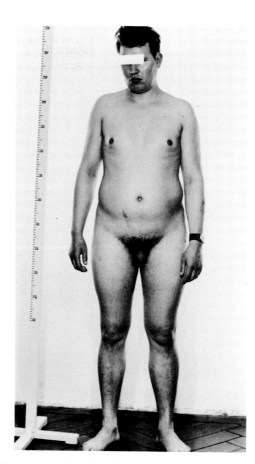

36 Patient with Klinefelter's syndrome, described by Moerchen.

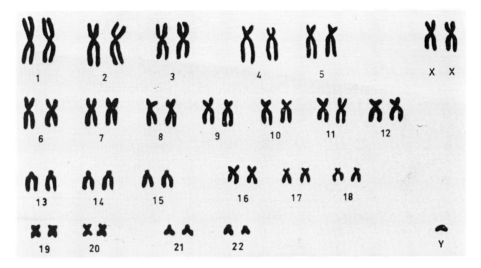

37 Karyotype of the patient with 47 chromosomes due to three sex chromosomes, two X chromosomes and one Y chromosome.

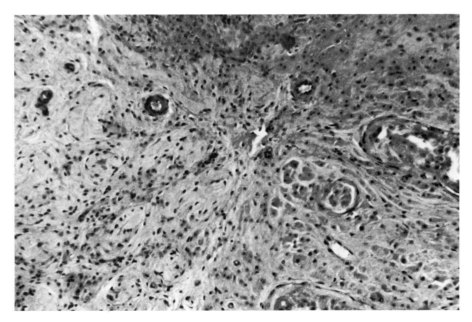

38 Testicular biopsy: nearly all the tubules are hyalinized; few atrophic seminiferous tubules are lined only by Sertoli cells. Focal increase of Leydig cells. (H + E. ×100)

Down's Syndrome (Mongolism) with Trisomy 21

Patient 35 years old.

History. Age of parents at birth of patient: mother 44 years old, father 41.

Findings. Regular menstrual periods. Congenital heart defect, clinically diagnosed as an interventricular septal defect with a right to left shunt, right ventricular hypertrophy, and pulmonary hypertension. Hands without simian line, but right hand with a distal triaxial triradius. Ears somewhat small and low set. Brushfield spots apparent. I.Q. 37.

The first description of the chromosome anomaly was given in J. Lejeune, M. Gautier, and R. Turpin, Etudes des chromosomes somatiques de neuf enfants mongoliens, *Compt. Rend. Acad. Sci. (Paris),* 248: 1721, 1959.

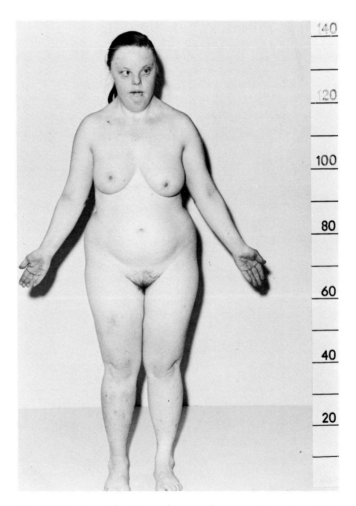

39 Patient with Down's syndrome, described by Breg.

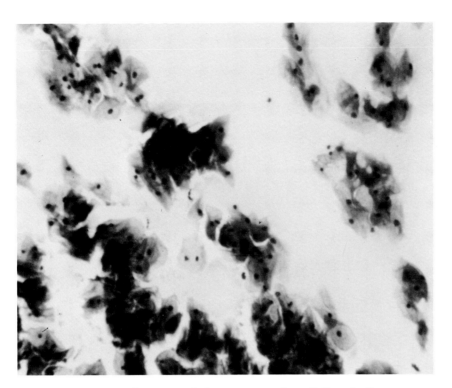

40 Vaginal smear of the patient taken 5 days before onset of menstrual bleeding, indicating progesterone effect. (×220)

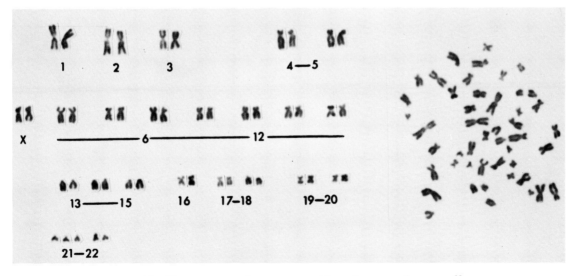

41 Karyotype of patient with trisomy of a small acrocentric autosome, suggesting trisomy 21.

CONCLUDING REMARKS

Sex chromatin determination and chromosome analysis have been applied in other areas of gynecology beside in the cases mentioned above.

The suspicion of chromosome anomalies in the tissues of *spontaneous abortions* has been confirmed by recent investigations. Aberrations in the chromosome set, such as trisomy 13–15, trisomy 17–18, trisomy 21, monosomy of the sex chromosomes (XO), and triploidy, have been found.[3, 5, 7, 29]

The incidence of *habitual abortions* also raised the suspicion of chromosomal aberrations in the parental gametes which could contribute to an early devitalization of the embryo by a defect chromosome set.

In a series of 10 couples with repeated abortions a chromosome aberration, a translocation, has been found in the male of one couple and in his father, both of whom were phenotypically normal.[34]

The examination of the sex chromatin in cells in the amniotic fluid which were shed from skin and mucous membranes of the fetus made possible a *prenatal sex determination.*[8, 18, 33, 36]

A report from Denmark pointed to the practical significance of this investigation. A legal interruption of pregnancy which was granted because of hemophilia in a previously born boy was withheld after the examination of the amniotic fluid showed chromatin-positive cells. This indicated that the child in utero was of female sex which was found to be correct after the birth of the child.[32]

The *malformations of the external genitalia* in the newborn are found to be either an incomplete masculinization of the male genitalia or a masculinization of the female genitalia.[10] Clinically these cases may show close similarities. The sex chromatin determination and the chromosome analysis may help to establish the correct diagnosis.

Some cases show intersexual external genitalia and a *positive* sex chromatin pattern: masculinization of female external genitalia due to the influence of a maternal arrhenoblastoma, due to the application of masculinizing drugs to the mother during pregnancy, and due to an adrenogenital syndrome of the child. All these newborns have a female chromosome complement (XX). In this group, cases with true hermaphroditism (XX) or with Klinefelter's syndrome (XXY) which mostly cannot be diagnosed at birth are rare because the male external genitalia ordinarily does not pose any problem at birth.

Cases with intersexual external genitalia and a *negative* sex chromatin pattern are seen rarely and may include hermaphrodites, e.g., with an XO/XY mosaic structure, or newborns with testicular failure. The testicular feminization syndrome is rarely diagnosed at birth because of the female external genitalia.

Difficulties in the differential diagnosis can be over-

SPONTANEOUS ABORTIONS

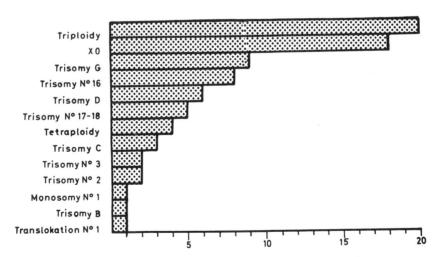

42 Abnormal chromosome findings in 80 out of 292 spontaneous abortions examined by nine groups of investigators.

583

come by applying the modern techniques of sex chromatin determination and chromosome analysis as is shown in the following case.[37]

A mother who had received stilbestrol during the 12th to 16th week of her pregnancy had borne a chromatin-positive baby who showed an enlarged clitoris with a terminal meatal dimple and a ventral chordee and with an opening for the urethra into a small vaginal vault. X-ray examination indicated a vagina, uterus, and tubes. At first one suspected a congenital adrenal hyperplasia. After obtaining the maternal history, these malformations were thought to have occurred as a result of the hormone treatment. But the chromosome analysis showed a mosaic structure with XX cells and XY cells. A true hermaphrodite was suspected, and a laparotomy which revealed an ovary and an ovotestis proved the diagnosis to be correct.

Besides the newborns with testicular feminization or Klinefelter's syndrome, those with Turner's syndrome (XO) may also be easily overlooked at birth unless routine examinations of buccal smears for sex chromatin are performed.

The number of newborns with differences between

anatomic and chromosomal sex has been determined by investigating the sex chromatin patterns and partly the karyotype in a large series of normal cases.[2, 19, 23] About 2 to 3 per cent of those with male external genitalia were chromatin-positive (XXY); 0.3 to 0.5 per mille showed female external genitalia and were chromatin-negative (XO); 1 per mille had female external genitalia and had a double sex chromatin, indicating the triple-X syndrome (XXX).

More recently, sex chromatin determination and chromosome analysis have been used in the investigation of cases with disturbed ovarian function causing *primary or secondary amenorrhea.* A large series of cases showed different chromosome abnormalities, even mosaic structures.[6, 11, 12, 15, 20, 30] Figs. 43 and 44.

It must be left to further investigations to indicate how far these results can be of value in the practice of gynecology.

Chromosomal studies have also been shown to be of value in the investigation of gonadal tumors.[31]

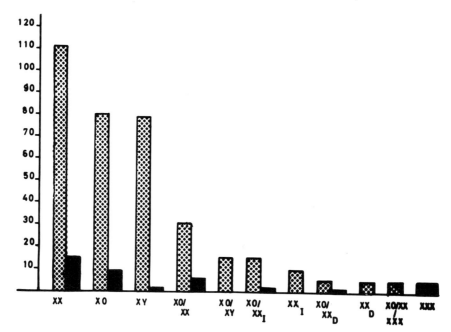

43 Distribution of chromosome findings in 386 cases with primary amenorrhea (dotted columns) and in 45 cases with pathologic secondary amenorrhea (black columns) as described in the literature.

Beside cases with one stemline (e.g. XO) there are cases with chromosomal mosaicism (e.g. XO/XY).

X_D is a deleted X-Chromosome. X_I is an X-isochromosome.

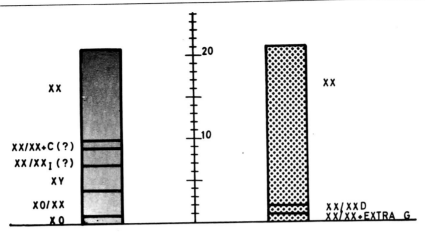

44 Results of chromosome analysis by using the lymphocyte culture of peripheral blood. 10 of 21 cases with primary amenorrhea (gray column) and 2 of 21 cases with pathologic secondary amenorrhea (dotted column) show cells with karyotypes differing from the normal female complement with two X-chromosomes (unpublished investigations).

ACKNOWLEDGEMENTS

Sincere gratitude is expressed herewith to the authors and publishers for permission to reprint the following illustrations, and thus for their support in compiling this material.

Fig. 4. Breg, W. Roy, Miller, O. J., and Schmickel, R. D., Chromosomal translocations in patients with mongolism and in their normal relatives, *New Engl. J. Med.*, 226: 845, 1962.

Fig. 8. Schmid, W., DNA replication patterns of human chromosomes, *Cytogenetics*, 2: 175, 1963. (S. Karger Basel, New York)

Figs. 9–17. Lindsten, J., "The Nature and Origin of X-chromosome Aberrations in Turner's Syndrome," Almquist & Wiksell, Stockholm, 1963.

Fig. 18–22. Hienz, H. A., Michael, C. M., Schulz, F. W., and Walter, K., Zur Trisomie des X-Chromosoms, *Klin. Wochschr.*, 41: 996, 1963. (Springer, Heidelberg)

Fig. 23–25. Lüers, Th., Nevinny-Stickel, J., and Struck, E., Ringchromosom bei Gonadendysgenesie, *Geburtsh. Frauenheilk.*, 24: 173, 1964. (G. Thieme, Stuttgart)

Fig. 26–28. Gropp, A., von Krosigk, H., Odunjo, F., Zander, J., Kern, E., and Buntru, G., Chromosomenmosaike bei primärer Amenorrhoe, *Klin. Wochschr.*, 41: 345, 1963. (Springer, Heidelberg)

Fig. 29–31. Rabau, E., David, A., Mashiah, S., Lunenfeld, B., and Leiba, S., Syndrome familial de feminisation testiculaire, *Compt. Rend. Soc. Française Gynécol.*, vol. 4, 1963.

Fig. 32–35. Dewhurst, C. J., Paine, C. G., and Blank, C. E., An XY female with absent gonads and vestigial pelvic organs, *J. Obstet. Gynaecol. Brit. Commonwealth*, 70: 675, 1963.

Fig. 36–38. Dr. Moerchen, doctoral thesis. Department of Dermatology, University of Frankfurt (Germany)

Figs. 39 and 41. Breg, W. Roy, M.D. Southbury Training School, Southbury, Conn., U.S.A.

Fig. 40. Tricomi, V., Valenti, C., and Hall, J. E., Ovulatory patterns in Down's syndrome, *Am. J. Obstet. Gynecol.*, 89: 651, 1964.

The support of the *Deutsche Forschungsgemeinschaft* is gratefully acknowledged.

Horst Naujoks

GLOSSARY

acrocentric. Relating to a centromere placed near one end of the chromosome. Acrocentric chromosomes in man are the autosomes 13–15 and 21–22 and the Y chromosome.

anaphase lag. Occurs when the daughter chromosomes move apart during anaphase and one lags and gets lost, thus causing one of the daughter cells to contain a deficient diploid chromosome set (2*n*-1), the other one being normal (2*n*).

aneuploidy. Numerical abnormality in the chromosome set due to lack or addition of chromosomes (see monosomy and polysomy).

autosome. Nonsex chromosome. In man there are 22 pairs of autosomes in somatic cells.

centromere. The point at which the fibers of the mitotic spindle contact the chromosome and which is the last part of it to divide. Synonym: primary or centric constriction, kinetochore.

chromatid. One of the two strands which after duplication of the chromosome are clearly seen at metaphase and which get separated after the division of the centromere. The chromatids form the daughter chromosomes.

chromatin. A component part of the nucleus forming the chromosomal material. Heterochromatin: condensed zones and heavier stained regions in the chromosome during interphase. Antonym: euchromatin.

deletion. Loss of a segment of the chromosome, either a terminal or an interstitial one.

diploid. Chromosome set in somatic cells (2*n*), in man 46 chromosomes.

drumstick. Small accessory nuclear lobule in polymorphonuclear leukocytes. Six drumsticks in 500 polymorphonuclear leukocytes indicate female chromosomal sex.

gonosomes. Sex chromosomes. In the human female two X chromosomes, in the human male one X and one Y chromosome.

haploid. The chromosome set in the gametes (*n*). In man, 22 autosomes and one sex chromosome.

inversion. Structural rearrangement of a chromosome segment which after two breaks becomes inverted 180 deg within the linear order of the chromosome.

isochromosome. A chromosome which is perfectly metacentric with two homologous arms. It has been formed out of a chromosome which went through a misdivision. Thus the chromatids did not separate longitudinally but transversely in the centromere.

metacentric. Relating to a centromere situated in the middle of the chromosome. In man, the autosomes 3, 16, 19, 20.

monosomy. One chromosome missing in the diploid chromosome set (2*n*-1). In man, e.g., monosomy of the sex chromosome (XO).

nondisjunction. Event during meiosis or mitosis leading to an anomaly of chromosome distribution and causing the formation of two daughter cells one with an extra chromosome, the other short of the chromosome. In nondisjunction during meiosis, either two paired chromosomes do not separate or two chromosomes do not pair and are distributed at random.

polyploidy. More than two sets of homologous chromosomes (2*n*), such as triploidy (3*n*), tetraploidy (4*n*), etc.

polysomy. Addition of one or more chromosomes to a diploid chromosome set, such as trisomy (2*n* + 1).

primary constriction. See centromere.

ring chromosome. Structural anomaly of the chromosome formed by interchange between the two arms of one chromosome.

satellites. Small segments which are separated from the end of a chromosome by a fine chromatic filament. In man, satellites are shown to exist on all acrocentric autosomes.

secondary constriction. Weakly stained parts of the chromosome which impress as constrictions. In man, used for the identification of certain chromosomes.

sex chromatin. A planoconvex deeply stained chromatin particle, measuring 0.8 by 1.1μ, which adheres to the nuclear membrane of the interphase nucleus. These cells are called chromatin-positive and point to the existence of two X chromosomes in the nucleus, one of which forms the sex chromatin (Barr body). Cells without the sex chromatin are chromatin-negative and indicate the presence of only one X chromosome in the diploid chromosome set.

submetacentric. Relating to a centromere situated between the middle and one of the ends of the chromosome.

translocation. Transfer of one segment of the chromosome to another part of the same chromosome or to another chromosome. This involves two chromosome breaks. The union of two chromosomes forms a translocation chromosome, e.g., the translocation between an autosome 15 and 21 (15/21 translocation) in some cases with Down's syndrome (mongolism). The small broken parts of these chromosomes get lost during mitosis if they lack a centromere.

trisomy. A form of polysomy. One chromosome in the diploid set is present in triplicate (2*n* + 1), e.g., in mongolism with a trisomy of autosome 21.

BIBLIOGRAPHY

1. Bergada, C., Cleveland, W. W., Jones, H. W., Jr., and Wilkins, L.: Gonadal histology in patients with male pseudohermaphroditism and atypical gonadal dysgenesis: relation to theories of sex differentiation, *Acta Endocrinol.*, 40: 493, 1962.

2. Bergemann, E.: Die Häufigkeit des Abweichens vom normalen Geschlechtschromatin and eine Familienuntersuchung bei Triplo X, *Helvetia Med. Acta*, 29: 420, 1962.

3. Carr, D. H.: Chromosome studies in spontaneous abortions. Obstet. & Gynecol. 26: 308 (1965).

4. Clarke, C. M.: Techniques in the study of human chromosomes, in J. L. Hamerton, "Chromosomes in Medicine," William Heinemann, Ltd., London, 1962.

5. Clendenin, Th. M., and Benirschke, K.: Chromosome studies on spontaneous abortions, *Lab. Invest.*, 12: 1281, 1963.

6. De la Chapelle, A.: Cytogenetical and clinical observations in female gonadal dysgenesis, *Acta Endocrinol. Suppl.*, vol. 65, 1962.

7. Delhanty, J. D. A., Ellis, J. R., and Rowley, P. T.: Triploid cells in human embryo, *Lancet*, 1: 1286, 1961.

8. Dewhurst, C. J.: Diagnosis of sex before birth, *Lancet*, 1: 471, 1956.

9. Edwards, J. H., Harnden, D. G., Cameron, A. H., Crosse, V. M., and Wolff, O. H.: A new trisomic syndrome, *Lancet*, 1: 787, 1960.

10. Gordon, R. R., and Dewhurst, C. J.: Ambiguous sex in the newborn, *Lancet*, 2: 872, 1962.

11. Gropp, A., Krosigk, H. v., Odunjo, F., Zander, J., Kern, E., and Buntru, G.: Chromosomenmosaike bei primärer Amenorrhoe, *Klin. Wochschr.*, 41: 345, 1963.

12. Grouchy, J. de, Lamy, M., Yaneva, H., Salomon, Y., and Netter, A.: Further abnormalities of the X-chromosome in primary amenorrhea or in severe oligomenorrhea, *Lancet*, 2: 777, 1961.

13. Hamerton, J. L.: "Chromosomes in Medicine," William Heinemann, Ltd., London, 1962.

14. Human Chromosomes Study Group: A proposal of nomenclature of human mitotic chromosomes, *Lancet*, 1: 1063, 1960.

15. Jacobs, P. A., Harnden, D. G., Buckton, K. E., Court-Brown, W. M., King, M. J., McBride, J. A., MacGregor, T. N., and MacLean, N.: Cytogenetic studies in primary amenorrhea, *Lancet*, 1: 1183, 1961.

16. Jacobs, P. A., Court-Brown, W. M., and Doll, R.: Distribution of human chromosome counts in relation to age, *Nature*, 191: 1178, 1961.

17. Jones, H. W., Jr., Ferguson-Smith, M. A., and Heller, R. H.: The pathology and cytogenetics of gonadal agenesis, *Am. J. Obstet. Gynecol.*, 87: 578, 1963.

18. Lin, T. J., Vasicka, A., and Bennett, A. E.: Prenatal determination of the sex of the baby, *Am. J. Obstet. Gynecol.*, 79: 938, 1960.

19. MacLean, N., Harnden, D. G., and Court-Brown, W. M.: Abnormalities of sex chromosome constitution in newborn babies, *Lancet*, 2: 406, 1961.

20. Miller, O. J.: The sex chromosome anomalies. *Am. J. Obstet. Gynecology* 90: 1078 (1964).

21. McKusick, V. A.: On the X-chromosome of man, *Am. Inst. Biol. Sci.*, 1964.

22. Montagu, M. F. Ashley: "Genetic Mechanism in Human Disease," Charles C Thomas, Publisher, Springfield, Ill., 1961.

23. Moore, K. L.: Sex reversal in newborn babies, *Lancet*, 1: 217, 1959.

24. Moorhead, P. S.: Chromosome preparations of leucocytes cultured from human peripheral blood, *Exptl. Cell Res.*, 20: 613, 1960.

25. Morris, J. McLean, and Mahesh, V. B.: Further observations on the syndrome of testicular feminization, *Am. J. Obstet. Gynecol.*, 87: 731, 1963.

26. Overzier, C.: Die Intersexualität, Georg Thieme Verlag KG, Stuttgart, 1961. ("The Intersexuality," Academic Press Inc., New York, 1963.)

27. Patau, K., Smith, D. W., Therman, E., Inhorn, S. L., and Wagner, H. P.: Multiple congenital anomalies caused by an extra autosome, *Lancet*, 1: 790, 1960.

28. Patau, K.: Chromosome identification and the Denver report, *Lancet*, 1: 933, 1961.

29. Penrose, L. S., and Delhanty, J. D. A.: Triploid cell cultures from a macerated fetus, *Lancet*, 1: 1261, 1961.

30. Philip, J., Sele, V., Trolle, D.: Primary amenorrhea. A study of 101 cases. *Fertility & Sterility*, 16: 795, 1965.

31. Philip, J., and Teter, J.: Significance of chromosomal investigation of somatic cells to determine the genetic origin of gonadoblastoma, *Acta Pathol. Microbiol. Scand.*, 61: 543, 1964.

32. Riis, P., and Fuchs, F.: Antenatal determination of foetal sex in prevention of hereditary diseases, *Lancet*, 2: 180, 1960.

33. Sachs, L., Serr, D. M., and Danon, M.: Analysis of amniotic fluid cells for diagnosis of foetal sex, *Brit. Med. J.*, 2: 795, 1956.

34. Schmid, W.: A familial chromosome abnormality associated with repeated abortions, *Cytogenetics*, 1: 199, 1962.

35. Schmid, W.: DNA replication patterns of human chromosomes, *Cytogenetics,* 2: 175, 1963.

36. Shettles, L. B.: Nuclear morphology of cells in human amniotic fluid in relation to the sex of the infant, *Am. J. Obstet. Gynecol.,* 71: 834, 1956.

37. Waxman, S. H., Gartler, S. M., and Kelley, V. C.: Apparent masculinization of the female fetus diagnosed as true hermaphroditism by chromosome studies, *J. Pediat.,* 60: 540, 1962.

Index

Italicized numbers refer to color illustrations

Special Index for Chapter 17, Chromosomal Aberrations in Gynecology, starts on page 610

Abortion, incomplete, retained, curetted tissue, 478, 480
  induced, curetted tissue, 484
  septic, kidney, 486
    myometrium, 484
    placentitis, 496
Abscess, Bartholin's gland, 14
  ovary, 288
    caused by Enterobius (Oxyuris) vermicularis, 290
Acanthosis nigricans, malignant, vulva, 28
Accessory oviduct, 250
Actinomycosis, pelvic tissue, 434
  vulva, 22
Adenoacanthoma, Bartholin's gland, 64
  cervix, 146
  endometrium, 198
  ovary, 326
Adenocarcinoma, Bartholin's gland, 62
  adenoid cystic type, 64
  mucus-secreting, 64
  cervix, cylindromatous, 148
    moderately differentiated, 144
    papillary, 144, 146
    poorly differentiated, 146, 34
    well differentiated, 144
  development in ovarian endometriosis, 302
  endometrium, early, 192
    effect of radiation, 208
    moderately well differentiated, 196
    papillary, 194, 198
    polypoid, 194
    poorly differentiated, 196
    transition into solid carcinoma, 198
    well differentiated, 194, 196
    with clear cells (helle Zellen, Feyrter), 49
    with lipid macrophages, 48
    with secretory changes, 196
  mesosalpinx, primary, 418
  oviduct, 268
    papillary, 268
    papillary, endometrioid type, 268
  vagina, adenoid cystic type, 96
    arising in endometriosis, 24
    cribriform type, 96
    mesonephric, 96
  vestibular glands, 96
Adenocystic carcinoma, cervix, 146, 148
Adenofibroma, endometrium, papillary, 43, 44
Adenoma, Bartholin's gland, 44
  development in struma ovarii, 392
  ovary, of adrenal cell rest, 356
  sebaceous, development in teratoma of ovary, 394
  Skene's glands, 78
  vulva, adnexal, 60
    papillary, 44
Adenomatoid tumor, myometrium, 226
  ovary, 352
  oviduct, 262

Adenomatous hyperplasia, cervix, 118, 120, 31
  endometrium, 182
    atypical, 184
    focal, 184
    in Stein-Leventhal syndrome, 184
    with squamous metaplasia, 184, 46
    with tubal epithelial metaplasia, 186
  in endometritis, 188
  endosalpinx, 262, 264
Adenomyoma, myometrium, 220
Adenomyosis, see endometriosis
Adenosis, cervix, circumscribed, 120
    diffuse, 120
  vagina, 21, 22
Adnexal adenoma, vulva, 60
Adnexal carcinoma, vulva, 60
    adenoid cystic type, 60
    mucus-secreting, 62
Adnexal papilloma, 44
Adrenal cell rest, adenoma, ovary, 356
  carcinoma, ovary, 356, 358
Adrenal cortical carcinoma, 454
Adrenal cortical hyperplasia, congenital, in adrenogenital syndrome, 454
Adrenal rest, mesosalpinx, 414, 99
  mesovarium, 412
Agenesis, ovary, 318
  umbilical cord, 520
Amniotic fluid embolism, 542
Amyloidosis, ovary, 310
  vulva, nodular, 30
Anaplastic carcinoma, cervix, 142
  endometrium, 198
  oviduct, 270
Androblastoma, ovary, mesenchymal type, 366
    mixed type, 366
    trabecular type, 364
    tubular type (Pick's adenoma), 362
    tubular type, feminizing, 368
    tubular type, moderately well differentiated, 364
    tubular type, well differentiated, with lipid storage, 364, 93
    tubular type, well differentiated, with lipid storage, feminizing, 362
    tubular type, with hilus cells, 364
    tubular type, with lipid storage, 364
Angiokeratoma of Mibelli, vulva, 50
Angiolipoma, vulva, 46
Angiomyoma, myometrium, 232
Angiomyxoma, umbilical cord, 520
Anovulatory endometrium, 174
Arteriosclerosis, myometrial vessels, 214
  ovary, calcific, 308
    medullary, 308
Arteritis, omentum, necrotizing, 430
Atrophy, endometrium, after radiation, 208
    in ovarial dysgenesis, 40
    in secondary amenorrhea, 174

593

Atrophy, endometrium, in Sheehan syndrome, 174
  senile, 168
    senile, with glandular dilatations, 168
  endosalpinx, postmenopausal, 248
    senile, 248
  vulva, senile, with hyperkeratosis, 32
Autograft ovary, in abdominal wall, 312

Bancroft's filariasis, vulva, 22
  with elephantiasis, 24
Bartholinitis, acute, suppurative, 14
  chronic, 16
  eosinophilic, 16
Bartholin's gland, abscess, 14
  adenoacanthoma, 64
  adenocarcinoma, 62
    adenoid cystic type, 64
    mucus-secreting, 64
  adenoma, 44
  cyst, 36
  cystic dilatation of acini, 34
  histology, 4
  mixed tumor, 54
Bartholin's gland duct, cyst, 36
  ectasia, 36
  inflammatory cyst, 14
  pseudoabscess, 14
  squamous metaplasia, epithelium, 36
Basal cell carcinoma, vulva, 58
Basal cell hyperplasia, exocervix, epithelium, 134, 546
Bilharziasis, cervix, 116
  vulva, 24
Blastomycosis, vulva, 22
Blighted ovum, 478
Boeck's sarcoid, cervix, 116
Bone marrow, in soap-intoxication syndrome, 488
Bony metaplasia, ovary, 278
Bowen's disease, vulva, 56, 15
Brain, in toxemia of pregnancy, 552
Breast tissue, vulva, 72
  lactating, 72
  lactating with cystic change, 36
Brenner tumor, ovary, cystic, 346, 348, 350
  epithelium, 346
  malignant, 350, 352
  miniature, 344, 346
  proliferating, 350
  solid, 346
  with edema, 348
  with mucinous epithelium, 348
  with stromal calcification, 348
Breus's mole, 478
Broad ligament, carcinosarcoma, 100
  granuloma, following talc powder administration, 418
  hemangioendotheliosarcoma, 420
  invading of choriocarcinoma, 536
  leiomyosarcoma, 420
  lipoma, 418
  reticulum sarcoma, 420, 422
  rhabdomyosarcoma, 102
  sarcoma, 101

Calcification, corpus albicans, 286
  endosalpinx, 254
  follicle, ovarian, 280
  glands of cervix, 122
  in Brenner tumor of ovary, 348
  in leiomyoma of myometrium, 234, 62
  ovary, cortical, 308
  placenta, 510
Candidiasis, vagina, 84
Carcinoid, arising in cystic benign teratoma of ovary, 392

Carcinoma, see also special histological types
  arising in, cystic benign teratoma of ovary, 394
    endometriosis of myometrium, 240
    endometriosis of vagina, 24
    glandular cystic hyperplasia of endometrium, 194
    lichen sclerosus et atrophicus of vulva, 30
    paramesonephric inclusion of pelvic lymph node, 448
    polyp of endometrium, 194
    struma ovarii, 392
  development after radiation, vulva, 72, 74
  of adrenal cell rest, ovary, 356, 358
  oviduct, in early stage, 266
Carcinomatosis, peritoneum, from cancer of ovary, 428
Carcinosarcoma, broad ligament, 100
  cervix, 150
  endometrium, 200
  ovary, 390
  oviduct, 270
Caruncle, urethral meatus, angiomatous, 76
  granulomatous, 76
  papillomatous, 74
  simulating carcinoma, 76
  with ectasia of a vein, 76
  with epithelial dysplasia, 78
Caruncula hymenalis, 80
Cerebellum, metastatic of choriocarcinoma, 538
Cervicitis, tuberculous, 116
Cervix, adenoacanthoma, 146
  adenocarcinoma, cylindromatous, 148
    moderately differentiated, 144
    poorly differentiated, 146, 34
    well differentiated, 144
  adenocystic carcinoma, 146, 148
  adenoma, mesonephric rest, 128
  adenomatous hyperplasia, 118, 120, 31
  adenosis, circumscribed, 120
    diffuse, 120
  anaplastic carcinoma, 142
  at term gestation, 466
  basal cell hyperplasia, epithelium, 134, 546
    epithelium, in pregnancy, 546, 548
  bilharziasis, 116
  Boeck's sarcoid, 116
  calcification of glands, 122
  carcinosarcoma, 150
  cervicitis, tuberculous, 116
  choriocarcinoma, metastatic from uterus, 152
  clear cell carcinoma, 33
  collision tumor, 35
  condyloma acuminatum, 118
  cyst, epidermal inclusion, 122
    mesonephric, 122
    paramesonephric, 122
  cytomegalic inclusion disease, 118
  dysplasia, epithelial, 134
    epithelial, in pregnancy, 546, 548
  endocervicitis, follicular, 114
    subacute with squamous metaplasia, 114
  endometriosis, 29
  eosinophilia of endocervix, 30
  epidermization in healed erosion, 27
  erosion, glandular, 108
    healed, 108
    healed with epidermization, 27
    healed with Nabothian cysts, 108
  exocervicitis, acute, non-specific, 114
  Gartner gang duct, 28
  gelatinous carcinoma, 148, 150
  glomus tumor, 126
  granulocytic leukemia, 154
  hamartoma, 124
  hemangioma, cavernous, 124

Cervix, hemangiopericytoma, 126
histology, in infant, 106, 110
in reproductive age, 106, 108, 110, 25
hyperkeratosis, 106
hyperplasia, of basal cells, 134, 546
of mesonephric rest, 128
in puerperal sepsis, 486
intraepithelial carcinoma, 136, 138
in pregnancy, 548
with glandular involvement, 138
leiomyoma, 126
leukemia, granulocytic, 154
lymphocytic, 152
leukoparakeratosis, 106
papillary, 106
tangential section, simulating carcinoma, 108
lipoma, 124
lymphoblastic lymphosarcoma, 152
lymphocytic leukemia, 152
lymphoma, malignant, 152
mesonephric adenoma, 128
mesonephric carcinoma, 130, 132
alveolar, 132
papillary, 132
mesonephric cyst, 122
mesonephric papilloma, 128, 130
proliferating, 130
mesonephric rest, hyperplasia, 128
metaplasia, squamous, epithelium of cervical polyp, 112
squamous, glandular epithelium, 110, 112, 26
metastatic choriocarcinoma, 152
microcarcinoma, 138, 140
occult carcinoma, 144
papilloma, 122
mesonephric, 128, 130
mesonephric, proliferating, 130
paramesonephric cyst, 122
polyp, 112
fibrous with squamous metaplasia of epithelium, 112
with inflammatory changes, 114
with Russell bodies, 114
with squamous metaplasia of epithelium, 112
pseudosarcomatous changes following radiation, 154
reticulum sarcoma, 36
sarcoidosis, 116
sarcoma botryoides, 150, 152
schistosomiasis, 116
scirrhous carcinoma, 142
sebaceous gland, heterotopic, 124
silver pigment deposition following treatment of erosion, 128
squamous cell carcinoma, 140, 142, 144, 32
effect of radiation, 154
poorly differentiated, 142
with lymphatic spread, 150
squamous epithelial nodule, 112
squamous metaplasia, in polyp, 112
glandular epithelium, 110, 112, 26
syphilitic lesion, secondary, 118
tuberculosis, 116
ulcer, decubital, 108
Chancroid, vulva, 10
Chocolate cyst, ovary, *see also* endometriosis of ovary
early stage, 300
end stage, 300
Chondrosarcoma, endometrium, 204
ovary, 388
Chordoma, retroperitoneal tissue, 444
Chorioadenoma destruens, 530
Chorioamnionitis, 496
Choriangioma, placenta, 510, 512
Choriocarcinoma, associated with, hyperplasia of breast tissue, 538

Choriocarcinoma, associated with, lutein cysts of ovary, 538
polycystic ovary, 538
finding in curetted tissue, 532, 534
invading in, myometrium, 534
veins of broad ligament, 536
metastatic, cerebellum, 538
cervix, 152
liver, 536
lung, 536
vagina, 102
primary, ovary, 398
oviduct, 538
Chorionic nodule, vagina, hemorrhagic, 100, 102
Chorionic villi, *see also* placenta
1 to 2 weeks, 460
3 to 4 weeks, 460
5 to 10 weeks, 460
10 to 16 weeks, 460
over 16 weeks, 462
at term, 462
Hofbauer's cells, hyperplasia, 462
hydropic degeneration, 478
in ectopic tubal pregnancy, 490
Clear cell carcinoma, cervix, 33
Clear cells (helle Zellen, Feyrter), endometrium, 168
Clitoris, corpus cavernosum, histology, 4
glomus tumor, 50
hypertrophy, 32
malignant melanoma, 68, 70
Pacinian corpuscle, histology, 4
Cloacogenic carcinoma, vulva, 78
Coccidiomycosis, placenta, 500
Collision tumor, cervix, 35
Condyloma acuminatum, cervix, 118
urethral meatus, 76
vagina, 86
vulva, 18
epithelial dysplasia, 18
Condyloma latum, vulva, 12
with ecthymalike changes, 12
Corpus albicans, 278, 286
calcification, 286
Corpus luteum, bloom stage, 282
cyst, 294
hemorrhage, 75
necrosis in thrombotic thrombocytopenic purpura, 290
pregnancy, 6 to 8 weeks gestation, 464, 466
proliferative stage, 282
regression stage, 282
rupturing, 284
vascularization stage, 282
Cortex, ovary, after menopause, 278
fetus, 276
neonatal, 276
prepubertal, 276
reproductive age, 278
Cortical fibrosis, in Stein-Leventhal syndrome, 298
Curetted tissue, in soap-intoxication syndrome, 486
finding in ectopic pregnancy, 490
inadequate fixation, invagination of endometrial glands, 170, 172
simulating carcinoma, 170
in choriocarcinoma of uterus, 532, 534
in induced abortion, 484
in placental polyp, 480
in retained incomplete abortion, 478, 480
menstrual endometrium, simulating carcinoma, 170
with epithelium of exocervix, 170
Cylindroma, dermal, eccrine, vulva, 60
Cyst, Bartholin's gland, 36
Bartholin's gland duct, 36
cervix, epidermal inclusion, 122

Cyst, cervix, mesonephric, 122
    paramesonephric, 122
  chocolate, ovary, 300
    ovary see also endometriosis of ovary
  lutein, multiple, ovary, associated with choriocarcinoma, 538
  mesosalpinx, mesonephric, 408
    paramesonephric, 410
  myometrium, epidermal inclusion, 222
    paramesonephric, 214
  of atretic ovarian follicle, luteinized, end stage, 294
  of corpus luteum, 294
  ovary, follicular, 292, 294
    not otherwise specified, 294
    with lutein cells, 294
  oviduct, peritoneal inclusion, 250
  paramesonephric, development, 408
    with inspissated secretion, 412
    with stalk, 410
  peritoneum, inclusion, 426
  placenta, 510
    chorionic, 118
  round ligament, unclassified, 414, 416
  sebaceous duct, 38
  vagina, epidermal inclusion, 86
    paramesonephric, 88
    with squamous metaplasia, 88
  vulva, epidermal inclusion, 38
    in ectopic lactating breast tissue, 36
    paramesonephric, 38
    peritoneal, 36
    sweat eccrine gland, 38
Cystadenocarcinoma, ovary, anaplastic, 326, 334
    mucinous, moderately well differentiated, 332, 334
    mucinous, poorly differentiated, 334
    mucinous, well differentiated, 332
    seromucinous, dimorphic, 338, 340
    seromucinous, dimorphic, poorly differentiated, 340
    serous, papillary, 324
    serous, papillary, moderately well differentiated, 324, 326
    serous, papillary, poorly differentiated, 326
    serous, papillary, well differentiated, 324
    serous, radiation effect, 326
Cystadenofibroma, developing from rete ovarii, 342
  ovary, 340
    malignant transformation, 342
    papillary, 342
    with metastatic lesion from cancer of breast, 342
Cystadenoma, mesosalpinx, papillary, serous, 412
  ovary, endometrioid, proliferating, without stromal invasion, 336
    mucinous, 328
    mucinous, complication with tuberculosis, 330
    mucinous, papillary, 328, 330
    mucinous, papillary, proliferating, without stromal invasion, 330
    mucinous, simple, 328
    mucinous, simple, malignant transformation, 332
    mucinous, pseudoglandular, 328
    mucinous, pseudoglandular, proliferating, without stromal invasion, 330
    seromucinous, dimorphic glazunow, 338
    serous, 320
    serous, coarse papillary, 320
    serous, fine papillary, 320
    serous, malignant transformation, 324
    serous, papillary, with psammoma bodies, 322
    serous, proliferating, without stromal invasion, 322
  papillary, development in ovarian endometriosis, 302
    development in ovarian endosalpingiosis, 304
Cystic glandular hyperplasia, see glandular cystic hyperplasia
Cystic dilatation, acini of Bartholin's gland, 34
Cytomegalic inclusion disease, cervix, 118
Cytotrophoblast, in a lymphatic channel, 532

Darier's disease, vulva, 28
Decidua, endometrium, 458
    Arias-Stella phenomenon, 458
    degenerative changes, 460
    hyalinization in postabortal endometritis, 482
Decidual polyp, 482
Decidual reaction, endometriosis of, myometrium, after enovid therapy, 218, 220
    ovary, during pregnancy, 470
    retrosigmoid, treated with enovid, 210
    uterus, during pregnancy, 470
  endometrium, following enovid therapy, 176
    in induced ovulation with clomiphen citrate, 41
  endosalpinx during pregnancy, 470, 472
  laparotomy scar, 104
  ovary, following nor-ethisterone administration, 85
    in pregnancy, 468, 470
    without pregnancy, 292
  pelvic lymph node, during pregnancy, 472
  peritoneum, in pregnancy, 472
  vermiform appendix, during pregnancy, 472
Dermatitis, vulva, acute, 24
    chronic, 24
Dermatofibroma, vulva, 44
Dermatofibrosarcoma, vulva, 68
Dermatophytosis, vulva, 22
Diabetes mellitus, placenta, 502
Diverticulum, suburethral, 74
    urethral, 74
Donovanosis, vulva, 10
Dysgenesis, gonadal, 314
    ovarian, atrophy of endometrium, 40
Dysgerminoma, ovary, 380, 382
Dyskeratosis, vulva, 54
Dysmenorrhea, membranous, 172
Dysplasia, epithelial, cervix, 134
    cervix, in pregnancy, 546, 548
    endosalpinx, 262, 264
    in condyloma acuminatum, 18
    in urethral caruncle, 78
    vagina, 94, 23
    vulva, 54

Ectasia, Bartholin's gland duct, 36
  vessels of endosalpinx, 250
Ecthyma, vulva, 8
Ectopic pregnancy, ovary, 490, 105
  oviduct, 488, 490
    finding in curetted tissue, 490
    hydropic degeneration of chorionic villi, 490
    peritubal hematoma with organization, 106
Eczema, vulva, acute, 24
    chronic, 24
Edema, endometrium, stromal, in fibrocongestive syndrome (Taylor), 172
Elephantiasis, vulva, 6
    in Bancroft's filariasis, 24
Embryonal carcinoma (Teilum), ovary, 396, 398
Endocervix, diseases see cervix, resp. special pathological changes of the cervix
Endometrial extension, oviduct, 260
Endometrioid carcinoma, ovary, moderately well differentiated, 336
    poorly differentiated, 336
    well differentiated, 336
    with acanthomatous change, 338
Endometrioid cystadenoma, ovary, proliferating, without stromal invasion, 336
Endometriosis, cervix, 29
  decidual changes in retrosigmoid treated with enovid, 210
  endosalpinx, 260, 67
  myometrium, 208, 216, 218, 58

Endometriosis, myometrium, after enovid therapy, 218, 220
    cancerous change, 240
    decidual reaction in pregnancy, 470
    sarcomatous change, 240
    stromal, 226, 228, 59
    with cyst formations, 218
    with secretory changes, 218
    with squamous metaplasia, 218
  omentum, 430
  ovary, *see also* chocolate cyst of ovary
    decidual reaction in pregnancy, 470
    development of adenocarcinoma, 302
    development of papillary cystadenoma, 302
    with formation of abortive endometrial cavity, 302
    with macrophages, 300, 79
    with secretory changes, 300
  oviduct, wall, 68
  pelvic lymph node, 446
  renal pelvis, 210
  round ligament, 416
  umbilicus, 210
  urinary bladder, 210
  vagina, 88
    carcinomatous change, 24
  vermiform appendix, 210
  vulva, 72
Endometritis, acute, 186
    with microabscess, 188
  after radiation, 206, 208
  chronic, 188
  postabortal, 480, 482, *120*
  pseudomembranous in puerperal sepsis, 486
  subacute, 188
  syncytial, 464
  tuberculous, 188, 190
  with focal adenomatous hyperplasia, 188
Endometrium, adenoacanthoma, 198
  adenocarcinoma, early, 192
    effect of radiation, 208
    moderately well differentiated, 196
    papillary, 194, 198
    polypoid, 194
    poorly differentiated, 196
    transition into solid carcinoma, 198
    well differentiated, 194, 196
    with clear cells (helle Zellen, Feyrter), *49*
    with lipid macrophages, *48*
    with secretory changes, 196
  adenofibroma, papillary, *43, 44*
  adenomatous hyperplasia, 182
    associated with endometritis, 188
    atypical, 184
    focal, 184
    in Stein-Leventhal syndrome, 184
    with squamous metaplasia, 184, *46*
    with tubal epithelial metaplasia, 186
  anaplastic carcinoma, 198
  Arias-Stella phenomenon, 458
  atrophy, after radiation, 208
    in ovarian dysgenesis, *40*
    in secondary amenorrhea, 174
    in Sheehan syndrome, 174
    senile, 168
    senile with glandular dilatations, 168
  carcinoma arising in, glandular cystic hyperplasia, 194
    polyp, 194
  carcinosarcoma, 200
    undifferentiated, 200
  chondrosarcoma, 204
  clear cells (helle Zellen, Feyrter), 168
  curetted tissue, inadequate fixation, simulating carcinoma, 170
    invagination of glands, produced by inadequate fixation, 170, 172

Endometrium, curetted tissue, menstrual phase, simulating carcinoma, 170
    with epithelium of exocervix, 170
  decidual reaction, following enovid therapy, 176
    in induced ovulation with clomiphen citrate, *41*
    pregnancy, 458
  dysmenorrhea, membranous, 172
  endometritis, acute, 186
    acute with microabscess, 188
    after radiation, 206, 208
    chronic, 188
    focal adenomatous hyperplasia, 188
    subacute, 188
    syncytial, 464
    tuberculous, 188, 190
  finding in ectopic pregnancy in curetted tissue, 490
  following enovid therapy, 176
  glandular cystic hyperplasia, 180
    associated with granulosa cell tumor, 174
    malignant change, 194
    secretory changes, 182
    with hemorrhage, 180, 182
    with oviduct-like epithelium, 182
  glycogen granules, *39*
  histology, child, cross section, 158
    infant, 158
    prepubertal, 158
    reproductive age, 158, 160, 162, 164, 166, 168, *37, 38, 39*
  hyperplasia, adenomatous, 182
    adenomatous, associated with endometritis, 188
    adenomatous, atypical, 184
    adenomatous, focal, 184
    adenomatous, in Stein-Leventhal syndrome, 184
    adenomatous, with squamous metaplasia, 184, *46*
    adenomatous, with tubal epithelial metaplasia, 186
  hyperplasia, stromal, 186, *45*
  hypoplasia in secondary amenorrhea, 174
  ichthyosis with lipid macrophages, *47*
  in anovulatory cycle, 174
  in fibrocongestive syndrome (Taylor), 172
  in first menstruation post partum, 474
  inadequately stimulated, 172
  inspissated corpus amylaceum-like secretion, 178
  lipoid macrophages in glands, 178
  lymphoblastic lymphosarcoma, 206
  lymphoma, malignant, 206
  mast cells, *37*
  melanotic progonoma (retinal anlage tumor), 204
  menstrual phase, 1st day, 166
    2nd day, 166
    3rd–4th day, 166
    established, 166
  mesonephric carcinoma, 206
  metaplasia, squamous, 178
    squamous, in adenomatous hyperplasia, 184, *46*
    squamous, in polyp, 190
    tubal epithelial, in adenomatous hyperplasia, 186
  mixed (irregular ripening), *42*
  neutral mucopolysaccharides, *38*
  polyp, adenomatous, 190
    adenomyomatous, 192
    development of carcinoma, 194
    stromal, 192
    with cystic changes of glands, 190, 192
    with squamous metaplasia, 190
  postabortal, endometritis, 480, 482, *120*
    fibrinoid nodule, 482
    hyalinization of decidua rest, 482
  proliferative phase, 5th–7th day, 158, 160
    8th–12th day, 160
    13th–15th day, 160
    mast cells, *37*
    neutral mucopolysaccharides, *38*

Endometrium, pseudodecidual reaction, associated with
    Krukenberg tumor, 176
  pseudosarcomatous changes, following norethindrone therapy,
      176
  regeneration after curettage, 168, 170
  reticulum cell sarcoma, 206
  sarcoma, mixed mesenchymal, 202
    stromal, 200, 202, 50, 51, 52, 53, 54
  secretory, delayed desquamation, 172
  secretory changes in adenocarcinoma, 196
  secretory phase, 16th day, 160, 162
    18th day, 162
    20th day, 162
    22nd day, 162, 164
    24th day, 164
    26th day, 164
    27th day, 164
    glycogen granules, 39
    in inadequate biphasic cycle, 172
  squamous cell carcinoma, 200
  squamous metaplasia, 178
    in adenomatous hyperplasia, 184, 46
    in polyp, 190
  stromal hyperplasia, 186, 45
  surface epithelium, participation in cycle, 166, 168
  with myelined nerve, 178
Endosalpingiosis, omentum, 430
  ovary, 302, 304
    development of papillary cystadenoma, 304
  oviduct, 260
  vermiform appendix, 272
Endosalpinx, diseases see oviduct resp. other special pathologi-
    cal changes of the oviduct
Endotoxin shock, fibrin thrombi in lung, 484
  finding in myometrium, 484
  pathological changes in kidney, 486
Eosinophilia, endocervix, 30
  myometrium, 57
Ependymoma, retroperitoneal tissue, 442
Epidermal inclusion cyst, myometrium, 222
Epidermization, in healed erosion, cervix, 27
Erosion, cervix, glandular, 108
    healed, 108
    healed, with epidermization, 27
    healed, with Nabothian cysts, 108
Erythema multiforme, vulva, 26, 28
Erythroblastosis fetalis, placenta, 504
Erythroplasia of Queyrat, vagina, 94
  vulva, 56
Exocervix, diseases see cervix, resp. special pathological changes
    of the cervix

Fallopian tube see oviduct
Fasciitis, vulva, 16
  nodular, round ligament, 414
Fat necrosis, omentum, 430
Fatty metamorphosis, liver in pregnancy, 542
Fetus papiraceus, 119
Fibrinoid nodule, in postabortal endometrium, 482
Fibroma, myometrium, 222
  ovary, 384
  vagina, 92
  vulva, 44, 46
Fibrosarcoma, myometrium, 238
  ovary, 386
  vulva, 66
Fibrosis, ovary, cortical, diffuse, 306
    cortical, nodular, 308
Follicle, Graafian, 280
    luteinization prior to rupture, 280
  ovarian, atretic, 284
    atretic, luteinized, early stage, 284

Follicle, ovarian, atretic, luteinized, end stage, 286
    atretic, with cystic change, 284
    growing, 73
    perifollicular hemorrhage, 74
    primordial, 280
    primordial with polynuclear ovum, 280
    with calcification, 280
    with perifollicular hyalinization, 280
Follicle cyst, ovary, 292, 294
    atretic, luteinized, end stage, 294
    intracystic hemorrhage, 294
Folliculitis, vulva, 8
Folliculoma lipidique of Lecène, ovary, 374
Funisitis, acute, 520

Ganglioneuroblastoma, pelvic tissue, 438, 440
Ganglioneuroma, pelvic tissue, 440
Gartner gang duct, cervix, 28
Gelatinous carcinoma, cervix, 148, 150
Germinal epithelium, ovary, 298
    mucinous metaplasia, 300
    squamous metaplasia, 298
Glandular cystic hyperplasia, endometrium, 180
    associated with granulosa cell tumor, 174
    malignant change, 194
    with hemorrhage, 180, 182
    with oviduct-like epithelium, 182
    secretory changes, 182
Glomerulonephritis, chronic, associated with pregnancy, 550
Glomus tumor, cervix, 126
    clitoris, 50
Gonadoblastoma, ovary, 378, 380
Gonads, agenesis, 318
    dysgenesis, 314
    in testicular feminization syndrome, 318, 80, 81, 82, 83, 84
Granular cell myoblastoma, vulva, 48
Granulation tissue, vagina, 86
Granulocytic leukemia, cervix, 154
    placenta, congenital, 514
Granuloma, broad ligament, following talc powder
        administration, 418
    ovary, cortical, 308, 310
    vagina, surgical, 86
    vulva, pyogenicum, 8
Granuloma inguinale, vulva, 10
Granulosa cell tumor, ovary, alveolar type, 372
    atypical, 374
    cystic, 370
    follicular type, 370
    mesenchymal type, 372, 374
    miniature, 370
    trabecular type, 372
    with luteinization, 374
Granulosa rest, ovary, 368, 370
Granulosa-theca cell tumor, ovary, 374, 376, 92
Gumma, vulva, 12, 14
Gynandroblastoma, ovary, 378

Hamartoma, cervix, 124
Hemangioendothelioma, myometrium, 66
  ovary, 386
Hemangioendotheliosarcoma, broad ligament, 420
  myometrium, 238, 240
Hemangioma, cervix, cavernous, 124
    myometrium, 220
    ovary, cavernous, 386
    vagina, 92
    vulva, capillary, 50
Hemangiopericytoma, cervix, 126
    ovary, 386
Hematoma, with organization, peritubal, ectopic tubal
      pregnancy, 106

Hemorrhage, in corpus luteum, 75
  in follicle cyst of ovary, 294
  perifollicular, *74*
Hemorrhagic mola (Breus's mole), 478
Hemosiderin deposition, ovary, 310
Hepatitis, viral, in pregnancy, 542
Herpes simplex, vulva, 20
Herpes zoster, vulva, 20
Hibernoma, vulva, 46
Hidradenoma, vulva, papilliferum, 42
Hilus cell hyperplasia, ovary, 358
Hilus cells, in tubular type androblastoma of ovary, 364
  ovary, 286, 288, *76, 77, 78*
    in hypoplasia, 314
Hilus cell tumor, ovary, 358, 360
    malignant, 362
    mesenchymal, 360
Histiocytes, accumulation in endosalpinx, 256, 258, *70, 71, 72*
Histiocytoma, vulva, 46
Histology, Bartholin's gland, 4
  cervix, infant, 106, 110
    reproductive age, 106, 108, 110, *25*
  clitoris, corpus cavernosum, 4
    Pacinian corpuscle, 4
  endometrium, cross section, child, 158
    glycogen granules, *39*
    infant, 158
    mast cells, *37*
    neutral mucopolysaccharides, *38*
    prepubertal, 158
    reproductive age, 158, 160, 162, 164, 166, 168, *37, 38, 39*
  endosalpinx, child, 246
    cyclical changes, 246
    reproductive age, 246
  female reproductive organs, fetus, 276
  hymen, imperforated, 4
  labium majus, 2
    sebaceous glands, 2
    sweat apocrine glands, 2
    sweat eccrine glands, 2
  labium minus, 2
  mesosalpinx, 408, *97, 98*
    fetus, 246
  mons veneris, 2
  myometrium, muscle content, reproductive age, *55*
  ovary, 246, 276, 278, 280, 282, 286, 288, 298, *73, 76, 77, 78*
    corpus luteum, 282
    cortex, after menopause, 278
    cortex, fetus, 276
    cortex, neonatal, 276
    cortex, prepubertal, 276
    cortex, reproductive age, 278
    fetus, 246
    follicle, 280, *73*
    germinal epithelium, 298
    hilus cells, 286, 288, *76, 77, 78*
    rete ovarii, 286
  oviduct, fetus, 246
    reproductive age, 246
  paraurethral glands, 4
  peritoneum, 426
  Skene's glands, 4
  urethral meatus, 4
  vagina, *19*
  vulva, 2, 4
Hodgkin's disease, cervix, 152
  vulva, 68
Hofbauer's cells, hyperplasia, 462
Hyalinization, decidua, in postabortal endometrium, 482
  myometrium, focal, 214
  ovarian follicle, 280
  ovary, cortical, 308

Hyalinization, placental site vessels, post partum, 552, 554, *109, 110*
Hydatid of Morgagni, 410
Hydatiform mole, in situ, 524
  lymphatic spread of throphoblasts, 532
  retained, 530, *111*
  with marked trophoblastic hyperplasia, 528
  with moderate trophoblastic hyperplasia, 526
  with slight trophoblastic overgrowth, 524
Hydropic degeneration, chorionic villi, 478
  in ectopic tubal pregnancy, 490
Hydrosalpinx, 254, 256
Hymen, caruncle, 80
  fibrosis, 80
  histology, 4
  imperforated, with hematocolpos, 80
Hyperkeratosis, cervix, 106
  vulva, in senile atrophy, 32
Hyperlipemic xanthoma, vulva, 30
Hyperplasia, adenomatous, in endometritis, 188
  apocrine sweat glands of vulva, 32
  basal cells, of exocervix, 134, 546
    of exocervix, in pregnancy, 546
  cervix, adenomatous, 118, 120, *31*
  endometrium, adenomatous, 182
    adenomatous, atypical, 184
    adenomatous, focal, 184
    adenomatous, in Stein-Leventhal syndrome, 184
    adenomatous, with squamous metaplasia, 184, *46*
    adenomatous, with tubal epithel metaplasia, 186
    stromal, 186, *45*
  endosalpinx, adenomatous, 262, 264
  hilus cells of ovary, 358
  Hofbauer cells of placental villi, 462
  mesonephric rest of cervix, 128
  mesonephric rest of mesosalpinx, 408
  sebaceous glands of vulva, 34
  stromal, subcortical, in polycystic ovary, 306
  vagina, pseudoepitheliomatous, 90
  vulva, pseudoepitheliomatous, simulating by tangential section, 32
Hyperthecosis, ovary, 306
  perifollicular, in Stein-Leventhal syndrome, 298
Hypertrophy, clitoris, 32
  myometrium, idiopathic, 214
Hypoplasia, endometrium, in secondary amenorrhea, 174
  endosalpinx, in Turner's syndrome, 248
  ovary, 314
    with hilus cells, 314

Ichthyosis, endometrium, with lipid storages, *47*
Impetigo herpetiformis, vulva, 8
Inadequately stimulated endometrium, 172
Inclusion, pelvic lymph node, paramesonephric, 446, 448
Inclusion cyst, oviduct, peritoneal, 250
  peritoneum, 426
  vagina, epidermal, 86
  vulva, epidermal, 38
Infarct, placenta, early, 506, 508
    old, 508
    red, *115, 116*
"Inflammatory" carcinoma, oviduct, 266
Intraepidermal carcinoma, vulva, 54, 56
    Bowenoid type, 56
    Bowen's disease, 56, *15*
    erythroplasia of Queyrat, 56
    urethral meatus, 78
Intraepithelial carcinoma, cervix, 136, 138
    in pregnancy, 548
    with glandular involvement, 138
  endosalpinx, 264
  vagina, 94

Intraepithelial carcinoma, vagina, erythroplasia of Queyrat, 94
Inverted follicular keratosis, vulva, 40
Inverted papilloma, vulva, 40

Keloid, vulva, 34
Keratoacanthoma, vulva, 40, 42
Keratosis follicularis, vulva, 28
Kidney, cortical necrosis post partum, 548
   glomerulonephritis, chronic, in pregnancy, 550
   in septic abortion with endotoxin shock, 486
   in toxemia of pregnancy, 550, *112, 113, 114*
   nephrosclerosis with pregnancy, 550
   pathological changes in soap-intoxication syndrome, 488
   pyelonephritis acute in pregnancy, 550
Krukenberg tumor, ovary, 400, 402, *95, 96*
   pseudodecidual reaction of endometrium, 176

Labium majus, histology, 2
Labium minus, histology, 2
Leiomyoma, broad ligament, 416, 418
   cervix, 126
   myometrium, 228
      cellular, 228
      intravascular, 230
      pseudosarcomatous changes following degeneration, 234, 236
      pseudosarcomatous changes following norethindrone therapy, 236
      serpentinous, 230
      with calcification, 234, *62*
      with cystic degeneration, 234
      with edema, 232, 234
      with fatty degeneration, 234
      with hyalinization, 232, *61*
      with lymphangiectatic degeneration, *65*
      with necrosis, 234
      with rhythmic nuclear pattern, 230
   ovary, 87
      with ossification, 88
   uterus, in pregnancy, 552
   vagina, 92
   vulva, 48
Leiomyosarcoma, broad ligament, 420
   metastatic in lung, from leiomyosarcoma(?) of uterus, *64*
   myometrium, 236, 238, *63*
   vagina, 100
   vulva, 66
Lentigo, vagina, 94
   vulva, 50
Leukemia, granulocytic, cervix, 154
      congenital, placenta, 514
   lymphocytic, cervix, 152
Leukoparakeratosis, cervix, 106
      papillary, 106
      tangential section, simulating carcinoma, 108
   vagina, 88
Lichen, chronicus simplex, vulva, 26
   planus, vulva, 26
      verrucosus, vulva, 26
   sclerosus et atrophicus, vulva, 30, *1, 2, 3, 4, 5, 6*
      vulva, development of carcinoma, 30
Lipid storage, endosalpinx, 252
Lipid tumor, ovary, undifferentiated, 354, 356
Lipogranuloma, vulva, traumatic, 34
Lipoid macrophages in endometrial glands, 178
Lipoma, broad ligament, 418
Lipoma, cervix, 124
   myometrium, 222
   oviduct, 262
Lipomatosis, myometrium, 216
Liposarcoma, retroperitoneal tissue, 436, 438
   vulva, 68

Listeriosis, placenta, 498
Liver, fatty metamorphosis in pregnancy, 542
   in soap-intoxication syndrome, *107*
   in toxemia of pregnancy, 552
   metastatic choriocarcinoma, 536
   viral hepatitis in pregnancy, 542
Lung, amniotic fluid embolism, 542
   fibrin thrombi in endotoxin shock, 484
   metastatic choriocarcinoma, 536
   metastatic leiomyosarcoma from leiomyosarcoma(?) of uterus, *64*
   secondary monilial infection in soap-intoxication syndrome, 488
Lupus vulgaris, vulva, 8, 10
Lutein cysts, associated with choriocarcinoma, 538
Luteinization, in granulosa cell tumor of ovary, 374
   in theca cell tumor of ovary, 376
   ovary, stromal, circumscribed, 292
      stromal, diffuse, 292
      stromal cells, in primary ovarian carcinoma, *94*
Luteoma gravidarum, ovary, 354
Lymphangiectasis, vulva, 6
Lymphangiocystic fibroma, myometrium, 224
Lymphangioma, myometrium, 220
   ovary, 388
   vulva, 50
Lymph node, pathological changes in lymphogranuloma venereum, vulva, 18
   pelvic, endometriosis, 446
      fatty tissue replacement, 448
      metastatic carcinoma from cancer of cervix, 450
      metastatic carcinoma from cancer of endometrium, 450
      metastatic carcinoma from cancer of ovary, 450
      metastatic dysgerminoma from ovary, 450
      metastatic malignant melanoma from vulva, 450
      paramesonephric inclusion, 446, 448
      paramesonephric inclusion with development of carcinoma, 448
      pseudosarcoid reaction, 446
   vulva, pathological changes in lymphogranuloma venereum, 18
Lymphoblastic lymphosarcoma, cervix, 152
   endometrium, 206
   ovary, 398
   oviduct, 272
   vulva, 68
Lymphocytic lymphosarcoma, ovary, 398, 400
Lymphogranuloma venereum, vulva, 18
   lymph node change, 18
Lymphoma, malignant, cervix, 152
   endometrium, 206
   ovary, 398, 400
   oviduct, 272
   vulva, 68

Malaria, placenta, 500, 502
Melanoma, malignant, clitoris, 68, 70
      metastatic in placenta, 512
      metastatic in urethral meatus, 80
      vagina, 100
      vulva, 70, *18*
Melanosis, placenta, 512
Melanotic progonoma (retinal anlage tumor), endometrium, 204
Membranes, amnion nodosum, 516
   amniotic, normal, 516
   chorioamnionitis, 496
   diamniotic, dichorionic, 516
      monochorionic, 516
Membranous dysmenorrhea, 172
Menstrual phase, endometrium, 1st day, 166
   2nd day, 166
   3rd–4th day, 166

Menstrual phase, endometrium, established, 166
Mesonephric adenocarcinoma, vagina, 96
Mesonephric adenoma, cervix, 128
Mesonephric carcinoma, cervix, 130, 132
    alveolar, 132
      papillary, 132
  endometrium, 206
  myometrium, 240
Mesonephric cyst, cervix, 122
  mesosalpinx, 408
Mesonephric papilloma, cervix, 128, 130
    proliferating, 130
  vagina, 90
Mesonephric rest, cervix, with hyperplasia, 128
  mesosalpinx, child, 408
    hyperplasia, 408
    reproductive age, 408, 97, 98
Mesonephric tumor (mesonephroma), mesosalpinx, 418, 420
  myometrium, 242
  ovary, 382, 384
Mesosalpinx, adenocarcinoma, primary, 418
  adrenal rest, 414, 99
  cyst, mesonephric, 408
    paramesonephric, 410
  cystadenoma, papillary, 412
  hyperplasia in mesonephric rest, 408
  histology, 408, 97, 98
    fetus, 246
  mesonephric cyst, 408
  mesonephric rest, child, 408
    hyperplasia, 408
    reproductive age, 408, 97, 98
  mesonephric tumor (mesonephroma), 418, 420
  paramesonephric cyst, 410
    with inspissated secretion, 412
  paramesonephric rest, child, 410
Mesothelioma, peritoneum, 428
Mesovarium, adrenal rest, 412
Metaplasia, bony, in ovary, 278
  epithelial, in chronic Skenitis, 74
  mucinous, in germinal epithelium of ovary, 300
  squamous, in adenomatous hyperplasia of endometrium, 184, 46
    in cervical polyp, 112
    in cyst of vagina, 88
    in endometrium, 178
    in endosalpinx, 248
    in epithelium of Bartholin's gland duct, 36
    in germinal epithelium of ovary, 298
    in glandular epithelium of cervix, 110, 112, 26
    in polyp of endometrium, 190
  tubal epithel-like, in adenomatous hyperplasia of endometrium, 186
Metastatic carcinoma, in cystadenofibroma of ovary, from cancer of breast, 342
  myometrium, from cancer of cervix, 242
    from cancer of ovary, 242
  omentum, from cancer of ovary, 430, 432
  ovary, from cancer of breast, 402
    from cancer of endometrium, 404
    from cancer of large intestine, 404
    from cancer of oviduct, 404
    from cancer of pancreas, 402
  oviduct, from cancer of ovary, 272
  parametrium, from cancer of cervix, 422
    from cancer of large intestine, 422
  pelvic lymph node, from cancer of cervix, 450
    from cancer of endometrium, 450
    from cancer of ovary, 450
  peritoneum, from cancer of ovary, 428
  placenta, from cancer of breast, 516
  vagina, from cancer of cervix, 100

Metastatic carcinoma, vagina, from cancer of kidney, 100
  vulva, from cancer of breast, 70
    from cancer of endometrium, 70
    from cancer of large intestine, 70
Metastatic choriocarcinoma, cervix, 152
  liver, 536
  lung, 536
  vagina, 102
Metastatic malignant melanoma, myometrium, 242
  ovary, 404
  pelvic lymph node from vulva, 450
  placenta, 512
  urethral meatus, 80
Metastatic mesonephroma, omentum, from ovary, 432
Metritis, phlegmonous, 214
Microcarcinoma, cervix, 138, 140
Mixed endometrium (irregular ripening), *42*
Mixed tumor, Bartholin's gland, 54
  ovary, mesodermal, 388
  vagina, benign, 90, 92
  vulva, 52
Mole, hemorrhagic (Breus's mole), 478
Molluscum contagiosum, vulva, 16
Mons veneris, histology, 2
Muscle content, myometrium, after menopause, 56
    in pregnancy, *103*
    reproductive age, 55
Myelined nerve, in endometrium, 178
Myometritis, syncytial, 464
  tuberculous, *60*
Myometrium, adenomatoid tumor, 226
  adenomyoma, 220
  adenomyosis *see* endometriosis of myometrium
  angiomyoma, 232
  arteriosclerosis of myometrial vessels, 214
  calcification in leiomyoma, 234, 62
  carcinoma, arising in endometriosis, 240
  cyst, epidermal inclusion, 222
    paramesonephric, 214
  decidual reaction in endometriosis following enovid therapy, 218, 220
  endometriosis, 208, 216, 218, 58
    change after enovid therapy, 218, 220
    decidual reaction in pregnancy, 470
    stromal, 226, 228, 59
    with cancerous change, 240
    with cyst formation, 218
    with sarcomatous change, 240
    with secretory changes, 218
    with squamous metaplasia, 218
  eosinophilia, 57
  epidermal inclusion cyst, 222
  fibroma, 222
  fibrosarcoma, 238
  hemangioendothelioma, 66
  hemangioendotheliosarcoma, 238, 240
  hemangioma, 220
  histology, muscle content, reproductive age, 55
  hyalinization, focal, 214
  hypertrophy, idiopathic, 214
  in pregnancy, 466, 468, *103*
  in puerperal sepsis, 486
  in septic abortion with endotoxin shock, 484
  invading of choriocarcinoma, 534
  leiomyoma, 228
    cellular, 228
    in pregnancy, 552
    intravascular, 230
    pseudosarcomatous changes following degeneration, 234, 236
    pseudosarcomatous changes following norethindrone therapy, 236

Myometrium, leiomyoma, serpentinous, 230
  with calcification, 234, 62
  with cystic degeneration, 234
  with edema, 232, 234
  with fatty degeneration, 234
  with hyalinization, 232, 61
  with lymphangiectatic degeneration, 65
  with necrosis, 234
  with rhythmic nuclear pattern, 230
 leiomyosarcoma, 236, 238, 63
 lipoma, 222
 lipomatosis, 216
 lymphangiocystic fibroma, 224
 lymphangioma, 220
 melanoma, malignant, 242
 mesonephric carcinoma, 240
 mesonephric tumor, 242
 metastatic carcinoma, from cancer of cervix, 242
  from cancer of ovary, 242
 metritis, phlegmonous, 214
 muscle content, after menopause, 56
  in pregnancy, 103
  reproductive age, 55
 myometritis, syncytial, 464
  tuberculous, 60
 paramesonephric cyst, 214
 pericytoma, 220
 pseudosarcomatous changes in leiomyoma, following degeneration, 234, 236
  following norethindrone therapy, 236
 sarcoma, developing in endometriosis, 240
  pleomorphic, 238
 secretory changes in endometriosis, 218
 squamous metaplasia in endometriosis, 218
 stromal endometriosis, 226, 228, 59
 subinvolution of placental site vessels post partum, 554
 xanthogranuloma, 216
Myxofibrosarcoma, ovary, 386
Myxoma, vulva, 46
Myxosarcoma, pelvic tissue, 436

Nephrosclerosis, associated with pregnancy, 550
Neurilemmoma, round ligament, 416
 vagina, 92
 vulva, 48
Neuroblastoma, congenital, placenta, 514
 pelvic tissue, 440
Neurodermatitis circumscripta, vulva, 26
Neurofibroma, pelvic tissue, 440, 442
 vulva, 48
Neurofibromatosis (v. Recklinghausen), vulva, 48, 50
Neuroma, vulva, 48
Nevus, blue, vulva, 52
 compound, vulva, 52
 epithelial, vulva, 34
 intradermal, vulva, 52
 junctional, vulva, 52

Occult carcinoma, cervix, 144
Omentitis, granulomatous, 430
Omentum, arteritis, necrotizing, 430
 carcinomatosis after yttrium therapy, 432, 434
 endometriosis, 430
 endosalpingiosis, 430
 fat necrosis, 430
 metastatic carcinoma from cancer of ovary, 430, 432
 metastatic mesonephroma from ovary, 432
 reticulum cell sarcoma, 432
Oophoritis, associated with infectious parotitis, 288
 tuberculous, 288
Ossification, in ovarian leiomyoma, 88
Ovary, 2 days post partum, 474

Ovary, abscess, 288
 caused by Enterobius (Oxyuris) vermicularis, 290
 adenoacanthoma, 326
 adenocarcinoma, development in endometriosis, 302
 adenocarcinoma see also endometrioid carcinoma
 adenoma, arising in ovarian struma, 392
  of adrenal cell rest, 356
  sebaceous, arising in teratoma, 394
 adenomatoid tumor, 352
 adrenal cell rest adenoma, 356
 adrenal cell rest carcinoma, 356, 358
 agenesis, 318
 amyloidosis, 310
 androblastoma, mesenchymal type, 366
  mixed type, 366
  trabecular type, 364
  tubular type, feminizing, 368
  tubular type, moderately well differentiated, 364
  tubular type (Pick's adenoma), 362
  tubular type, well differentiated with lipid storage, 364, 93
  tubular type, well differentiated with lipid storage, feminizing, 362
  tubular type with hilus cells, 364
  tubular type with lipid storage, 364
 arteriosclerosis, calcific, 308
  medullary, 308
 bony metaplasia, 278
 Brenner tumor, cystic, 346, 348, 350
  epithelium, 346
  malignant, 350, 352
  miniature, 344, 346
  proliferating, 350
  solid, 346
  with mucinous epithelium, 348
  with stromal calcification, 348
  with stromal edema, 348
 calcification, cortical, 308
  in Brenner tumor, 348
  in corpus albicans, 286
  in Graafian follicle, 280
 carcinoid, arising in cystic ovarian teratoma, 392
 carcinoma, arising in cystic benign teratoma, 394
  arising in struma ovarii, 322
  of adrenal cell rest, 356, 358
 carcinosarcoma, 390
 chocolate cyst, early stage, 300
  end stage, 300
 chondrosarcoma, 388
 choriocarcinoma, primary, 398
 corpus albicans, 278, 286
  calcification, 286
 corpus luteum, bloom stage, 282
  necrosis in thrombotic thrombocytopenic purpura, 290
  proliferative stage, 282
  regression stage, 282
  rupturing, 284
  vascularization stage, 282
  with hemorrhage, 75
 corpus luteum cyst, 294
 cortex, after menopause, 278
  fetus, 276
  neonatal, 276
  prepubertal, 276
  reproductive age, 278
 cortical fibrosis in Stein-Leventhal syndrome, 298
 cyst, chocolate, 300
  not otherwise specified, 294
  of atretic luteinized follicle, end stage, 294
  of corpus luteum, 294
  of Graafian follicle, 292, 294
  with theca lutein cells, 294
  lutein, multiple, associated with choriocarcinoma, 538

Ovary, cystadenocarcinoma, anaplastic, 326, 334
  mucinous, moderately well differentiated, 332, 334
  mucinous, poorly differentiated, 334
  mucinous, well differentiated, 332
  seromucinous, dimorphic, 338, 340
  seromucinous, dimorphic, poorly differentiated, 340
  serous, effect of radiation, 326
  serous, papillary, 324
  serous, papillary, moderately well differentiated, 324, 326
  serous, papillary, poorly differentiated, 326
  serous, papillary, well differentiated, 324
cystadenofibroma, 340
  developing from rete ovarii, 342
  malignant transformation, 342
  papillary, 342
  with metastatic lesion from cancer of breast, 342
cystadenoma, endometrioid, proliferating without stromal invasion, 336
  mucinous, 328
  mucinous, malignant transformation, 332
  mucinous, papillary, 328, 330   [330
  mucinous, papillary, proliferating, without stromal invasion,
  mucinous, pseudoglandular, 328
  mucinous, pseudoglandular, proliferating, without stromal invasion, 330
  mucinous, simple, 328
  mucinous, with tuberculosis in the wall, 330
  papillary, development in endometriosis, 302
  papillary, development in endosalpingiosis, 304
  seromucinous, dimorphic, 338
  serous, 320
  serous, coarse papillary, 320
  serous, fine papillary, 320
  serous, malignant transformation, 324
  serous, papillary, proliferating, without stromal invasion, 322
  serous, papillary, with psammoma bodies, 322
decidual reaction, following nor-ethisterone administration, 85
  in pregnancy, 468, 470
  without pregnancy, 292
dysgenesis, 314
  atrophy of endometrium, 40
dysgerminoma, 380, 382
ectopic pregnancy, 490, 105
embryonal carcinoma Teilum, 396, 398
endodermal sinus tumor—Teilum see embryonal carcinoma
endometrioid carcinoma, moderately well differentiated, 336
  poorly differentiated, 336
  well differentiated, 336
  with acanthomatous change, 338
endometrioid cystadenoma, proliferating, without stromal invasion, 336
endometriosis, decidual reaction in pregnancy, 470
  development of adenocarcinoma, 302
  development of papillary cystadenoma, 302
  with cystic change see chocolate cyst
  with formation of abortive endometrial cavity, 302
  with macrophages, 300, 79
  with secretory changes, 300
endosalpingiosis, 302, 304
  development of papillary cystadenoma, 304
fibroma, 384
fibrosarcoma, 386
fibrosis, cortical, diffuse, 306
  cortical, nodular, 308
follicle, atretic, 284
  atretic, luteinized, early stage, 284
  atretic, luteinized, end stage, 284, 286
  atretic with cystic change, 284
  cyst, 292, 294
  cyst, intracystic hemorrhage, 294
  Graafian, 280
  Graafian, luteinization prior to rupture, 280

Ovary, follicle, growing, 73
  perifollicular hemorrhage, 74
  primordial, 280
  primordial with polynuclear ovum, 280
  with calcification, 280
  with perifollicular hyalinization, 280
folliculoma lipidique (Lecène), 374
germinal epithelium, 298
  mucinous metaplasia, 300
  squamous metaplasia, 298
gonadoblastoma, 378, 380
granuloma, cortical, 308, 310
granulosa cell tumor, alveolar type, 372
  atypical, 374
  cystic, 370
  follicular type, 370
  mesenchymal type, 372, 374
  miniature, 370
  trabecular type, 372
  with luteinization, 374
granulosa rest, 368, 370
granulosa theca cell tumor, 374, 376, 92
gynandroblastoma, 378
gyratum, 278
hemangioendothelioma, 386
hemangioma, cavernous, 386
hemangiopericytoma, 386
hemorrhage, in corpus luteum, 75
  in follicle cyst, 294
  perifollicular, 74
hemosiderin deposition, 310
hilus cells, 286, 288, 76, 77, 78
  hyperplasia, 358
  in ovarian hypoplasia, 314
  in tubular type androblastoma, 364
hilus cell tumor, 358, 360
  malignant, 362
  mesenchymal, 360
histology, 246, 276, 278, 280, 282, 286, 288, 298, 73, 76, 77, 78
  corpus luteum, 282
  cortex after menopause, 278
  cortex, fetus, 276
  cortex, neonatal, 276
  cortex, prepubertal, 276
  cortex, reproductive age, 278
  fetus, 246
  follicle, 280, 73
  germinal epithelium, 298
  hilus cells, 286, 288, 76, 77, 78
  rete ovarii, 286
hyalinization, cortical, 308
  of follicle, 280
hyperplasia, hilus cells, 358
  stromal, subcortical in polycystic ovary, 306
hyperthecosis, 306
  perifollicular in Stein-Leventhal syndrome, 298
hypoplasia, 314
  with hilus cells, 314
in adrenogenital syndrome, 312
  infant, 312
in included ovulation with clomiphen citrate, 316
in pregnancy, 466
Krukenberg tumor, 400, 402, 95, 96
  pseudodecidual reaction of endometrium, 176
leiomyoma, 87
  with ossification, 88
lipid tumor, undifferentiated, 354, 356
lutein cysts, associated with choriocarcinoma, 538
luteinization, in granulosa cell tumor, 374
  in theca cell tumor, 376
  of stromal cells in ovarian carcinoma, 94
  stromal, circumscribed, 292

Ovary, luteinization, stromal, diffuse, 292
   luteoma gravidarum, 354
   lymphangioma, 388
   lymphoblastic lymphosarcoma, 398
   lymphocytic lymphosarcoma, 398, 400
   lymphoma, malignant, 398, 400
   mesonephric tumor (mesonephroma), 382, 384
   metaplasia, bony, 278
      mucinous, germinal epithelium, 300
      squamous, germinal epithelium, 298
   metastatic carcinoma, from cancer of breast, 402
      from cancer of endometrium, 404
      from cancer of large intestine, 404
      from cancer of oviduct, 404
      from cancer of pancreas, 402
      from cancer of sigmoid, 404
      in cystadenofibroma from cancer of breast, 342
   mixed mesodermal tumor, 388
   myxofibrosarcoma, 386
   oophoritis, associated with infectious parotitis, 288
      tuberculous, 288
   ossification in leiomyoma of ovary, 88
   papilloma, surface, 344
   papillomatous proliferation, surface epithelium, 306
   paragonadal spleen, 312
   perifollicular hyperthecosis in Stein-Leventhal syndrome, 298
   perioophoritis, chronic, 290
      healed with adhesions, 292
   polycystic, 296
      associated with choriocarcinoma, 538
      in Stein-Leventhal syndrome, 298
      with atrophic granulosa cell layer, 296
      with hyperplasia of granulosa cell layer, 296
      with subcortical stromal hyperplasia, 306
   psammoma bodies, 86
      pseudomyxoma, 330
   radiation, effect, 314
      effect on cystadenocarcinoma, 326
   rete ovarii, 286
   reticulum cell sarcoma, 400
   rhabdomyosarcoma, 396
   sarcoma, pleomorphic, undifferentiated, 388
   secretory changes in endometriosis, 300
   Sertoli cell tumor, 362, 368
   splenogonadal fusion, 312
   squamous metaplasia of germinal epithelium, 298
   stromal subcortical hyperplasia in polycystic ovary, 306
   struma ovarii, development of adenoma, 392
      development of carcinoma, 392
   syphilis, 290
   teratocarcinoma, 394, 396
   teratoma, cystic, benign, 390
      cystic, benign, with cerebellar tissue, 390
      cystic, benign, with chorioid plexus, 390
      cystic, benign, with foreign bodies reaction, 390
      cystic, development of carcinoid, 392
      cystic, development of carcinoma, 394
      development of sebaceous adenoma, 394
      solid, benign, 392
   theca cell tumor, 376, *91*
      malignant, 376, 378
      sclerosing, *89, 90*
      with edema, 376
      with luteinization, 376
   theca lutein cyst, 294
   tuberculosis, 288
      in mucinous cystadenoma, 330
   undifferentiated carcinoma, 344
Oviduct, accessory, 250
   adenocarcinoma, 268
      endometrioid type, 268
      papillary, 268

Oviduct, adenomatoid tumor, 262
   anaplastic carcinoma, 270
   carcinoma, early stage, 266
   carcinosarcoma, 270
   choriocarcinoma, primary, 538
   cyst, peritoneal inclusion, 250
   ectopic pregnancy, 488, 490
      chronic, peritubal hematoma with organization, *106*
      finding in curetted tissue, 490
      hydropic degeneration of chorionic villi, 490
   endometrial extension, 260
   endometriosis in tubal wall, 68
   endosalpingiosis, 262
   endosalpingitis, acute, 252
      chronic, 254
      chronic with hemosiderin macrophages, 254
      tuberculous, 258
   endosalpinx, accumulation of histiocytes, 256, 258, *70, 71, 72*
      adenomatous hyperplasia, 262, 264
      at term gestation, 468
      atrophy, postmenopausal, 248
      atrophy, senile, 248
      calcification, 254
      cyclical changes, 246
      decidual reaction, 470, 472
      dysplasia of epithelium, 262, 264
      ectasia of vessels, 250
      endometriosis, 260, 67
      histology, child, 246
      histology, reproductive age, 246
      hypoplasia in Turner syndrome, 248
      intraepithelial carcinoma, 264
      lipid storage, 252
      squamous metaplasia, 248
   histology, endosalpinx, child, 246
      endosalpinx, reproductive age, 246
      fetus, 246
      reproductive age, 246
   hydrosalpinx, 254, 256
   inclusion cyst, peritoneal, 250
   "inflammatory" carcinoma, 266
   lipoma, 262
   lymphoblastic lymphosarcoma, 272
   lymphoma malignant, 272
   metastatic carcinoma from cancer of ovary, 272
   papilloma, 262
   perisalpingitis, chronic, 256
   primary choriocarcinoma, 538
   pyosalpinx, 252
   reticulum cell sarcoma, 270, 272
   salpingitis, caused by Enterobius (Oxyuris) vermicularis, 258
      granulomatous, 254
      healed, 254
      pseudofollicular, 254
      pseudoxanthomatous, 256, 69
   squamous cell carcinoma, 268, 270
   thrombosis of a vein with organization, 248
   tuberculosis, 258, 472
   Walthard's cell rest, child, 250
      development, 246
      fetus, 250
      reproductive age, 250, 252
Ovotestis, 316
Ovum, 10 days old, 460
   blighted, 478

Paget's disease, vulva, 56, 58, *7, 8, 9, 10, 11, 12, 13, 14*
Papilloma, cervix, 122
   mesonephric, 128, 130
      mesonephric, proliferating, 130
   ovary, surface, 344
   oviduct, 262

Papilloma, urethral meatus, 76
  vagina, mesonephric, 90
  vulva, adnexal, 44
    fibroepithelial, 40
    fibroepithelial, congenital, 40
    inverted, 40
Papillomatosis, vagina, 88, 90
Papillomatous proliferation, ovary, surface, 306
Paraganglioma, pelvic tissue, 438
Paragonadal spleen, 312
Paramesonephric appendix, 410
Paramesonephric cyst, cervix, 122
  development, 408
  mesosalpinx, 410
    with inspissated secretion, 412
  myometrium, 214
  vagina, 88
  vulva, 38
  with stalk, 410
Paramesonephric inclusion, pelvic lymph node, 446, 448
    development of carcinoma, 448
Paramesonephric rest, mesosalpinx, child, 410
Parametrium, metastatic carcinoma, from cancer of cervix, 422
    from cancer of large intestine, 422
  pelvic ganglion, effect of radiation, 422
Paraurethral glands, histology, 4
Pelvic ganglion, parametrium, effect of radiation, 422
Pelvic lymph node, decidual reaction, in pregnancy, 472
  development of carcinoma in paramesonephric inclusion, 448
  endometriosis, 446
  fatty tissue replacement, 448
  metastatic carcinoma, from cancer of cervix, 450
    from cancer of endometrium, 450
    from cancer of ovary, 450
  metastatic dysgerminoma from ovary, 450
  metastatic malignant melanoma from vulva, 450
  paramesonephric inclusion, 446, 448
  pseudosarcoid reaction, 446
Pelvic peritoneum see peritoneum
Pelvic tissue, actinomycosis, 434
  ganglioneuroblastoma, 438, 440
  ganglioneuroma, 440
  myxosarcoma, 436
  neuroblastoma, 440
  neurofibroma, 440, 442
  paraganglioma, 438
Pemphigus vulgaris, vulva, 26
Pericytoma, myometrium, 220
Perifollicular hyperthecosis in Stein-Leventhal syndrome, 298
Perifolliculitis, vulva, 8
Perioophoritis, chronic, 290
  healed, with adhesions, 292
Perisalpingitis, chronic, 256
Peritoneum, carcinomatosis from cancer of ovary, 428
  cyst, inclusion, 426
  decidual reaction in pregnancy, 472
  histology, 426
  inclusion cyst, 426
  mesothelioma, 428
  metastatic carcinoma from cancer of ovary, 428
  peritonitis, acute, 426
    organizing, 426
  pseudomyxoma, 426
  tuberculosis, 426
Peritonitis, acute, 426
  organizing, 426
  tuberculous, 426
Pituitary gland, at full term pregnancy, 474
Pituitary necrosis, intra partum, 544
  post partum, 544
Pituitary scarring, post partum, with Sheehan syndrome, 544
Pityriasis rubra pilaris, vulva, 28

Placenta see also chorionic villi
Placenta, accreta, 496
  calcification, 510
  chorioangioma, 510, 512
  congenital granulocytic leukemia, 514
  congenital neuroblastoma, 514
  cyst, 510, 118
  extrauterine, full term, 494
  fibrosis, nonspecific, 508
    subchorionic, 508
  in coccidiomycosis, 500
  in diabetes mellitus, 502
  in erythroblastosis fetalis, 504
  in interstitial pregnancy, 496
  in listeriosis, 498
  in malaria, 500, 502
  in sickle cell anemia, 502, 504
  in syphilis, 498, 500
  in toxemia of pregnancy, 504, 506
  increta, 496
  infarct, early, 506, 508
    old, 508
    red, 115, 116
  melanosis, 512
  membranacea, 494
  metastatic carcinoma from cancer of breast, 516
  metastatic of melanoma malignant, 512
  rupture of marginal sinus, 117
  teratoma, 512
  thrombosis of marginal sinus, 506
Placental polyp, 480
Placental site vessels, hyalinization post partum, 552, 554, 109, 110
Placentar villi see chorionic villi
Placentitis, advanced acute, 498
  early, 496
  in septic abortion, 496
  tuberculous, 498
Pleomorphic undifferentiated sarcoma, ovary, 388
Polycystic ovary, 296
  associated with choriocarcinoma, 538
  in Stein-Leventhal syndrome, 298
  with atrophic granulosa cell layer, 296
  with hyperplasia of granulosa cell layer, 296
  with subcortical stromal hyperplasia, 306
Polyp, adenomatous, endometrium, 190
  adenomyomatous, endometrium, 192
  cervix, 112
    fibrous with squamous metaplasia of epithelium, 112
    with inflammatory changes, 114
    with Russell bodies, 114
    with squamous metaplasia of epithelium, 112
  decidual, 482
  endometrium, cystic changes of glands, 190, 192
    malignant change, 194
    squamous metaplasia, 190
    stromal, 192
  placental, 480
  vagina, 90
  vulva, fibroepithelial, 44
Pregnancy, diseases see special pathological changes of ovum, fetus, placenta, umbilical cord, membranes, resp. of the maternal genital and extragenital organs
Proliferative phase, endometrium, 5th–7th day, 158, 160
    8th–12th day, 160
    13th–15th day, 160
    mast cells, 37
    neutral mucopolysaccharides, 38
Psammoma bodies, ovary, 86
Pseudoabscess, Bartholin's gland duct, 14
Pseudodecidual reaction, endometrium, associated with Krukenberg tumor, 176

Pseudoepitheliomatous hyperplasia, vagina, 90
  vulva, 32, 40
    simulating by tangential section, 32
Pseudomyxoma, ovary, 330
  peritoneum, 426
Pseudosarcoid reaction, pelvic lymph node, 446
Pseudosarcomatous changes, cervix, following radiation, 154
  endometrium, following norethindrone therapy, 176
  in leiomyoma of myometrium, following degeneration, 234, 236
    following norethindrone therapy, 236
  simulating by fasciitis, vulva, 16
Pseudotumor, vagina, inflammatory, 84
  vulva, inflammatory, 16
Psoriasis, vulva, 26
Pyelonephritis, acute, in pregnancy, 550
Pyosalpinx, 252

Radiation, atrophy of endometrium, 208
  effect on, adenocarcinoma of endometrium, 208
    ovary, 314
    pelvic ganglion, 422
    serous cystadenocarcinoma of ovary, 326
    squamous cell carcinoma of cervix, 154
  endometritis, 206, 208
  pseudosarcomatous changes of cervix, 154
  vaginitis, 102
  vascular change, vagina, 102
Radiation ulcer, vulva, 72
Radiodermatitis, vulva, 72
Radiotherapy, vulva, development of carcinoma, 72, 74
Regeneration, endometrium, after curettage, 168, 170
Renal pelvis, endometriosis, 210
Rete ovarii, 286
Reticulum cell sarcoma, broad ligament, 420, 422
  cervix, *36*
  endometrium, 206
  omentum, 432
  ovary, 400
  oviduct, 270, 272
Retroperitoneal sclerosis, idiopathic (Ormon's disease), 436
Retroperitoneal tissue, chordoma, 444
  ependymoma, 442
  idiopathic sclerosis (Ormon's disease), 436
  liposarcoma, 436, 438
  teratocarcinoma, 444
  xanthogranuloma, 434
Retrosigmoid, endometriosis, decidual changes treated with enovid, 210
Retrovaginal septum, rhabdomyosarcoma, 438
Rhabdomyosarcoma, broad ligament, *102*
  ovary, 396
  retrovaginal septum, 438
  vulva, 66
Round ligament, cyst, unclassified, 414, 416
  endometriosis, 416
  fasciitis, nodular, 414
  leiomyoma, 416, 418
  neurilemmoma, 416

Salpingitis, caused by Enterobius (Oxyuris) vermicularis, 258
  granulomatous, 254
  healed, 254
  pseudofollicular, 254
  pseudoxanthomatous, 256, *69*
Sarcoidosis, cervix, 116
Sarcoma *see also* special histological types
Sarcoma, arising in endometriosis of myometrium, 240
  botryoides, cervix, 150, 152
    vagina, 98
  broad ligament, *101*
  mixed mesenchymal, endometrium, 202

Sarcoma, pleomorphic, myometrium, 238
  stromal, endometrium, 200, 202, *50, 51, 52, 53, 54*
Schistosomiasis, cervix, 116
  vulva, 24
Scin tag, vulva, 44
Scirrhous carcinoma, cervix, 142
Sebaceous adenoma, arising in teratoma of ovary, 394
Sebaceous duct cyst, 38
Sebaceous gland, heterotopic, cervix, 124
  hyperplasia, vulva, 34
  labium majus, histology, 2
Sebaceous gland carcinoma, vulva, 64
  anaplastic, 66
  well differentiated, 66
Seborrheic keratosis, vulva, 40
Secretion, inspissated, in endometrial glands, 178
Secretory changes, in adenocarcinoma of endometrium, 196
  in endometriosis of, myometrium, 218
    ovary, 300
  in glandular cystic hyperplasia of endometrium, 182
Secretory endometrium, delayed desquamation, 172
  glycogen granules, *39*
  in inadequate biphasic cycle, 172
Secretory phase, endometrium, 16th day, 160, 162
  18th day, 162
  20th day, 162
  22nd day, 162, 164
  24th day, 164
  26th day, 164
  27th day, 164
Sertoli cell tumor, ovary, 362, 368
Sheehan syndrome, 544
Sickle cell anemia, placenta, 502, 504
Silver pigment deposition, cervix, following treatment of erosion, 128
Skene's glands, 4
  adenoma, 78
Skenitis, chronic, 74
  with epithelial metaplasia, 74
Soap-intoxication syndrome, curetted tissue, 486
  hypoplasia of bone marrow, 488
  lung, secondary monilial infection, 488
  pathological changes in, kidney, 488
    liver, *107*
  thrombosis of an ovarian vein, 488
Spleen, paragonadal, 312
Splenogonadal fusion, 312
Squamous cell carcinoma, cervix, 140, 142, 144, 32
  effect of radiation, 154
  poorly differentiated, 142
  with lymphatic spread, 150
  endometrium, 200
  oviduct, 268, 270
  urethral meatus, 78
  vagina, 94, 96
  vulva, 62, *16, 17*
Squamous epithelial nodule, cervix, 112
Squamous metaplasia, endometrium, 178
  endosalpinx, 248
  germinal epithelium of ovary, 298
  glandular epithelium of cervix, 110, 112, *26*
  in adenomatous hyperplastic endometrium, 184, *46*
  in cervical polyp, 112
  in endometriosis of myometrium, 218
  in polyp of endometrium, 190
Stromal endometriosis, myometrium, 226, 228, *59*
Stromal hyperplasia, endometrium, 186, *45*
  subcortical, in polycystic ovary, 306
Stromal sarcoma, endometrium, 200, 202, *50, 51, 52, 53, 54*
Struma ovarii, development of adenoma, 392
  development of carcinoma, 392
Subhymenal annular sclerosis (Halban), 80

Index

Surface epithelium, endometrium, participation in cycle, 166, 168
Surgical granuloma, vagina, 86
Sweat apocrine gland, labium majus, histology, 2
    vulva, carcinoma, 66
        hyperplasia, 32
Sweat eccrine gland, labium majus, histology, 2
    vulva, cystic change, 38
Syncytiotrophoblasts in lymphatic channel, 532
Syphilis, ovary, 290
    placenta, 498, 500
Syphilitic chancre, vulva, 12
Syphilitic lesion, cervix, secondary, 118
Syringoma, vulva, 42

Teratocarcinoma, ovary, 394, 396
    retroperitoneal tissue, 444
Teratoma, ovary, cystic benign, 390
        cystic benign, with cerebellar tissue, 390
        cystic benign, with chorioid plexus, 390
        cystic benign, with foreign bodies reaction, 390
        cystic, development of carcinoid, 392
        cystic, development of carcinoma, 394
        development of sebaceous adenoma, 394
        solid benign, 392
    placenta, 512
Theca cell tumor, ovary, 376, 91
    malignant, 376, 378
    sclerosing, 89, 90
    with edema, 376
    with luteinization, 376
Theca-lutein cyst, ovary, 294
Thrombosis, ovarial vein, in soap-intoxication syndrome, 488
    vein of oviduct, with organization, 248
Toxemia of pregnancy, brain, 552
    kidney, 550, 112, 113, 114
    liver, 552
    placenta, 504, 506
Trichomoniasis, vagina, 84
Tubal pregnancy see ectopic pregnancy
Tuberculosis, cervix, 116
    in mucinous cystadenoma of ovary, 330
    myometrium, 60
    ovary, 288
    oviduct, 258, 472
    peritoneum, 426
    placenta, 498
Tuberculosis cutis luposa, vulva, 8, 10
Tumors see special histological types of benign resp. malignant tumors

Ulcer, decubital, cervix, 108
    vagina, due to potassium permanganate, 84
    vulva, following radiotherapy, 72
Ulcus durum, vulva, 12
Ulcus molle, vulva, 10
Ulcus vulvae acutum (Lipschütz), 16
Umbilical cord, agenesis of artery, 520
    angiomyxoma, 520
    funisitis, acute, 520
    normal, 520
    thrombosis of the vein, 520
Umbilicus, endometriosis, 210
Undifferentiated carcinoma, ovary, 344
Urethral meatus, caruncle, angiomatous, 76
        granulomatous, 76
        papillomatous, 74
        simulating carcinoma, 76
        with epithelial dysplasia, 78
    condyloma acuminatum, 76
    histology, 4
    intraepidermal carcinoma, 78

Urethral meatus, metastatic malignant melanoma, 80
    papilloma, 76
    squamous cell carcinoma, 78
    with ectasia of a vein, 76
Urinary bladder, endometriosis, 210
Uteroplacental apoplexia (Couvelaire's uterus), 108
Uterus, histology, cross section, child, 158
    subinvolution, puerperal, 554
    subseptus, 180

Vagina, adenocarcinoma, adenoid cystic type, 96
        arising in endometriosis, 24
        cribriform type, 96
        mesonephric, 96
    adenosis, 21, 22
    candidiasis, 84
    carcinoma arising in endometriosis, 24
    choriocarcinoma, metastatic from uterus, 102
    chronic nodule, hemorrhagic, 100, 102
    condyloma acuminatum, 86
    cyst, epidermal inclusion, 86
        paramesonephric, 88
        with squamous metaplasia, 88
    dysplasia of vaginal epithelium, 94, 23
    emphysematous vaginitis, 86, 20
    endometriosis, 88
        carcinomatous change, 24
    epidermal inclusion cyst, 86
    erythroplasia of Queyrat, 94
    fibroma, 92
    granulation tissue, 86
    hemangioma, 92
    histology, 19
    hyperplasia, epithelial, pseudoepitheliomatous, 90
    intraepithelial carcinoma, 94
        erythroplasia of Queyrat, 94
    leiomyoma, 92
    leiomyosarcoma, 100
    lentigo, 94
    leukoparakeratosis, 88
    melanoma malignant, 100
    mesonephric papilloma, 90
    metaplasia, squamous in a cyst, 88
    metastatic carcinoma from, cancer of cervix, 100
        cancer of kidney, 100
    metastatic choriocarcinoma, 102
    mixed benign tumor, 90, 92
    neurilemmoma, 92
    papilloma, mesonephric, 90
    papillomatosis, 88, 90
    paramesonephric cyst, 88
    polyp, 90
    pseudoepitheliomatous hyperplasia, 90
    pseudotumor, inflammatory, 84
    radiation, vaginitis, 102
        vascular change, 102
    sarcoma botryoides, 98
    squamous cell carcinoma, 94, 96
    surgical granuloma, 86
    trichomoniasis, 84
    ulcer, due to potassium permanganate, 84
    vaginitis, acute, nonspecific, 84
        emphysematosa in pregnancy, 546
        erosive in pregnancy, 546
        following radiation, 102
    varicose vein, 86
    vascular change, following radiation, 102
Vaginitis, acute, nonspecific, 84
    emphysematosa, 86, 20
        in pregnancy, 546
    erosive in pregnancy, 546
    following radiation, 102

Varicella, vulva, 20
Varicose vein, vagina, 86
  vulva, 6
Vascular change, vagina, following chronic radiation, 102
Vermiform appendix, endometriosis, 210
  endosalpingiosis, 272
  decidual reaction in pregnancy, 472
Verruca vulgaris, vulva, 18
Viral hepatitis in pregnancy, 542
Vulva, abscess, Bartholin's gland, 14
  acanthosis nigricans, malignant, 28
  adenoacanthoma, Bartholin's gland, 64
  adenocarcinoma, adenocystic type, Bartholin's gland, 64
    Bartholin's gland, 62
    mucus-secreting, Bartholin's gland, 64
  adenoma, adnexal, 60
    Bartholin's gland, 44
    papillary, 44
    Skene's glands, 78
  adnexal adenoma, 60
  adnexal carcinoma, 62
    adenoid cystic type, 60
    mucus-secreting, 60
  adnexal papilloma, 44
  actinomycosis, 22
  amyloidosis, nodular, 30
  angiokeratoma of Mibelli, 50
  angiolipoma, 46
  atrophy, senile, with hyperkeratosis, 32
  Bancroft's filariasis, 22
    with elephantiasis, 24
  Bartholinitis, acute, suppurative, 14
    chronic, 116
    eosinophilic, 16
  Bartholin's gland, abscess, 14
    adenoacanthoma, 64
    adenocarcinoma, 62
    adenocarcinoma, adenocystic type, 64
    adenocarcinoma, mucus-secreting, 64
    adenoma, 44
    cyst, 36
    cystic dilatation of acini, 34
    mixed tumor, 54
  Bartholin's gland duct, cyst, 36
    ectasia, 36
    inflammatory cyst, 14
    pseudoabscess, 14
    squamous metaplasia of epithelium, 36
  basal cell carcinoma, 58
  bilharziasis, 24
  blastomycosis, 22
  Bowen's disease, 56, *15*
  breast tissue, 72
    lactating, 72
    lactating with cystic change, 36
  carcinoma, arising in lichen sclerosus et atrophicus, 30
    development after radiation, 72, 74
  caruncle of urethral meatus, angiomatous, 76
    granulomatous, 76
    papillomatous, 74
    simulating carcinoma, 76
    with ectasia of a vein, 76
    with epithelial dysplasia, 78
  chancroid, 10
  clitoris, glomus tumor, 50
    hypertrophy, 32
    malignant melanoma, 68, 70
  cloacogenic carcinoma, 78
  condyloma acuminatum, epithelial dysplasia, 18
    urethral meatus, 76
  condyloma latum, 12
    with ecthymalike changes, 12

Vulva, cylindroma, dermal eccrine, 60
  cyst, Bartholin's gland, 36
    Bartholin's gland duct, 36
    epidermal inclusion, 38
    in ectopic lactating breast tissue, 36
    inflammatory, Bartholin's gland duct, 14
    paramesonephric, 38
    peritoneal, 36
    sebaceous duct, 38
    sweat eccrine gland, 38
  cystic dilatation of acini, Bartholin's gland, 34
  Darier's disease, 28
  dermatitis, acute, 24
    chronic, 24
  dermatofibroma, 44
  dermatofibrosarcoma, 68
  dermatophytosis, 22
  diverticulum, suburethral, 74
    urethral, 74
  donovaniosis, 10
  dyskeratosis, 54
  dysplasia, epidermal, 54
    epithelial in condyloma acuminatum, 18
    epithelial in urethral caruncle, 78
  ectasia, Bartholin's gland duct, 36
  ecthyma, 8
  eczema, acute, 24
    chronic, 24
  elephantiasis, 6
    in Bancroft's filariasis, 24
  endometriosis, 72
  erythema multiforme, 26, 28
  erythroplasia of Queyrat, 56
  fasciitis, 16
  fibroma, 44, 46
  fibrosarcoma, 66
  fibrosis, 80
  folliculitis, 8
  glomus tumor, clitoris, 50
  granular cell myoblastoma, 48
  granuloma inguinale, 10
  granuloma pyogenicum, 8
  gumma, 12, 14
  hemangioma, capillary, 50
  herpes simplex, 20
  herpes zoster, 20
  hibernoma, 46
  hidradenoma, papilliferum, 42
  histiocytoma, 46
  histology, 2, 4
    Bartholin's gland, 4
    clitoris, corpus cavernosum, 4
    clitoris, Pacinian corpuscle, 4
    labium majus, 2
    labium minus, 2
    mons veneris, 2
    paraurethral glands, 4
    urethral meatus, 4
  Hodgkin's disease, 68
  hymen, imperforated, with hematocolpos, 80
  hyperkeratosis, in senile vulva atrophy, 32
  hyperlipemic xanthoma, 30
  hyperplasia, apocrine sweat glands, 32
    pseudoepitheliomatous, simulating by tangential section, 32
    sebaceous gland, 34
  hypertrophy, clitoris, 32
  impetigo herpetiformis, 8
  in neurofibromatosis (v. Recklinghausen), 48, 50
  inclusion cyst, epidermal, 38
  intraepidermal carcinoma, 54, 56
    Bowenoid type, 56
    Bowen's disease, 56, *15*

Vulva, intraepidermal carcinoma, erythroplasia of Queyrat, 56
    urethral meatus, 78
  inverted follicular keratosis, 40
  inverted papilloma, 40
  keloid, 34
  keratoacanthoma, 40, 42
  keratosis follicularis, 28
  leiomyoma, 48
  leiomyosarcoma, 66
  lentigo, 50
  lichen, chronicus simplex, 26
    planus, 26
    planus, verrucosus, 26
    sclerosus et atrophicus, 30, *1, 2, 3, 4, 5, 6*
    sclerosus et atrophicus, development of carcinoma, 30
  lipogranuloma, traumatic, 34
  liposarcoma, 68
  lupus vulgaris, 8, 10
  lymphangiectasis, 6
  lymphangioma, 50
  lymph node, pathological changes in lymphogranuloma venereum, 18
  lymphoblastic lymphosarcoma, 68
  lymphogranuloma venereum, 18
    lymph node change, 18
  malignant lymphoma, 68
  malignant melanoma, 70, *18*
    clitoris, 68, 70
    metastatic, urethral meatus, 80
  metaplasia, epithelial, chronic skenitis, 74
    squamous, Bartholin's gland duct, 36
  metastatic carcinoma from, cancer of breast, 70
    cancer of endometrium, 70
    cancer of large intestine, 70
  metastatic malignant melanoma, urethral meatus, 80
  mixed tumor, 52
    Bartholin's gland, 54
  molluscum contagiosum, 16
  myxoma, 46
  neurilemmoma, 48
  neurodermatitis circumscripta, 26
  neurofibroma, 48
  neuroma, 48
  nevus, blue, 52
    compound, 52
    epithelial, 34
    intradermal, 52
    junctional, 52
  Paget's disease, 56, 58, *7, 8, 9, 10, 11, 12, 13, 14*
  papilloma, adnexal, 44
    fibroepithelial, 40
    fibroepithelial, congenital, 40
    inverted, 40
    urethral meatus, 76
  paramesonephric cyst, 38
  pemphigus vulgaris, 26
  perifolliculitis, 8
  pityriasis rubra pilaris, 28
  polyp, fibroepithelial, 44
  pseudoabscess, Bartholin's gland duct, 14
  pseudoepitheliomatous hyperplasia, 32, 40
    simulating by tangential section, 32
  pseudosarcomatous changes, simulating by fasciitis, 16

Vulva, pseudotumor, inflammatory, 16
  psoriasis, 26
  radiation ulcer, 72
  radiodermatitis, 72
  radiotherapy, development of carcinoma, 72, 74
  rhabdomyosarcoma, 66
  schistosomiasis, 24
  scin tag, 44
  sebaceous duct cyst, 38
  sebaceous gland carcinoma, 64
    anaplastic, 66
    well differentiated, 66
  sebaceous gland hyperplasia, 34
  seborrheic keratosis, 40
  Skene's gland, adenoma, 78
  skenitis, chronic, 74
    chronic, with transitional cell metaplasia, 74
  squamous cell carcinoma, 62, *16, 17*
    urethral meatus, 78
  subhymenal annular sclerosis (Halban), 80
  sweat apocrine glands, carcinoma, 66
    hyperplasia, 32
  sweat eccrine gland, cyst, 38
  syphilitic chancre, 12
  syringoma, 42
  tuberculosis cutis luposa, 8, 10
  ulcer following radiotherapy, 72
  ulcus durum, 12
  ulcus molle, 10
  ulcus vulvae acutum (Lipschütz), 16
  urethral meatus, caruncle, angiomatous, 76
    caruncle, granulomatous, 76
    caruncle, papillomatous, 74
    caruncle, simulating carcinoma, 76
    caruncle, with ectasia of a vein, 76
    caruncle, with epithelial dysplasia, 78
    condyloma acuminatum, 76
    intraepidermal carcinoma, 78
    papilloma, 76
    squamous cell carcinoma, 78
  varicella, 20
  varicose vein, 6
  verruca vulgaris, 18
  vulvitis, acute, nonspecific, 6
    chronic, hyperkeratotic, 6
    chronic, nonspecific, 6
    diabetic, 8
  xanthoma, diabeticorum, 30
    hyperlipemic, 30
Vulvitis, acute, nonspecific, 6
  chronic, nonspecific, 6
    nonspecific, hyperkeratotic, 6
  diabetic, 8

Walthard's cell rest, oviduct, child, 250
    development, 246
    fetus, 250
    reproductive age, 250, 252

Xanthogranuloma, myometrium, 216
  retroperitoneal tissue, 434
Xanthoma, diabeticorum, vulva, 30
  hyperlipemic, vulva, 30

Index

Chromosomal Aberrations
in Gynecology

Aberration, chromosomal, 559
    numerical, 559, 562
    structural, 559, 562
Abortion, habitual, 583
  spontaneous, 583
Acrocentric, 589
  chromosomes, 561
Anaphase lag, 559, 589
Aneuploidy, 559, 589
Autoradiography, 563
Autosomes, 559, 560, 561, 562, 563, 589
Barr body, 563
Centromere, 561, 589
Chromatid, 589
Chromatin, 589
Deletion, 559, 562, 589
  X-chromosome, 559, 572
Diploid, 559, 589
Drumsticks, 589
  Klinefelter-syndrome (XXY), 578
  ringchromosome, 570
  triple X- female (XXX), 568, 569
Gonosomes see sex chromosomes
Haploid, 589
Inversion, 559, 562, 589
Isochromosome, 559, 589
  X-chromosome, 559, 566
Karyotype, 561
  female (XX), 561
  male (XY), 561
  ringchromosome, 570
  trisomy 21 (Down's syndrome), 562, 580
  XX_D (deleted X-chromosome), 572
  XO, 563, 564, 584
  XO/XX-isochromosome, 566
  XO/XY, 583
  XY (testicular feminization), 574
  XY (vestigial pelvic organs, absent gonads), 576
  XXX, 568, 569, 584
  XXY (Klinefelter's syndrome), 578, 584
Klinefelter's syndrome, 578, 583, 584
Malformation, newborns, 583
Masculinization, adrenogenital syndrome, 583
  drugs during pregnancy, 583
  female genitalia, 583
  incomplete, 583
Metacentric, 589
Metaphase, 559, 560
Mongolism (Down's syndrome), 562, 580
Monosomy, 559, 589
Mosaicism, chromosomal, 559, 584
  XO/XX-isochromosome, 566
  XO/XX/X + ringchromosome, 570
  XO/XY, 583

Mosaicism, chromosomal, XX/XX_D, 572
Nondisjunction, 559, 589
Phytohemagglutinin, 560
Polyploidy, 589
Polysomy, 589
Primary constriction see centromere
Ringchromosome, 570, 589
Satellites, 589
Secondary constriction, 589
Sex chromatin, 559, 563, 589
  Klinefelter's syndrome(XXY), 578
  negative, 563
  newborns, 584
  positive, 563
  prenatal sex determination, 583
  testicular feminization (XY), 574
  triple X- female (XXX), 568, 569
  Turner's syndrome (XO), 564
    (XO/XX-isochromosome), 566
  vestigial pelvic organs (XY), 576
  XO/XX/X + ringchromosome, 570
  XX_D (deleted X-chromosome), 572
Sex chromosome (gonosome), 559, 561, 583, 589
Sex determination, prenatal, 583
Submetacentric, 589
Testicular feminization, 574, 583, 584
Translocation, 559, 562, 583, 589
  15/21, 562
Triploidy, 559, 589
  spontaneous abortion, 583
Trisomy, 559, 589
  D (Patau's syndrome), 562, 583
  E (Edward's syndrome), 562, 583
  G (Down's syndrome), 562, 580, 583
  spontaneous abortion, 583
Turner's syndrome, XO, 564, 584
  XO/XX-isochromosome, 566
Vestigial pelvic organs, 576
X-chromosome, 559, 561, 563
  "cold," 563
  deletion, 572
  "hot," 563
  monosomy, 564
XO, 563
  newborns, 584
  spontaneous abortions, 583
  Turner's syndrome, 564
XO/XY, 583
XX, 559, 561, 563, 570, 572, 583, 584
XX/XX_D, 572
XX/XY, 584
XXX, 568, 569, 584
XY, 559, 561, 563, 574, 576
Y-chromosome, 559, 561